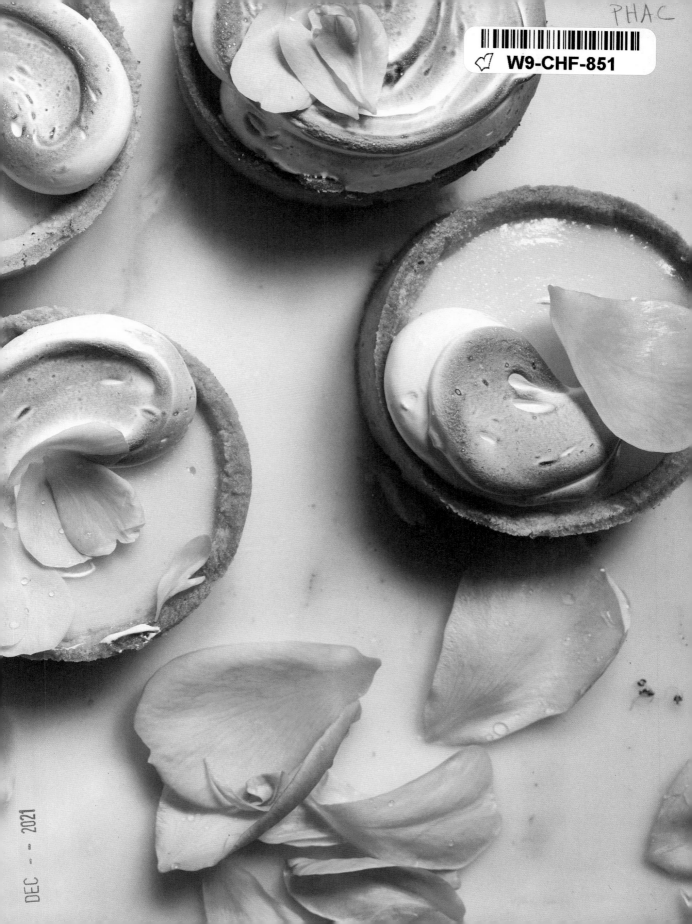

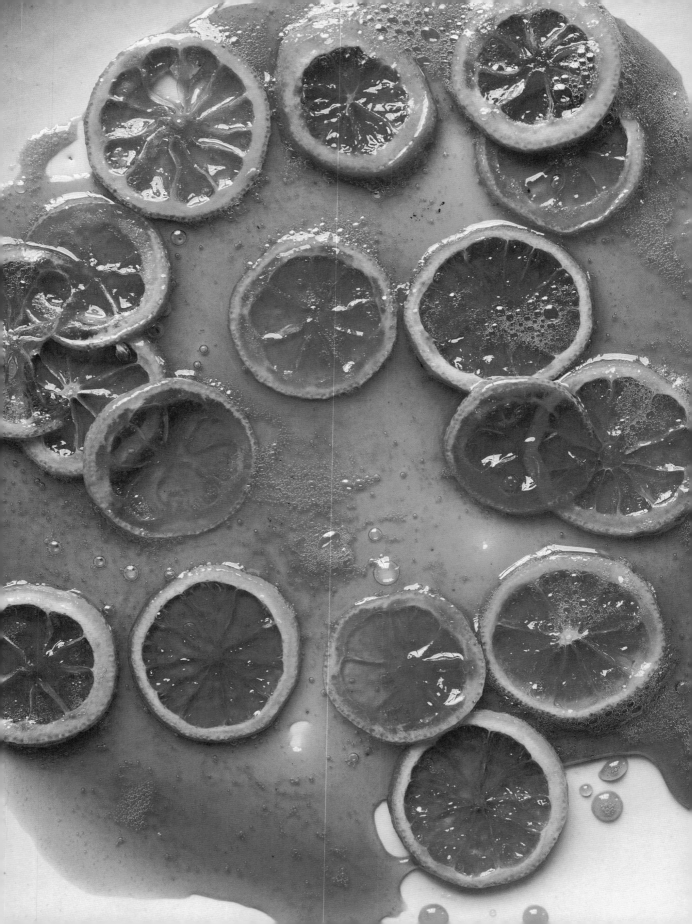

Cannelle et Vanille
BAKES SIMPLE

"Aran's book, filled with beauty and an abundance of staples, breads, and pastries, is the baker's companion for those who long for artisanal, gluten-free delights."

—**LAUREL GALLUCCI**, author of *Sweet Laurel*
and *Sweet Laurel Savory*

"Aran writes about baking with an ease that is simultaneously soothing, inspiring, and empowering—each page will make you want to bake . . . now! . . . You needn't be avoiding gluten to fall in love with this book . . . it is for anyone who loves to spend time baking, especially if they love to share their bakes with others."

—**ERIN JEANNE McDOWELL**, author of *The Book on Pie*

"*Cannelle et Vanille Bakes Simple* is the gluten-free baking bible we all need. Aran has done an incredible job of making a subject that can be overwhelming and mysterious simple and accessible. . . . You feel like Aran is in the kitchen calmly guiding, inspiring, and answering all your baking questions."

—**ODETTE WILLIAMS**, author of *Simple Cake*

"Whether you're looking for gluten-free recipes or just baking inspiration, this wonderful book is for you."

—**KERRY DIAMOND**, founder of *Cherry Bombe*

"The timeless recipes and techniques illustrated . . . are truly valuable—not only to those that are gluten-free but to all of us who enjoy delicious baked goods made with alternative flours. The combination of Aran's talents as a pastry chef (and baker) along with her heartachingly beautiful styling and photographs makes for a spellbinding book that may never leave your kitchen."

—**AMY CHAPLIN**, James Beard Award–winning author of
Whole Food Cooking Every Day

"Aran offers up an array of desserts without gluten that will satisfy any cravings, even if you're not gluten-free. The bread recipes ensure that beautiful loaves of bread (and even bagels!) are within the reach of all, and cookie-lovers will find something delicious and satisfying."

—**DAVID LEBOVITZ**, author of *My Paris Kitchen*

"Aran Goyoaga is truly a master of gluten-free baking, which she elevates to an art. . . . The soothing practice of baking is celebrated on every page of this useful and beautiful book."

—**SUSAN SPUNGEN**, author of *Open Kitchen*

"Aran uses classic, time-honored techniques but with a gluten-free twist, using whole food ingredients that both nourish and dazzle. There are countless recipes in this book that I know I will fold into my repertoire, in the hopes that Aran's poetic connection to baking will be infused into my own."

—**SARAH BRITTON**, holistic nutritionist and founder of *My New Roots*

"I am not experienced with gluten-free baking. . . . But, reading Aran's recipes made me believe that I could excel at all of these efforts."

—**CARLA LALLI MUSIC**, author of *Where Cooking Begins*

"These recipes manage to pull off the rare and difficult feat of being simultaneously beautiful, delicious, and truly approachable for the home baker. That they're also gluten-free, and in many cases vegan, gives them a touch of the magical, a quality Aran herself possesses."

—**CLAIRE SAFFITZ**, author of *Dessert Person*

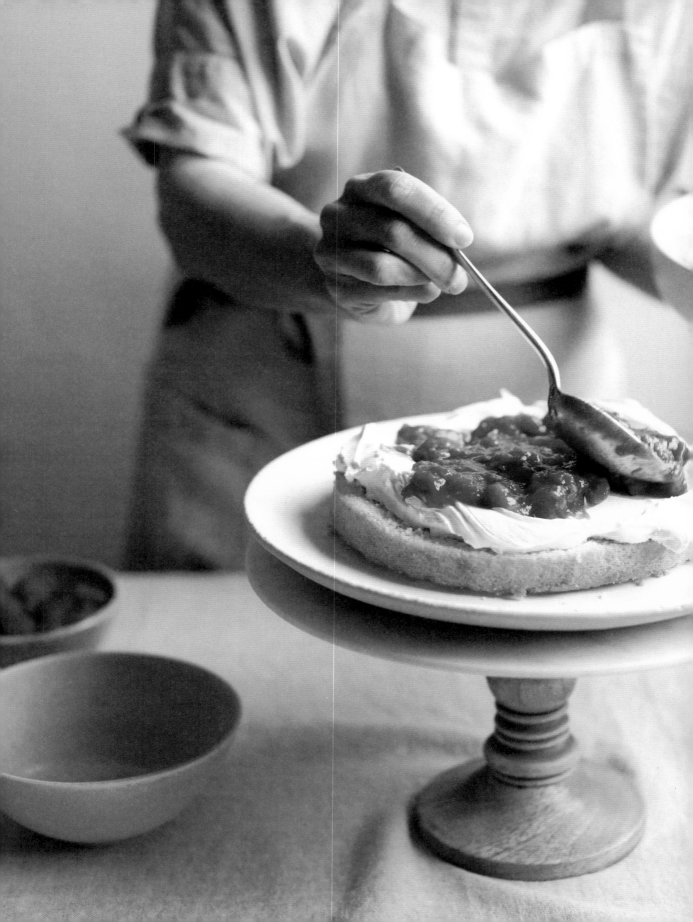

Cannelle et Vanille BAKES SIMPLE

A New Way to Bake
GLUTEN-FREE

Written and photographed by

Aran Goyoaga

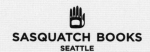

SASQUATCH BOOKS

SEATTLE

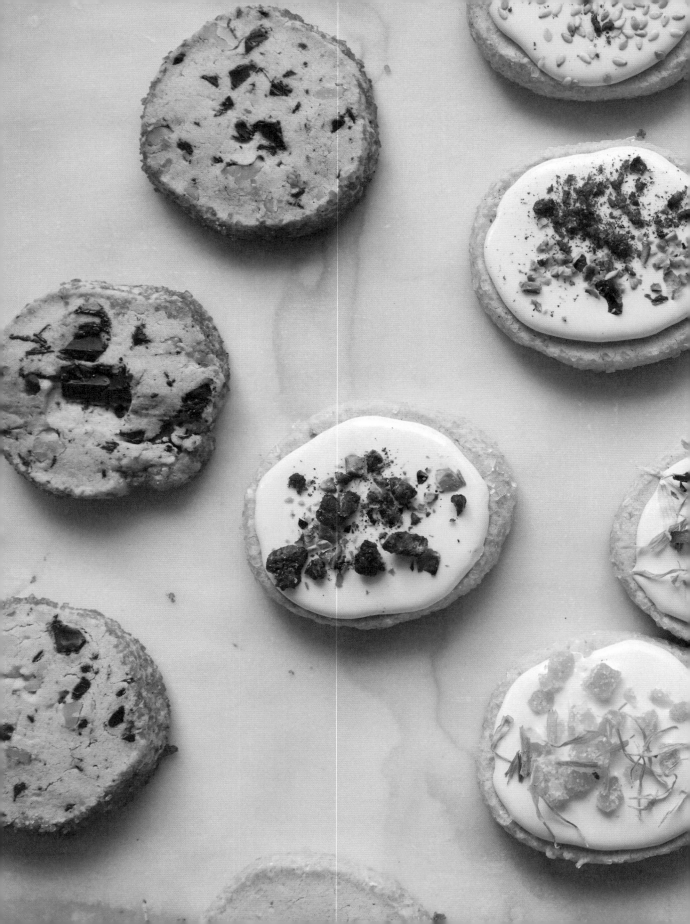

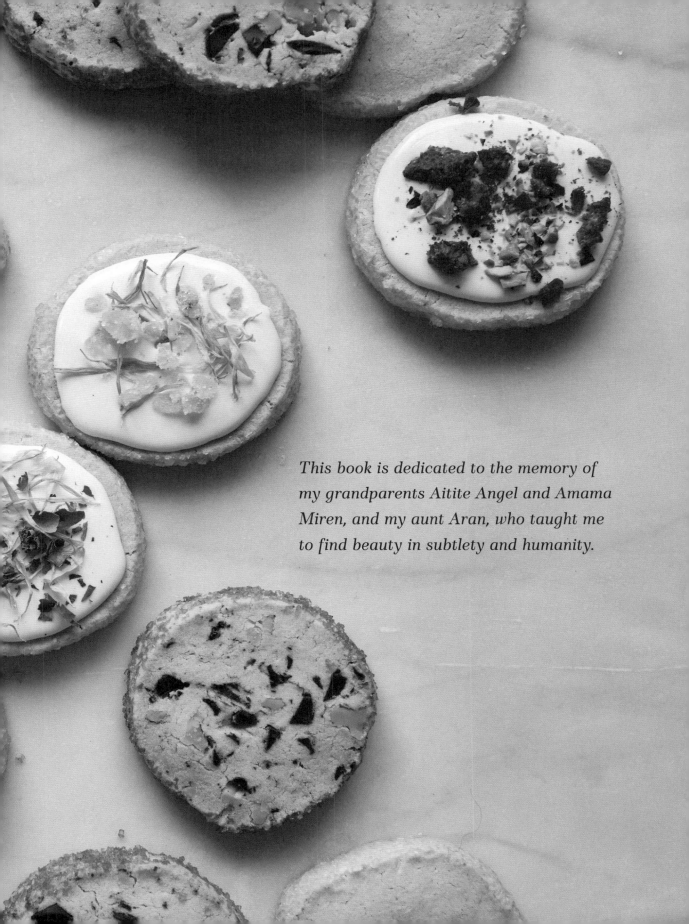

This book is dedicated to the memory of my grandparents Aitite Angel and Amama Miren, and my aunt Aran, who taught me to find beauty in subtlety and humanity.

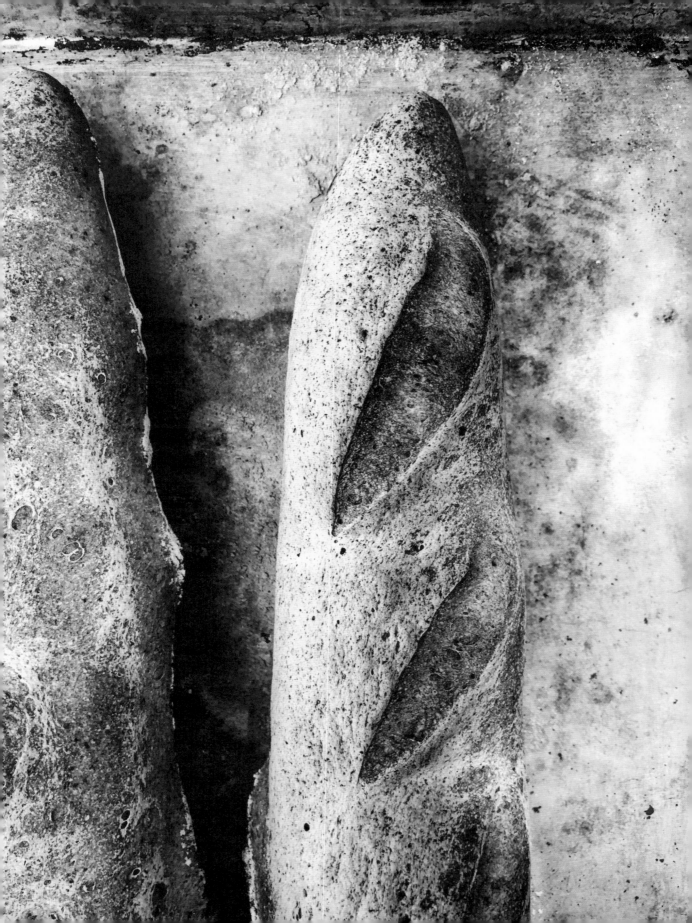

Contents

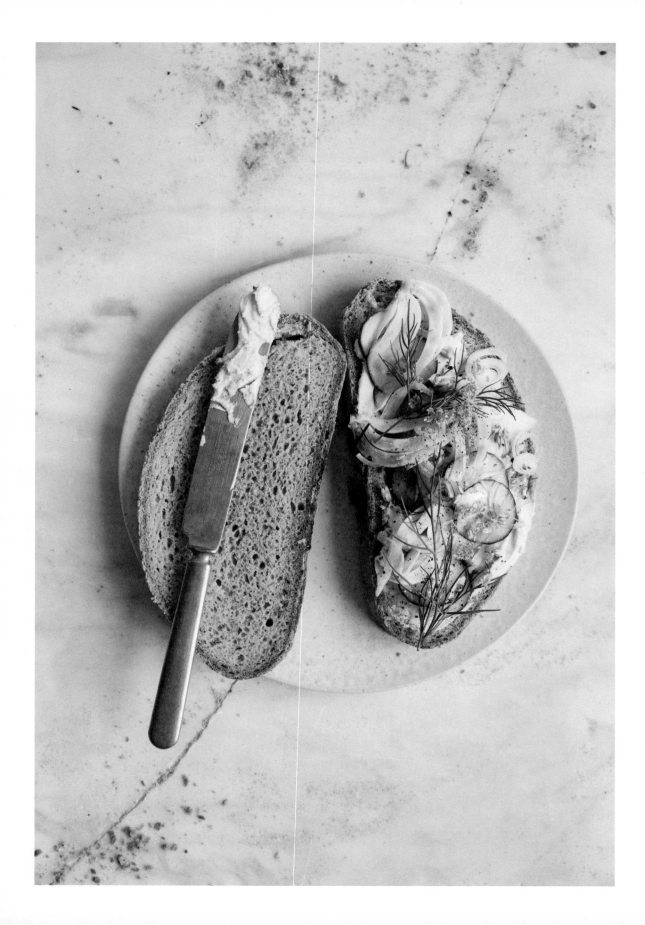

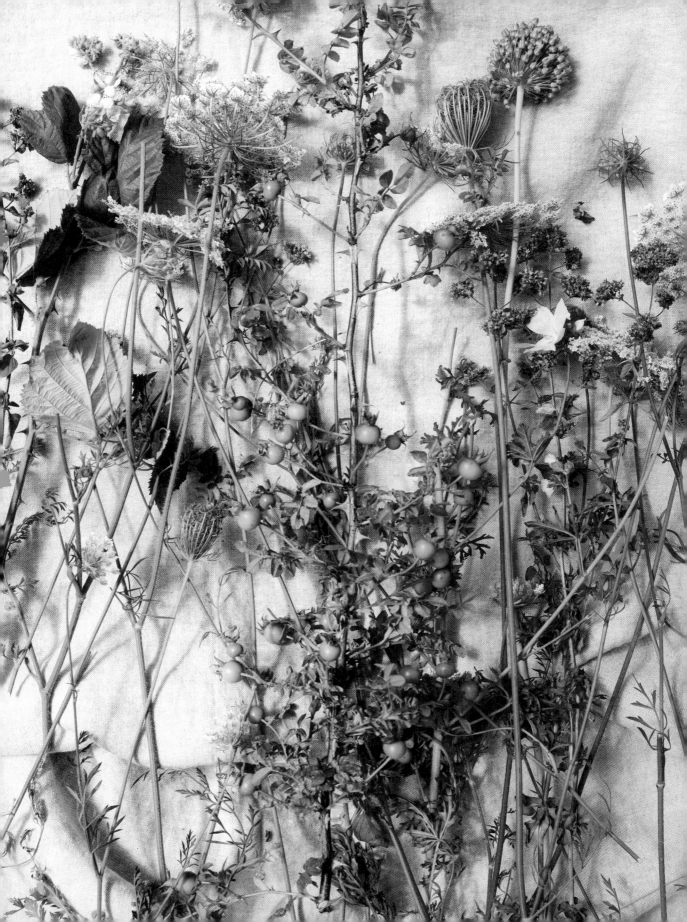

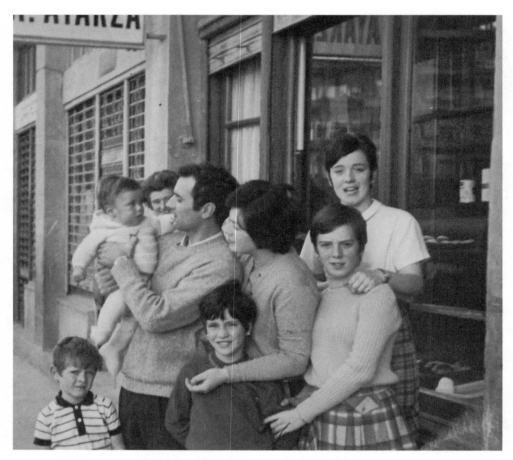

Pastelería Ayarza, circa 1970
Amorebieta, Basque Country

Family Heirlooms Made Mine

AN INTRODUCTION

It was November 16, 2001. The house was dark and it was an unseasonably warm day in Denver, where we were living at the time. It was two months after September 11, when the world felt unstable and strange. My grandfather had passed away in the morning, and while I was mourning his loss, I received a letter informing me that I was being laid off from my marketing job at a big corporation. My husband, Chad, had lost his job weeks before. I sat alone on the kitchen floor, resting my head on my knees, anxious and worried about the future. Then I stood up, pulled out jars of flour and sugar, and started baking. Since childhood, this is how I have calmed myself. Later that evening, sharing a piece of the marble cake I had made, I said to Chad, "I really think I want to pursue this." As always, he nodded.

I called my parents the following morning. My hands were shaking. Even though I was twenty-seven, married, and living half a world away, I was afraid they would be disappointed with my decision and that they would remind me of all the money they had spent on my education or ask me why I had never shown any interest in our family's pastry business. Of course, they didn't say either. They were surprised but understood that I was to find my own path in my own time, as I'd always been one to go against the grain. A few short weeks later, we moved to Florida and I enrolled in culinary school.

I am a fourth-generation baker. My family says it all started with my great-great-uncle Julian Mugida, who worked as a baker and store manager at Martina de Zuricalday in Bilbao, in the Basque Country in northern Spain. When my grandfather Angel Ayarza turned fourteen, Julian secured an apprenticeship for him. He excelled and worked at Martina de Zuricalday until 1936, when the Spanish Civil War broke out. At sixteen, Angel was sent to war. We know very little about this time. He worked as a radio operator and told me, just once, about a stormy night of battle where he witnessed tremendous death. After that night, my grandfather could not bear nights of wind and thunder. No one knows much about his years immediately after the war, but he married my grandmother Miren Gaztelu in 1946 after being introduced by one of his aunts, and they settled in Amorebieta. My mother was born shortly after, and another seven children followed. In early 1949, while working at a local factory making vacuum cleaners, my grandfather decided to lease a small storefront and adjacent workshop on Luis Urrengoetxea, number 11. He opened a bakery called Pastelería Ayarza that September. The family slept in a small room next to the workshop. He taught my grandmother everything he knew. She prepped for him during the day while also tending to the children. Sometime in the late 1950s, my grandfather quit the factory job and dedicated his life to the pastry shop. They bought a flat right above it and moved in. We called this flat "upstairs" and the pastry shop "downstairs."

I grew up across the street from the pastry shop and my grandparents' flat. I often waved at my grandmother from my bedroom window. The pastry shop was our world. My mother worked front of the house along with my uncles and aunts. I spent my time there before and after school. On weekends, I delivered pastries all around town on foot and helped my grandmother peel fruit, fill brioche with buttercream, or glaze shortbread cookies. The pastry shop was always warm—literally and figuratively. It was a gathering place for friends, relatives, or anyone who needed a place to rest and converse. I remember my grandmother stepping outside the shop to greet strangers and familiar faces, always with her apron on.

I was encouraged to study and to be curious. From the age of eleven, my parents enrolled me in foreign exchange programs and I traveled all over Europe and the United States. They wanted to show me there was a vast world outside of our small town of Amorebieta. I studied business and economics in university, and in 1998 I moved to the US. I married my American boyfriend and found work in the corporate world. Those years were marked by a secret eating disorder, anxiety, and disconnection from my own path and self. All along, I baked. I baked to feel connected to my family and I baked to find purpose. On that unseasonably warm day in November 2001, everything changed.

My professional career in pastry was short lived, but it was tremendously educational and intense. I learned and worked under some of the best pastry chefs in the US, most of them European men. I worked from dawn till dusk; sometimes from dusk till dawn. I went to school in the morning, then headed to one of the several restaurants where I worked during the evening. Once I graduated from culinary school, I landed a job at a five-star hotel. I continued to work my way up the ladder. I was consumed by the work, and the pastry team became my family. But in 2006, when Chad and I started a family, I left the professional kitchen. At the time, raising children and my life as a pastry chef felt incompatible. Eventually I began creating and sharing recipes on my blog, *Cannelle et Vanille*. It became a vehicle to channel my creativity and my love for pastry. I began experimenting with photography and taught myself about light and composition, always with the goal of creating an emotional response in my readers. I realized that a recipe could be so much more than a mere list of ingredients and steps—it was a tool for the creative expression I had longed for.

I come from a close-knit family of pastry chefs but developed my own career trajectory on a different continent. My uncles, aunts, and cousins have carried on my grandparents' torch. Their spirit is always with me, and we maintain a strong connection through our shared memories. My goal has always been to mesh the world of traditional pastry with the new horizons of alternative baking. To take the knowledge I was given and honor my family, yet transform the recipes through my filter and experiences with gluten intolerance. And with this, it is my hope, dear reader, that the recipes in this book will become part of your life. Share them with your family, with your neighbors, and create heirlooms to pass along to those you love.

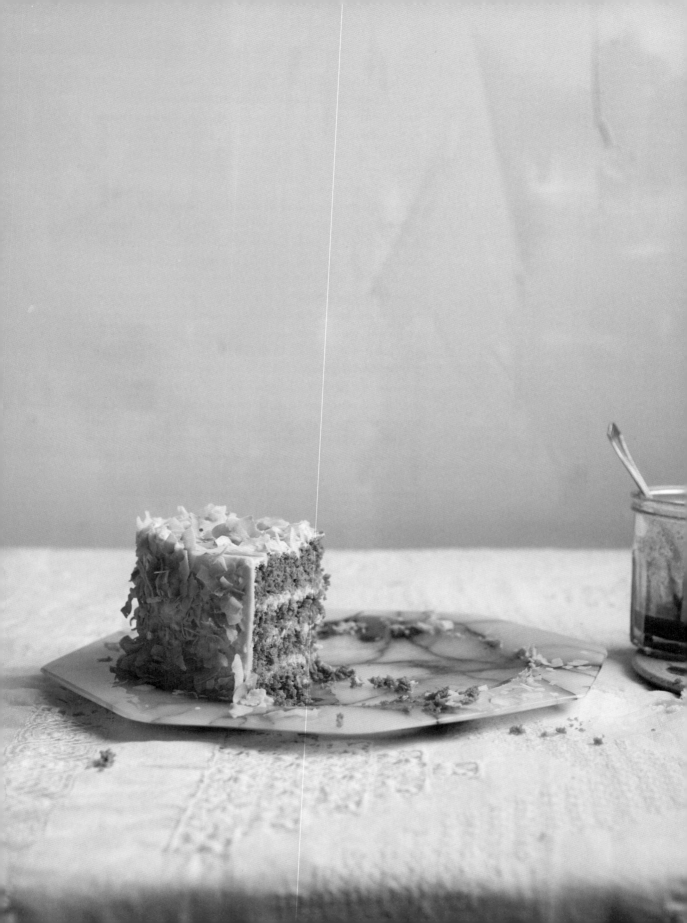

How to Use This Book

This book is divided into six chapters, each one organized by type of baked good. Please take a moment to read the sidebars sprinkled throughout as they include important information about ingredients, processes, and substitutions.

A note about the word *simple*. In my mind, simple doesn't always mean quick or short recipes. Sometimes simplicity requires understanding why we do what we do. So even if a recipe is longer, know that I wrote it in a detailed way so you understand the goal of every step. Some recipes are in fact fairly easy to make, like the Chocolate Sourdough Cake with Chocolate Glaze (page 147), Cheddar and Herb Scones (page 197), and Quick Crusty Boule (page 69). Other recipes require time to ferment or set but aren't inherently complex, such as Sourdough Boules (page 62), Chocolate–Olive Oil Babkas (page 101), or Lemon Meringue Tartlets (page 175).

All the recipes in this book are gluten-free and also offer dairy-free options. As I get older, I have noticed that my tolerance for dairy has decreased. My son has a casein intolerance, which has forced me to make most of what we eat at home without using cow's milk products. There are so many great products available these days that it is easy to substitute non-dairy ingredients.

If gluten is not an issue for you, you can use all-purpose wheat flour in place of the total weight of the gluten-free flours and starches in many of my recipes. This works well for cakes, tarts, and cookies. For example, if a recipe calls for 140 grams of superfine brown rice flour, 100 grams of sorghum, and 60 grams of tapioca starch, you can use 300 grams of all-purpose wheat flour instead. Remember that gluten is a very elastic protein though, so the texture might be slightly different. However, wheat flour substitution won't work for the yeast breads, which were formulated to use psyllium and flaxseed as an alternative to gluten.

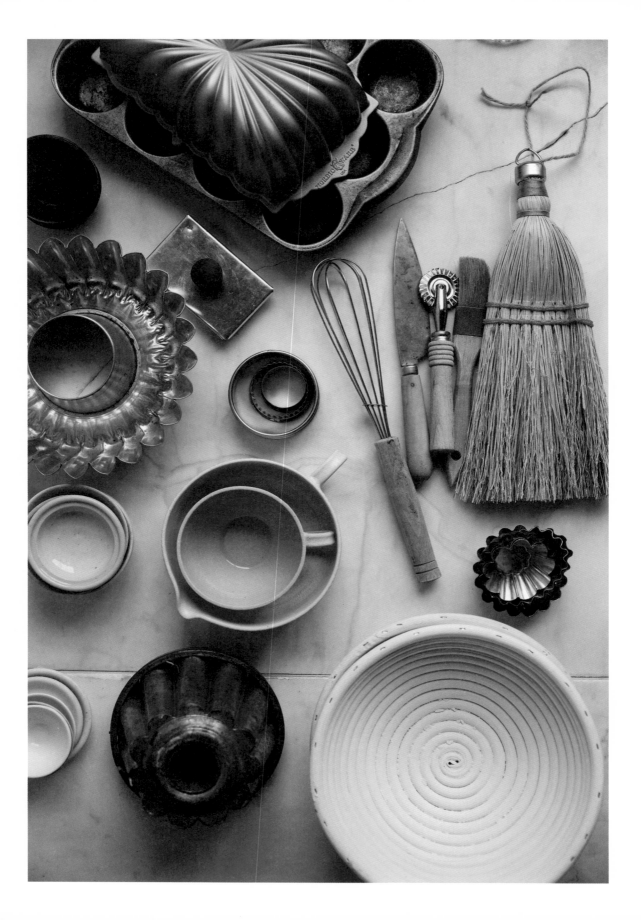

Stocking the Pantry and Tools to Use

PANTRY INGREDIENTS

I store all of my flours, spices, and other pantry ingredients in labeled clear mason jars. It allows me to keep my kitchen organized and clean. At my studio, the jars live on the open shelves above the counter, but at home, they are put away in deep pull-out drawers. What follows is a list of gluten-free flours and other staples used in recipes throughout the book.

Flours

BUCKWHEAT FLOUR. Despite its name, buckwheat is actually not a grain nor related to wheat. It is a fruit seed with an earthy flavor, so it is apt for grain-free baking. If you are trying to maintain a low-grain or low-starch diet, buckwheat is perfect for you. In general, I prefer light buckwheat flour, and since the raw groats are quite soft, I grind them at home in a high-speed blender. Some of the commercially packaged buckwheat flours in the US, such as Bob's Red Mill and Arrowhead Mills, are darker and earthier, which is not my preference, but they do work—the flavor will just be more distinct.

NUT FLOUR. Nut flour adds fat and loads of flavor to baked goods, particularly cakes, tarts, and cookies. I love a bit of almond or hazelnut flour in my recipes. However, if you are avoiding almond flour, you can substitute tigernut flour, which is technically not a nut despite its name. I grew up with tigernuts (*chufas*) as they are what *horchata* is made from in Spain. The flour is delicious, good for you, works just like almond flour does, and is now readily available in most health-food stores.

OAT FLOUR. In the US, it is easy to find certified gluten-free oats (meaning oats that have been processed in a facility not cross-contaminated with wheat). However, it is possible to be allergic to avenin, the protein in oats, just as you are to gluten. If you cannot tolerate oat flour, I recommend substituting it with light buckwheat flour.

POTATO STARCH. Potato starch is used in baked goods to create a soft and tender crumb. If you cannot have potatoes, you can substitute tapioca or arrowroot starch.

SORGHUM FLOUR. This slightly sweet and yellow-colored flour is high in protein and works well with other whole-grain and nut flours. I tend to use it a lot in breads. If you cannot find sorghum, you can use millet flour.

SUPERFINE BROWN RICE FLOUR. This is the base of many of my baking recipes because it's quite neutral in flavor and its finely milled texture allows doughs to hydrate well. This results in baked goods that are not as crumbly and have better mouthfeel. You can use stone-ground brown rice flour, but expect a bit crumblier texture. If you are using stone-ground brown rice flour and the bread doughs are too wet, reduce the amount of water by 10 percent and see if that helps.

SWEET WHITE RICE FLOUR. This flour is made from sticky short-grain rice that is very glutinous. Sometimes it can make baked goods a bit too gummy, but it works well in certain pastries, such as brioche or puff pastry. It is mild and sweet in flavor.

TAPIOCA STARCH. Also known as tapioca flour, tapioca starch is extracted from the cassava root. It helps bind and create crisp baked goods. You can use cornstarch or arrowroot in its place.

Binding Agents

FLAXSEED MEAL. Flaxseed is a great thickener when mixed with water. It gels and expands. I use it in bread-baking to create structure and also to replace eggs. It's important that the flaxseeds are ground as finely as possible so they can absorb water well. You can easily pulverize them at home to make a flour or meal—use a clean coffee grinder or high-speed blender.

PSYLLIUM HUSK POWDER. Psyllium husks come from the seed of the plantago plant, which is native to India and Pakistan. It is a great source of soluble fiber and absorbs large amounts of water. Be sure to use finely milled psyllium husk powder and not whole psyllium husks or flakes. You can pulverize whole husks in a coffee grinder or high-speed blender. If you do this, it is important to weigh the powder because freshly ground husk powder will be less dense.

XANTHAN GUM. I use xanthan gum only when necessary as it can be hard to digest. I typically reserve it for pastry that requires lamination, stretch, and handling. There are a couple of recipes in this book where it is called for but optional. You will be able to make the recipe without it, but the pastry might fall apart a bit more than if you include it.

Chocolate

I use bars of chocolate, which I chop by hand. I hardly ever use chocolate chips, not even for cookies. I usually keep 70 percent and 85 percent cacao bars in my pantry. Theo Chocolate, a Seattle-based company, is one of my favorite chocolate makers. All of their chocolates are free of soy, which I also try to avoid.

Eggs

I use large eggs in my recipes, which weigh approximately 1½ ounces (45 g) without the shell. I try to buy eggs at my local farmers' market.

Replacing Eggs

Most of the breads in the book are egg-free except the richer ones, such as brioche dough, but I do rely on eggs for cakes and cookies. You can replace the eggs using "flax egg" or aquafaba.

To make one flax egg, combine 1 tablespoon of flaxseed meal with 2 tablespoons of hot water until it gels, then add to your recipe as you would eggs. This works well when eggs are used simply to bind but not when they need to be whipped like meringue. When using flax eggs for cakes, add ¼ teaspoon baking powder to the dry ingredients to help with aeration.

Aquafaba is the liquid left over from cooking chickpeas (and other beans). It is thick and full of protein. Drain chickpeas from a can and reserve the liquid. It can replace eggs for binding, such as in breads or cakes, but also when they need to be whipped. Use 3 tablespoons of aquafaba to replace 1 large egg; 2 tablespoons for 1 large egg white; or 1 tablespoon for 1 large egg yolk. I have tested this method for various recipes in the book and it works well.

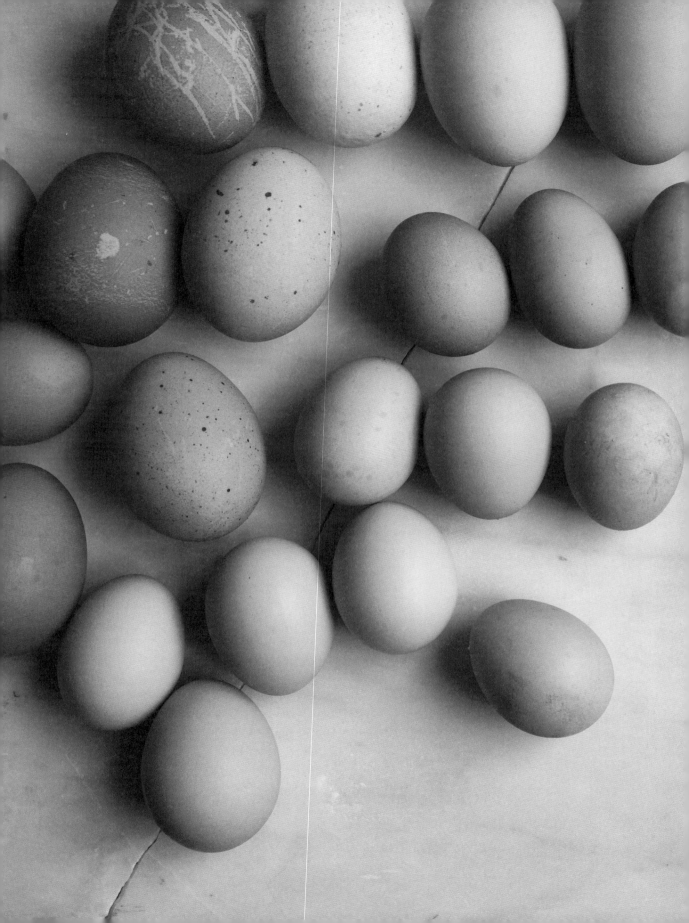

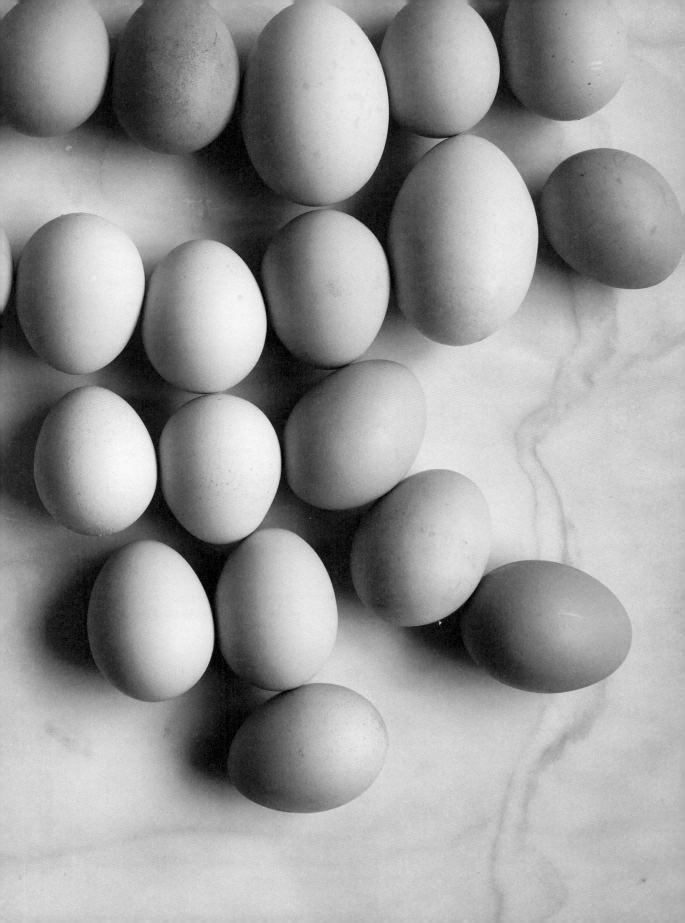

Sweeteners

BROWN SUGAR. Brown sugar adds moisture to baked goods. It is simply white sugar with molasses added back into it, so it has a bit more viscosity, richer flavor, and color. Light brown sugar has slightly less molasses than the dark variety.

COCONUT SUGAR. Coconut sugar, also called coconut palm sugar, is a natural sugar made from coconut palm sap. It is dark in color and is a great substitute for light or dark brown sugar.

HONEY. Honey is the perfect sweetener, really: antibacterial, antifungal, full of antioxidants, and it provides lots of moisture to baked goods, helping to preserve them. For these recipes, I like to use runny honey because it mixes better with the rest of the ingredients.

MAPLE SYRUP. Maple syrup is a syrup made from boiling the sap of sugar maple. It has similar sweetening power as sugar but adds a distinct flavor.

MOLASSES. Molasses is a thick dark-brown syrup obtained from refining raw sugar cane. It adds moisture, color, and slight bitterness to baked goods. If don't have molasses, you can use honey, but the color and flavor will be slightly different.

POWDERED SUGAR. Powdered sugar, also called confectioners' sugar, is produced by milling granulated sugar into a powder. Oftentimes, a bit of cornstarch is added to help absorb moisture and prevent clumping. Using powdered sugar helps dough retain its shape, like with cutout cookies or shortbread.

SUGAR. When an ingredient list calls for simply *sugar*, I am referring to white granulated sugar or natural cane sugar. Natural cane sugar is slightly coarser than white sugar but works similarly.

Leavenings

BAKER'S YEAST. This is the common name given to strands of yeast used in commercial bread-baking. It is much faster-acting than wild yeast cultivated through the process of growing a sourdough starter. In the US, the most common types are active dry yeast and instant yeast. In general, you may substitute active dry for instant in the same amount; however, active dry yeast needs to be activated in a warm liquid, whereas instant yeast, which is added straight into the flour, does not.

BAKING POWDER. Baking powder is a mixture of baking soda, cream of tartar, and sometimes cornstarch. The cream of tartar, an acid, neutralizes the baking soda, and therefore it is most often used when a recipe does not call for an additional acidic ingredient.

BAKING SODA. Baking soda is an alkali that needs an acid to react and create carbon dioxide, which in turn allows baked good to rise. Baking soda is much more powerful than baking powder, so you don't need as much.

Fats

BUTTER. High-fat-content butters, often labeled as European-style butters, have a deeper yellow color, tend to contain less water, and are more pliable. I prefer these for pastries and cookies where the butter flavor is predominant. I will also use dairy-free or vegan butters in my recipes. Look for formulations that are sold in sticks, as these have less water than those in containers and are better suited for pastry. On page 33, you can find a recipe for Cultured Cashew-Coconut Butter that works great for baking and as a spread.

COCONUT OIL. I didn't grow up with coconut oil, so I don't tend to use it unless I am working on a recipe where coconut is the main ingredient. I refer to two different kinds in the book—virgin and refined. Virgin (unrefined) has a very distinct coconut flavor and aroma, while refined coconut oil is much more neutral.

OLIVE OIL. Extra-virgin olive oil is my go-to oil for baking. It adds beautiful flavor and moisture to cakes and breads. Not all olive oils are equal—some are peppery, some are fruity—so make sure you taste them and decide what you love best.

Milks

COCONUT MILK AND CREAM. All recipes that call for coconut milk use canned full-fat coconut milk. If the recipe calls for coconut cream, you can used canned coconut cream or collect the cream that solidifies at the top of a can of full-fat coconut milk after it has been refrigerated (see page 39). My go-to brands are Native Forest and 365 by Whole Foods Market.

OAT MILK. My go-to plant-based milk is oat milk, especially the brands Oatly and Califia Farms. I particularly love the Barista line because it's thick and works just like rich whole milk or even half-and-half. Oat milk has a naturally sweet flavor that works very well in baking. You can also use nut milks in place of oat milk, but make sure they are unsweetened and thick.

WHOLE COW'S MILK. I grew up with raw milk that my grandmother and mother pasteurized daily. I remember its deeply rich yellow with a thick layer of cream on top. Today I look for pasteurized and unhomogenized cow's milk (the kind that says "cream on top"). Whole milk contains between 3½ and 4 percent fat content, which is how many countries label it.

Salt

FLAKY SEA SALT. I use flaky sea salt mostly for finishing to add crunch and texture to a recipe. I prefer Maldon sea salt flakes and Brittany Sea Salt fleur de sel.

KOSHER SALT. Kosher salt is my everyday salt, even for baking (I like Morton brand). If you only have fine iodized or sea salt, reduce the volume by 20 percent.

KITCHEN TOOLS

I am really a minimalist when it comes to baking equipment. I believe in purchasing a small number of high-quality tools that will endure beatings and years of baking. Here is a list of my must-haves and favorite brands.

BENCH SCRAPER. A bench scraper is always at my side when I am making bread and pastry doughs. It allows you to cut, scrape a surface of stuck dough, or move pieces around easily. I have a stainless steel one and also a plastic one from my grandfather that I use to scrape dough from bowls or meringues into pastry bags.

BREAD LAME. A lame is a double-sided blade that is used to slash or score bread dough right before it goes into the oven. It helps create beautiful designs on the crust but also allows the dough to expand without cracking the surface when it bakes. There are many lame tools in the market, but I use a simple razor blade that I hold gently between my fingers when scoring. You can also use a very sharp knife, but the small razor blade allows you to cut more intricate designs.

BREAD-PROOFING BASKET OR _BANNETON_. Bread-proofing baskets or _bannetons_ are used to perfectly shape boules. They are inexpensive and come in different sizes, but I use 8-inch round _bannetons_. You can use a plain bowl for proofing, but make sure it is not wider than 8 inches.

CAKE AND LOAF PANS. Seek out cake and loaf pans that are heavy and sturdy, as they will last a lifetime. In general, gluten-free breads need extra support when rising, so I prefer loaf pans that are narrow and tall. My favorite brands are Nordic Ware, USA Pan, and Chicago Metallic; all three make beautiful and high-quality products. I have many different shapes and sizes, but if I were to only have three, I would recommend an 8- or 9-inch-wide and 3-inch-deep heavy-duty cake pan; a 9-cup Bundt pan; and a 1-pound loaf pan.

CANDY THERMOMETER. Candy thermometers are indispensable when cooking sugar. Taylor makes a 12-inch thermometer with a clip on the back that has been my preferred for years. It marks different sugar cooking stages, which is helpful.

CAST-IRON DUTCH OVEN. Many of the crusty breads in this book call for baking in a cast-iron Dutch oven, which works as a steam chamber. When the dough goes into the pot and is exposed to very high heat, it releases large amounts of steam, and when this steam is trapped in the hot vessel, it creates a crispy and beautifully caramelized crust. My preferred size for bread-baking is approximately 5 quarts. Alternatively, you can use a clay pot, also known as a cloche.

Creating Steam in the Oven

If you don't have a Dutch oven, you can bake bread dough directly on a baking sheet, but the crust will be paler and not as crispy. To address this, you can create steam in your oven by using boiling water. Put a shallow metal pan on the bottom rack of the oven while it preheats. When you put the baking sheet with dough into the oven, add 1 to 2 cups of boiling water to the empty pan and close the oven door immediately. The resulting steam helps develop a crust closer to one achieved with a Dutch oven. Of course, if you have a steam-injection oven, use it: add three cycles of steam about 5 minutes apart.

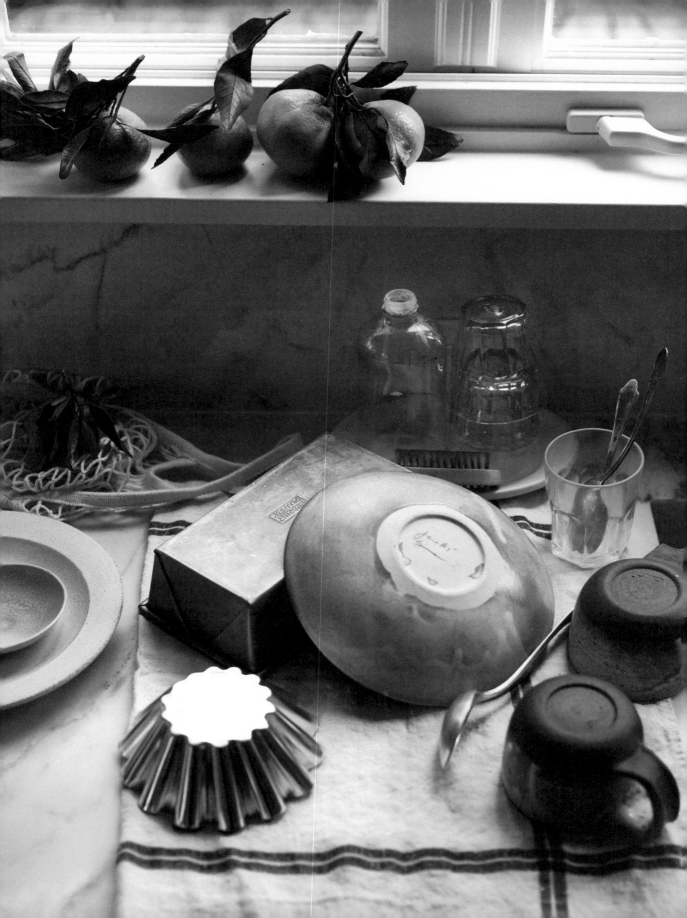

HIGH-SPEED BLENDER OR FOOD PROCESSOR. High-speed blenders and food processors can be used interchangeably sometimes, but not always. The only time I recommend a high-speed blender in this book is for blending cashews to a very fine paste to use for yogurt, butter, or cream. The pastry doughs call for a food processor, but you can easily make them by hand, simply breaking up the butter pieces into the flour between your fingers or using a pastry cutter.

KITCHEN SCALE. Digital scales are inexpensive and a must when baking. Choose one that measures both ounce and gram units. They are simple to use—put a bowl on the digital scale, zero (tare) it out, and add the ingredients to the bowl for an accurate weight.

STAND MIXER. My stand mixer is a refurbished 6-quart KitchenAid, and I use it for mixing bread, whipping meringue, and creaming butter. If you don't have one, you can mix the bread recipes by hand. For meringue or cookies, whip with a balloon whisk and some elbow grease, or use handheld electric beaters.

TART PANS. A 9-inch stainless steel tart pan with removable bottom is all you really need when making tarts. For tartlets, I use 3-inch stainless steel rings that are usually designed to make English muffins. These can be a bit harder to find, so search at restaurant supply shops.

The Importance of Weighing, Especially in Gluten-Free Baking

If you have baked from my previous books, you have already read my pleas to weigh your ingredients! Weighing will give you consistent results every time, and this is especially important in gluten-free baking, where there is wide variance in products. As a test, I weighed 1 cup of flour using different volume measuring cups, and every single one read a different amount in grams. As little as 25 grams more (or less) flour in a bread recipe can affect the texture of the dough significantly.

I develop my recipes using grams and then convert each amount to a volume measure to stay as standard as possible. For example, you will notice that 1 cup of superfine brown rice flour is always listed as 140 grams, 1 cup of almond flour is 100 grams, and so on.

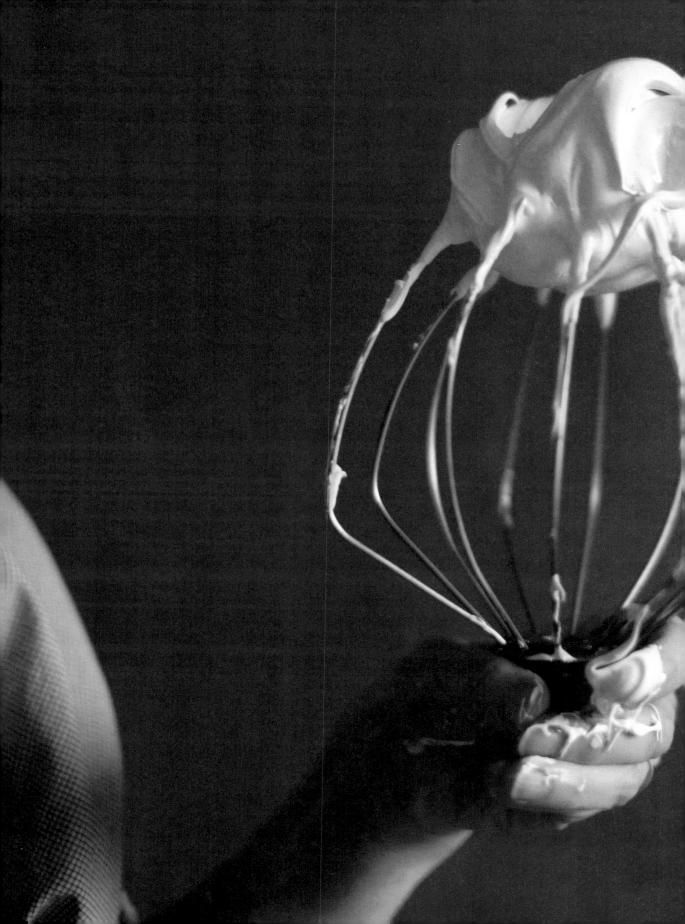

CHAPTER ONE

Staples

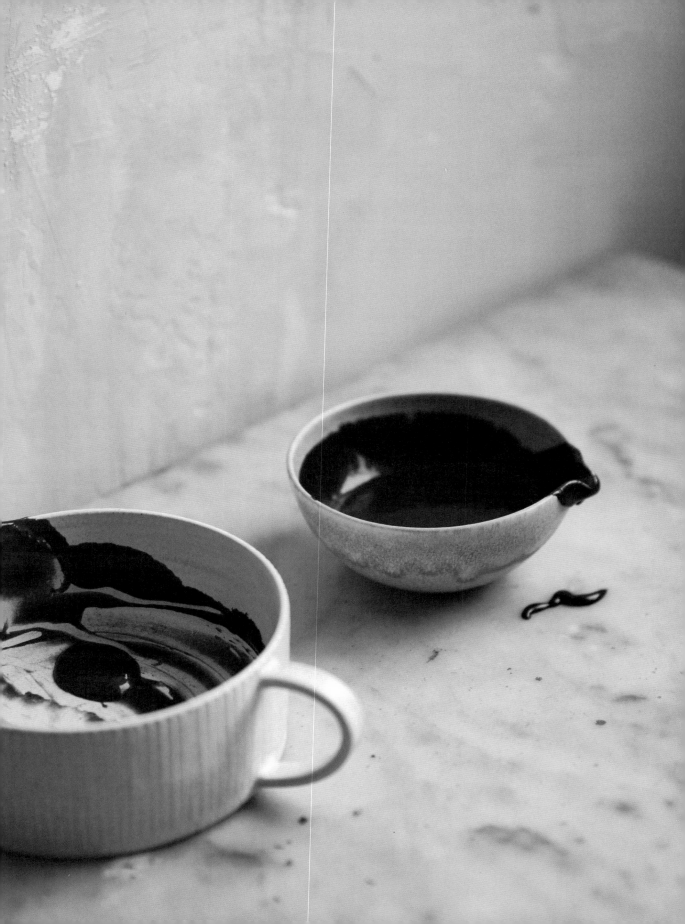

One thing I learned from my professional pastry chef days is the importance of building blocks in your baking repertoire. In this chapter, you will find many of my basic recipes that I use as foundational elements for baking, such as Cultured Cashew-Coconut Butter (page 33) in tarts and cookies, Coconut-Miso Caramel (page 46) to drizzle over fruit or cookies, or my favorite multipurpose frosting, Swiss Buttercream (page 42). Many of these staples are a base for other recipes throughout the book, and you can also use them as a base for your own creations. For example, bake Streusel (page 49) and sprinkle it on top of lightly poached ripe peaches, or whip up some Chocolate Pastry Cream (page 34) and serve it in a small ramekin with a dollop of whipped cream for a last-minute dessert.

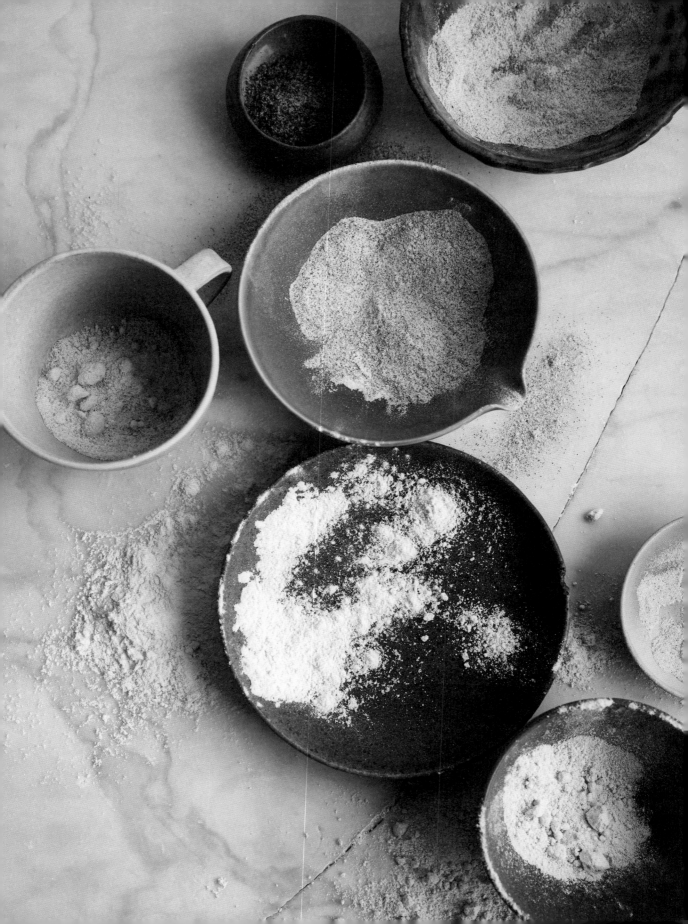

All-Purpose Gluten-Free Flour Mix

_____

4¾ cups (665 g) superfine brown
    rice flour
1½ cups (240 g) potato starch
¾ cup plus 1 tablespoon (95 g)
    tapioca starch

This is a good neutral-flavor gluten-free flour mix. It contains the ratio of whole grains and starches that I use in many baking recipes, especially for tender-crumb cakes and cookies. I don't add any xanthan gum to my all-purpose mix (unlike many commercial brands), and this is because I don't believe most of my cake and cookie recipes need it. I understand the popularity of ready mixes: it's convenient to open a bag or jar and measure directly. My preference is to consider the texture and flavor profile of an individual recipe and tailor my flours to it, which I've done throughout the book. However, if you prefer to use this mix, simply add up the weights of all flours and starches in the recipe and substitute the same total number of grams. This is true for most recipes except my sourdough starter, which needs to be made with whole-grain flour.

MAKES ABOUT 7 HEAPING CUPS (1,000 G)

1   Whisk all the ingredients together in a large bowl and store in a large flour jar. The flour mix will last for several months stored at room temperature.

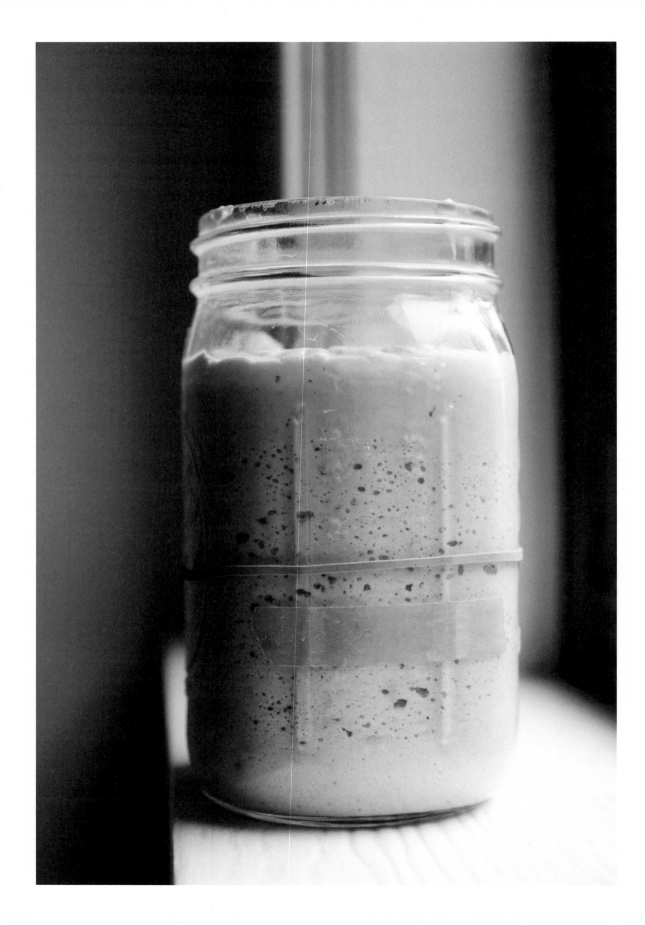

Gluten-Free Sourdough Starter

Wild yeast and bacteria exist all around us: on our hands, on fruit skins, on your kitchen counter, and in flour. A sourdough starter is a process of cultivating and harvesting these micro-organisms that create a process of fermentation when they eat sugars and carbohydrates. That fermentation releases alcohol and gases, which leaven bread.

If you have been following my work for a while or baked from *Cannelle et Vanille*, you likely will have created a gluten-free sourdough starter already. Since that book was published, I have been troubleshooting and coaching many of you through this process on social media, which has been such a community of support and learning. The recipe for the starter I am sharing here is similar to that one, but I wanted to include some new ideas about how I manage mine these days. The main difference is that I have reduced the hydration level and introduced a discard process while building the starter to help maintain even fermentation.

What is hydration level, you may ask? It is the ratio of flour and water in a starter, which is noted as a percentage. My original starter recipe was approximately 135 percent hydration, meaning that for every 100 grams of flour, there were 135 grams of water. For context, most wheat starters are around 100 percent hydration, so my starter was, and still is, much wetter. But this version is less so at 120 percent hydration, which results in a slightly more acidic flavor profile in the final bread. If you already have an established starter, there is no need to start over, but you may want to experiment with reducing the hydration level to see if you prefer the resulting texture and flavor.

Each starter is unique. Yours will be a result of your own blend of yeast and bacteria that has evolved based on your environment, feeding schedule, and type of flour. It will change throughout the seasons, and most definitely when you feed it a different kind of flour. As delicate as this seems, sourdough starters are hardy—it takes a lot to kill them. Be sure to read the troubleshooting tips on page 27.

My favorite flour continues to be superfine brown rice flour because it is mild in flavor and suitable for many different recipes, but you can also make a starter with teff, buckwheat, sorghum, millet, or quinoa flours.

1 cup (140 g) superfine
  brown rice flour
¾ cup (170 g) filtered water,
  at room temperature

FIRST FEEDING

In a medium ceramic or glass bowl, whisk together the flour and water until the mixture forms a pourable paste. Cover the bowl with a clean linen towel and set aside at room temperature for 16 to 24 hours, until you see some small bubbles form on the surface. Ideally the room should be around 75 degrees F.

⅓ cup (45 g) superfine
  brown rice flour
¼ cup (55 g) filtered water,
  at room temperature

SECOND FEEDING

Add the flour and water to the bowl and whisk to combine. Cover again with the towel and set aside at room temperature for another 16 to 24 hours.

⅓ cup (45 g) superfine
  brown rice flour
¼ cup (55 g) filtered water,
  at room temperature

THIRD FEEDING

By now the mixture should bubble up slightly and smell sour, like yogurt. Discard ¼ cup (75 g) of the starter, then add the flour and water, whisk, re-cover, and set aside at room temperature. As the starter becomes more active and larger in volume, it will eat through its food much faster, so you might have to feed it sooner than 16 to 24 hours. Check it after 12 hours and then every 2 hours from then on. When it bubbles up really nicely and begins to deflate, feed it—otherwise it will become watery.

⅓ cup (45 g) superfine brown
  rice flour
¼ cup (55 g) filtered water, at
  room temperature

FOURTH FEEDING

Discard another ¼ cup (75 g) of the starter. Whisk in the flour and water, re-cover, and set aside at room temperature again to ferment until it bubbles and puffs up. Because it might be ready for a feeding sooner than 16 to 24 hours, depending on the environment, keep an eye on it. As before, check it after 12 hours and then every 2 hours from then on.

½ cup (70 g) superfine
  brown rice flour
⅓ cup (85 g) filtered water,
  at room temperature

FIFTH AND FINAL FEEDING

Discard ½ cup (150 g) of the starter. Whisk in the flour and water, cover with a clean linen towel, and set aside at room temperature until it bubbles up nicely. This can take anywhere from 6 to 12 hours. At this point, you have enough established starter to begin making recipes. I store mine in a lidded 1-quart glass mason jar and keep it in the refrigerator until ready to use.

Sourdough Starter Troubleshooting Tips

Your Starter Falls Flat

If your starter was initially very bubbly and then suddenly falls flat and collects water (also called *hooch*) on top or sometimes the bottom, the starter is typically hungry. Don't be alarmed: it is normal for starters to collect hooch. Unless the hooch is dark brown—in which case discard it—I stir the hooch back into the starter when I am about to use it and feed it. If your starter falls flat during the building process or because it has been neglected for weeks, discard one-quarter of the starter and feed it again. You are trying to reduce a bit of the yeast and bacteria population and increase the amount of carbohydrates. Ideally, use your starter twice a week, but you can keep it in the refrigerator for up to 3 weeks without feeding (possibly longer, but try to discard and feed it before then!).

Your Starter Doesn't Bubble

If your starter isn't bubbling after the first two feedings and your room temperature is colder than 70 degrees F, put the bowl in a lukewarm water bath to aid fermentation. Also make sure the filtered water you add to the starter is around 75 degrees F and not any cooler.

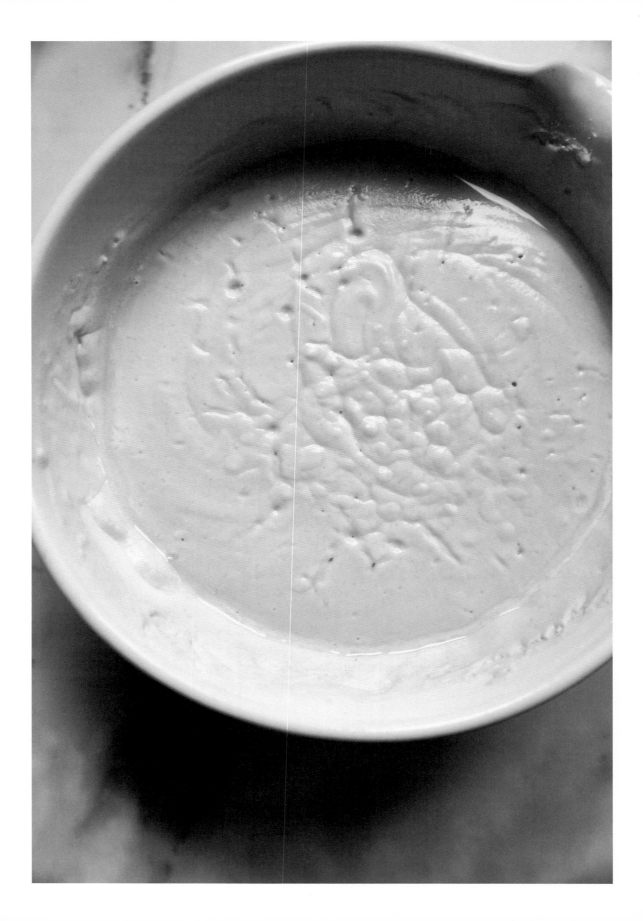

USING SOURDOUGH STARTER

All recipes that call for sourdough starter should begin with cold starter straight from the refrigerator because this allows for longer fermentation, which helps develops flavor and results in a better crumb. If you are excited to make bread as soon as your starter is ready to use, you will likely have to reduce the fermentation time stated in the recipe. Otherwise, when you proceed with a recipe, stir and then measure out the amount of cold starter called for, then transfer the remaining starter to a large bowl. Proceed with the cold starter as directed by the recipe. The remaining starter will need to be fed if you plan to use it within a few days.

FEEDING SOURDOUGH STARTER

Another frequent question is how much flour and water do I feed my starter? Well, it all depends on how much starter you will need the next time you use it and what the hydration ratio is. The sum of flour and water you are feeding should equal the amount of starter you will be taking out, plus a little more to compensate for transfer loss. For example, because I mostly make the sourdough boules that require ¾ cup plus 1 tablespoon (255 g) of starter, I replenish it with 1 cup (140 g) of superfine brown rice flour and ¾ cup (165 g) room-temperature filtered water (a combined 305 g total), which maintains the 120-percent hydration ratio.

Once you have determined how much to feed your starter, whisk in the flour and water until smooth, then transfer the mixture back into its mason jar and ferment, uncovered, at room temperature for anywhere from 6 to 12 hours. Once the starter bubbles up again, cover with the lid and return it to the refrigerator until the next use. The starter will likely deflate some and even develop a bit of hooch on top, which is completely normal.

Cashew-Coconut Yogurt

1 cup (150 g) raw cashews

3 cups (675 g) canned coconut cream

1 tablespoon maple syrup

½ teaspoon (about 2 capsules) probiotic powder (50 billion CFU)

This dairy-free yogurt is tangy, creamy, and thick without relying on stabilizers. The process is fairly simple, but allot at least 24 hours, as you must first soak the cashews to make the milk, then ferment the yogurt. Note that if you prefer a thinner yogurt, you can substitute 1 cup (225 g) of the coconut cream with either water or light coconut milk. I recommend serving the yogurt with fresh fruit and chopped nuts, or with chamomile-poached quince (page 191) and Streusel (page 49), as seen on the opposite page.

MAKES 1 QUART

1   Put the cashews in a medium bowl and cover them with abundant cold water. Put in the refrigerator to soak for 8 to 12 hours, then drain.

2   Puree the soaked cashews, coconut cream, and maple syrup in a high-speed blender until very smooth. You might have to stop, stir, and blend several times to ensure there are no gritty cashew pieces. Gently heat the mixture in a small saucepan over low heat until it reaches 100 degrees F. Do not let the mixture get too hot or it will kill the bacteria.

3   Put the probiotic powder in a medium bowl and whisk in about 1 cup of the cream mixture until it's smooth and lump-free. Pour in the remaining cream and whisk to combine.

4   Pour the yogurt into eight 4-ounce glass jars or a 1-quart mason jar. Put them, uncovered, on a baking sheet inside the oven with the oven light on for 8 to 12 hours. The yogurt will thicken. Lid the jars and chill in the refrigerator for at least 2 hours before using. The yogurt will keep, refrigerated, for up to 1 week.

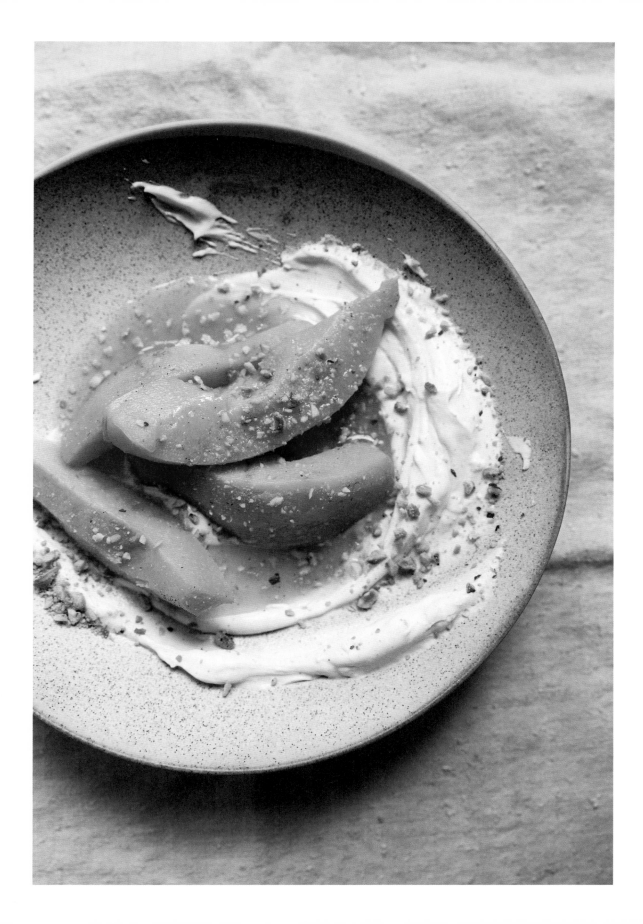

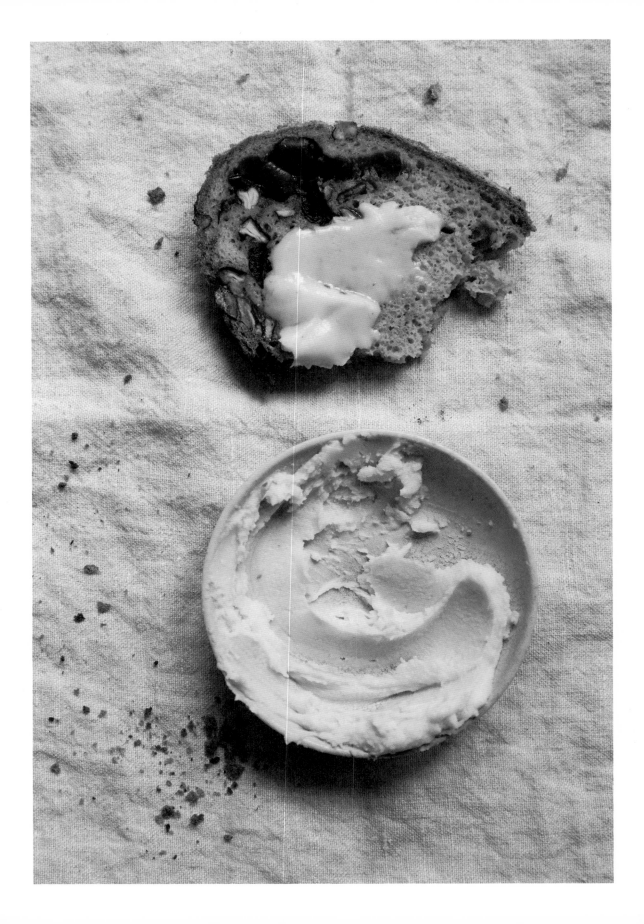

Cultured Cashew-Coconut Butter

In my book *Cannelle et Vanille*, I shared a recipe for cultured butter made by fermenting cream and then churning it. The tang resulting from fermentation adds much more depth of flavor, and it is particularly important in this dairy-free version. This butter works well in baking, especially for pastry doughs where you use cold butter. Keep it refrigerated since it changes texture after sitting at room temperature for an extended period of time. You can purchase silicone butter molds online in ½-cup sizes, which makes for especially easy measuring.

MAKES ABOUT 1 POUND (454 G)

½ cup (115 g) Cashew-Coconut Yogurt (page 30) or store-bought unsweetened dairy-free yogurt

½ cup (50 g) almond flour

¼ cup (55 g) extra-virgin olive oil

1 cup plus 2 tablespoons (225 g) refined coconut oil, melted and cooled to room temperature

¾ teaspoon kosher salt

1　Prepare a 1-pound butter mold or a small glass storage container by lining it with a sheet of parchment paper with enough overhang to easily pull the butter out later, or use individual stick molds.

2　Blend the yogurt, almond flour, and olive oil in a high-speed blender for 2 minutes, until smooth and airy. Add the coconut oil and salt. Blend for a few seconds to combine. Pour the mixture into the mold and refrigerate for at least 4 hours or preferably overnight. The butter will keep in the refrigerator for up to 1 week.

Pastry Cream

2 cups (450 g) whole milk,
   oat milk, or canned full-fat
   coconut milk
½ cup (100 g) sugar, divided
1 vanilla bean, split lengthwise
   and seeds scraped
1 large whole egg plus 2 egg yolks
¼ cup (30 g) cornstarch
2 tablespoons unsalted butter
   or dairy-free butter, cut
   into ½-inch pieces, at room
   temperature

Pastry cream is a classic in traditional baking. It is the cream that I remember most from my youth as it was the preferred filling for fruit tarts, profiteroles, or eating by the spoonful at my family's pastry shop. To make this dairy-free, use oat milk and dairy-free butter. I offer some flavor variations below, but you can use a variety of warming spices when steeping the milk, if desired.

MAKES 3 CUPS

1 In a medium saucepan, combine the milk, ¼ cup (50 g) of the sugar, and vanilla bean and seeds. Bring the milk to a low simmer over medium heat, turn off the heat, and steep for 5 minutes to infuse the milk.

2 In a medium bowl, whisk together the egg, egg yolks, remaining ¼ cup (50 g) sugar, and cornstarch until smooth and lump-free. Pour the warm milk mixture into the eggs, whisking constantly. Pour the entire mixture back into the saucepan. Whisk constantly over medium-high heat until the cream starts bubbling and thickens, 1 to 2 minutes.

3 Strain the pastry cream through a fine-mesh strainer into a clean bowl. Discard the vanilla bean. The cream will be steaming hot. Continue whisking until it cools slightly. Once the pastry cream has cooled to room temperature, whisk in the butter one piece at a time.

4 Cover the surface of the cream with a sheet of plastic wrap to prevent it from forming a skin. Store in the refrigerator for up to 3 days.

CHOCOLATE

Add 4 ounces (115 g) chopped 70 percent chocolate to the hot pastry cream after removing the vanilla bean, stirring until it melts and the mixture is smooth. Proceed as directed.

TOASTED-COCONUT

Toast ½ cup (40 g) unsweetened finely grated coconut in a dry pan over medium heat, stirring occasionally, for about 3 minutes. In step 1, steep the coconut in the milk with the vanilla bean for 15 minutes, strain, then proceed as directed.

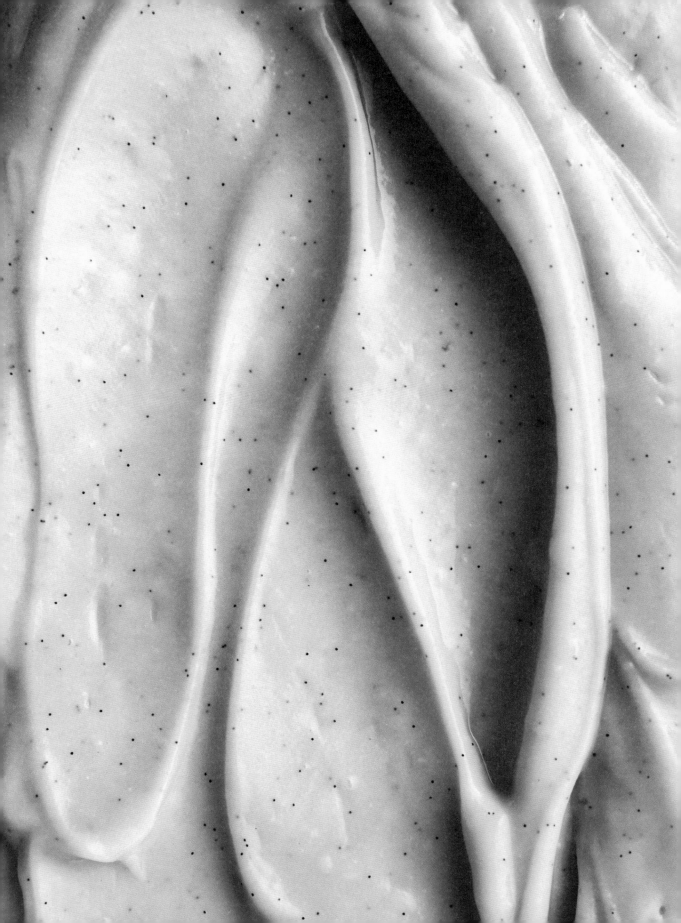

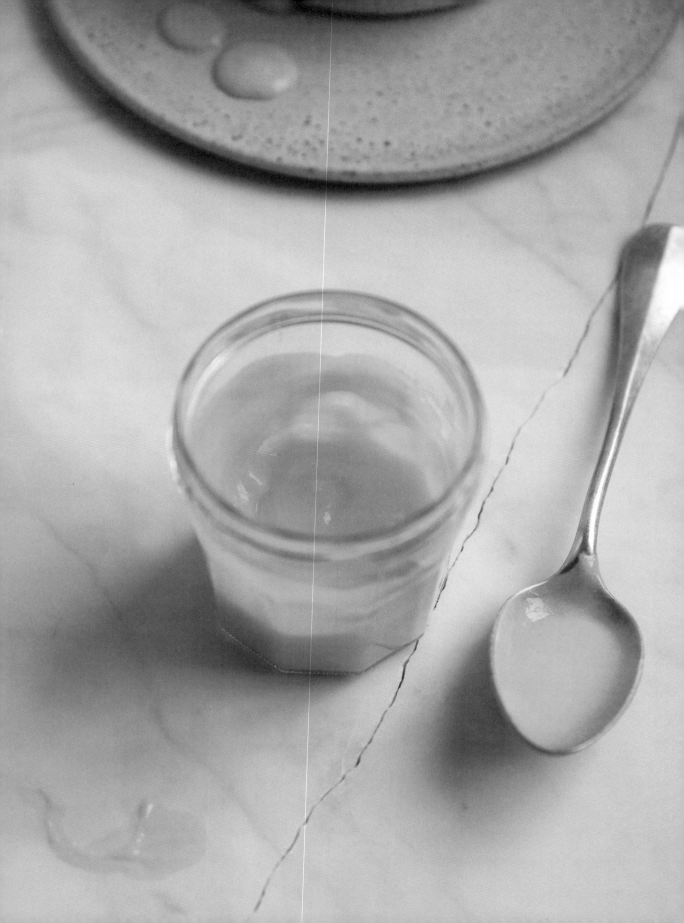

Lemon Curd

3 to 4 medium lemons
5 large eggs
½ cup (100 g) sugar
½ cup (115 g) unsalted butter
   or dairy-free butter, cut
   into ½-inch pieces, at room
   temperature

Every winter, when my friend Terisa sends me lemons from her orchard in California, I make a large batch of lemon curd to enjoy spread on toast or mixed into yogurt. This curd is quite tart (you can increase the amount of sugar to ¾ cup, if desired). You can also make the curd with different citrus, like blood orange or grapefruit. With sweeter citrus, such as mandarins or oranges, use half lemon juice to increase the acidity.

MAKES 2 CUPS

1   Fill a medium saucepan one-quarter full with water and bring it to a simmer over medium heat.

2   Using a vegetable peeler, cut strips of zest from 3 lemons (avoiding the pith) and put them in a large heatproof bowl. Juice the lemons until you have ¾ cup (170 g) of juice—you might need the fourth lemon. Add the juice to the bowl. Whisk in the eggs and sugar.

3   Place the bowl over the simmering water and continue whisking until the curd thickens, which should take 8 to 10 minutes.

4   Strain the curd through a fine-mesh strainer into a clean bowl. Whisk the curd to release much of the steam, and let it cool for about 15 minutes, or until it's warm to the touch but not hot.

5   Add the pieces of butter, whisking until the curd is smooth and shiny. If the curd is too hot, the butter will melt too quickly. The goal is to create a nice emulsion, so the butter and curd need to be approximately the same temperature. Cover the surface of the curd with a sheet of plastic wrap to prevent it from forming a skin. Refrigerate for at least 2 hours. The curd can be covered and refrigerated for up to 1 week.

Basic Frangipane

1 cup (100 g) nut flour (almond, hazelnut, pistachio, pecan)
½ cup (100 g) sugar
7 tablespoons (100 g) very soft unsalted butter or dairy-free butter
1 large egg
1 vanilla bean, split lengthwise and seeds scraped (optional)
½ teaspoon kosher salt

I shared a recipe for basic frangipane in *Cannelle et Vanille*, but I wanted to include it here so I could also offer dairy-free and nut-free versions. It is my favorite tart and galette filling because it's so moist, rich, and versatile. The sunflower-coconut variation below was inspired by my friend Naomi Devlin, but you can simply use tigernut flour in place of the nut flour to make this frangipane nut-free.

MAKES ENOUGH FOR ONE 9-INCH TART

1 Mix the nut flour, sugar, butter, egg, vanilla seeds, and salt together in a medium bowl using a wooden spoon or spatula until smooth. The frangipane can be used right away or refrigerated for up to 3 days. If chilled, let it sit at room temperature for a couple of hours and whisk it before using.

SUNFLOWER-COCONUT

In a food processor, pulverize ½ cup (60 g) raw sunflower seeds, ½ cup (45 g) unsweetened finely grated coconut, and the ½ cup (100 g) sugar. (Omit the flour entirely.) Add just 6 tablespoons of the butter, the egg, vanilla seeds, and salt, and mix until creamy and smooth.

CHOCOLATE, BROWN SUGAR, AND RUM

Use hazelnut flour and brown sugar (in place of granulated white), along with 1 tablespoon unsweetened cocoa powder and 1 tablespoon dark rum, and mix with the butter, egg, and salt until creamy and smooth.

Whipped Cashew-Coconut Cream

This cream is a great substitute for whipped mascarpone or crème fraîche. It is airy, tangy, and mildly sweet. It needs to be very cold to whip, so be sure to give it plenty of chilling time. You really need a high-power blender for this recipe, as a food processor is unlikely to puree the cashews to a fine cream. Also note that it needs to be started the night before, so plan ahead.

MAKES 2 CUPS

1 cup (225 g) canned
   coconut cream
1 cup (150 g) raw cashews
5 to 6 tablespoons freshly
   squeezed lemon juice
2 tablespoons maple syrup
¼ teaspoon kosher salt
1 vanilla bean, split lengthwise
   and seeds scraped

1   Put the coconut cream in the refrigerator overnight. Put the cashews in a medium bowl and cover them with abundant cold water. Soak at room temperature overnight (unless it's very warm in your kitchen, then put in the refrigerator).

2   Drain the cashews and transfer them to a high-speed blender with 5 tablespoons of the lemon juice, maple syrup, and salt. Blend until very creamy and smooth. You might have to stop the blender a few times, especially in the beginning, to help redistribute the cashews and grind them better. Add another tablespoon of lemon juice if needed. You want the cream to be the consistency of very smooth, creamy hummus. It should not be gritty or grainy at all. Once you have the right texture, transfer the mixture to a bowl, and chill in the refrigerator for at least 2 hours. You need the base to be very cold in order to whip it.

3   Add the chilled coconut cream into the bowl of a stand mixer fitted with the whisk attachment. Add the cashew cream and vanilla seeds and whip on high speed until thick, 2 to 3 minutes. If it doesn't whip well, refrigerate for another hour and try again. The cream will keep in the refrigerator for up to 3 days. If it deflates at all, whisk it vigorously again before using.

How to Collect Coconut Cream

I reference canned full-fat coconut milk and canned coconut cream throughout the book. You can buy canned coconut cream as is, but you can also collect it from canned full-fat coconut milk. Put a can of coconut milk in the refrigerator for at least 4 hours. In that time, the cream will have risen to the top and separated from the coconut water—scoop out the cream and use it in recipes as directed. The remaining water can be used in smoothies.

Swiss Meringue

4 large egg whites
1 cup (200 g) sugar
⅛ teaspoon kosher salt

Meringue is one of the easiest things to make without a recipe. Essentially you need one part egg whites and two parts sugar by weight. If you have leftover egg whites after making a custard or something that requires lots of yolks, this is a great use for them. It is very important to ensure that your egg whites don't contain any bits of yolk and also that your bowl and whisk are squeaky clean, otherwise the whites won't whip properly.

MAKES 3 CUPS

1   Fill a medium saucepan about one-quarter full with water and bring it to a simmer over medium heat.

2   In the bowl of a stand mixer, combine all the ingredients. Place the bowl over the saucepan and whisk constantly until the sugar has dissolved and the whites feel warm to the touch. You can rub the mixture between your fingers to check both.

3   Immediately attach the bowl to the mixer fitted with the whisk attachment and whip on medium-high speed until the meringue is stiff and forms glossy peaks, about 5 minutes. The meringue must be used immediately.

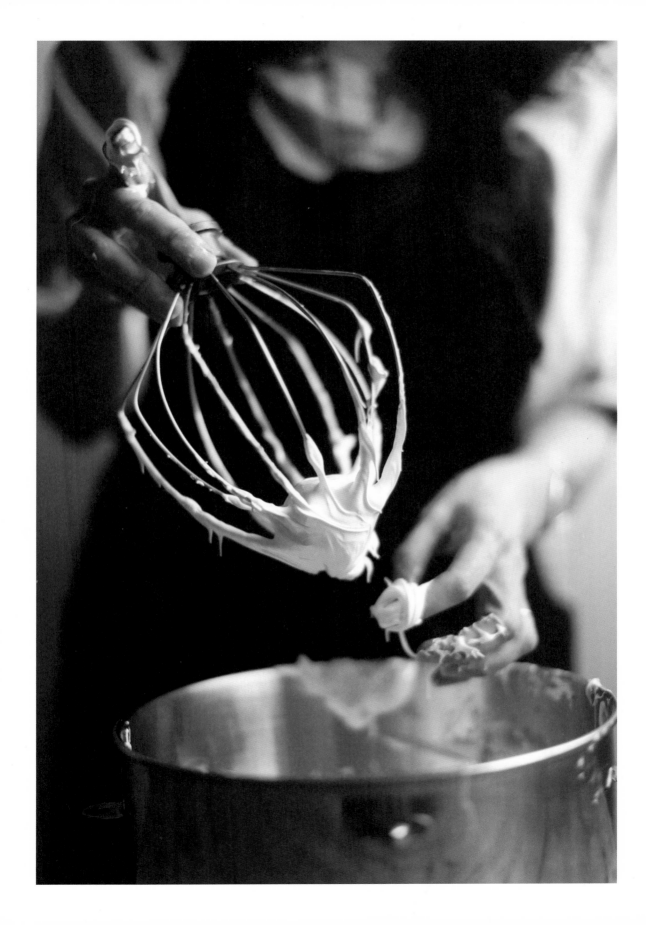

Swiss Buttercream

5 large egg whites
1½ cups (300 g) sugar
¼ teaspoon kosher salt
1 pound (454 g) unsalted
  butter, cut into tablespoons,
  at room temperature

VANILLA BEAN

Mix in the seeds scraped
from 1 vanilla bean
plus 1 teaspoon vanilla
extract at the end of
step 4.

HONEY-LEMON

Beat in 3 tablespoons
honey and 2 tablespoons
freshly squeezed lemon
juice until smooth at the
end of step 4.

CHOCOLATE

Fold in 4 ounces (115 g)
melted and cooled
70 percent chocolate at
the end of step 4.

Swiss meringue is the base for Swiss buttercream. Meringue is one part egg whites and two parts sugar, and buttercream has a third element: three parts butter, always by weight. You need approximately 3 cups of buttercream for a double-layer 9-inch cake, or 4 cups for a triple-layer cake, so adjust accordingly.

A note about making a dairy-free version: Some dairy-free butter brands tend to have a higher water content and can make this buttercream curdled rather than emulsified and smooth. If you need to make a dairy-free buttercream, I recommend the American-Style Buttercream on page 45 instead.

MAKES 3 CUPS

1   Fill a medium saucepan about one-quarter full with water and bring it to a simmer over medium heat.

2   In the bowl of a stand mixer, combine the egg whites, sugar, and salt. Place the bowl over the saucepan and whisk constantly until the sugar has dissolved and the whites feel warm to the touch. You can rub the mixture between your fingers to check both.

3   Immediately attach the bowl to the mixer fitted with the whisk attachment and whip on high speed until the whites are stiff and glossy and the bottom of the bowl feels cool, about 7 minutes. This is important because if the meringue is warm when you add the butter, the butter will simply melt, making the buttercream runny. This is also why the butter should be at room temperature—to create an emulsion, both elements need to be at approximately same temperature.

4   Reduce the speed to medium and add the butter a few tablespoons at a time, mixing well after each addition and scraping down the sides of the bowl as needed, until all the butter is incorporated. Don't worry if the meringue has deflated and the buttercream looks curdled. It will eventually come together. Switch to the paddle attachment and continue mixing for another 2 minutes, until smooth.

5   Keep the buttercream at room temperature if you will use it the same day. If not, transfer to an airtight container and refrigerate for up to 5 days. Let it sit at room temperature for at least 4 hours and beat with the paddle attachment on low speed to smooth it again.

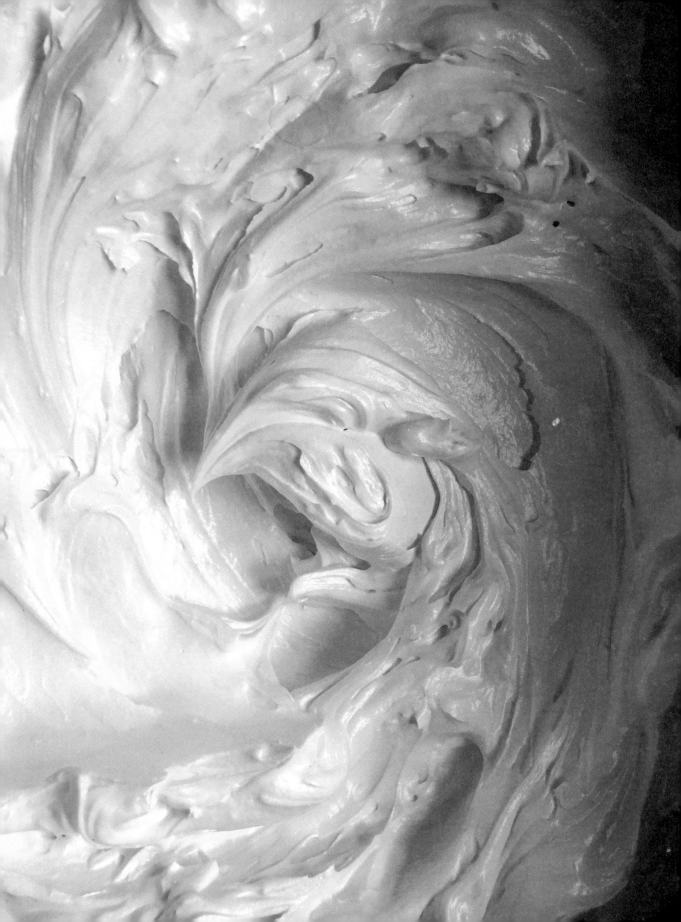

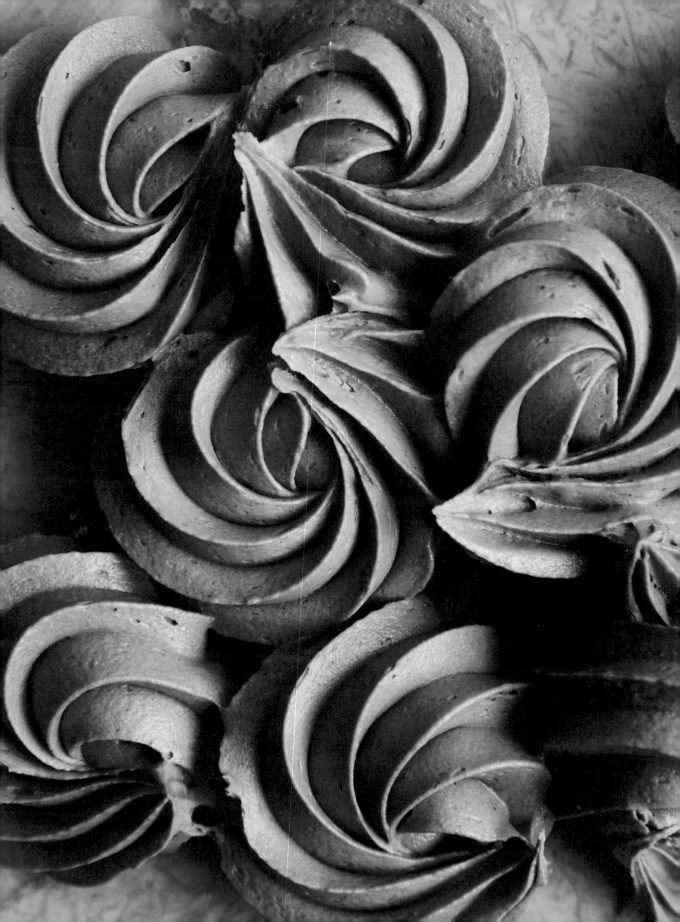

American-Style Buttercream

This is a quick and simple alternative to Swiss Buttercream (page 42). It is quite a bit sweeter than the Swiss version, so I prefer not to pair it with very sweet cakes. If you are making this with dairy-free butter, start with just 1 tablespoon of milk as the butter has a higher water content. Refrigerate after whipping so that it hardens slightly before use.

MAKES 2 CUPS

2 cups (240 g) powdered sugar
½ cup (115 g) unsalted butter or dairy-free butter, at room temperature
1 to 2 tablespoons whole milk, oat milk, or canned full-fat coconut milk
1 teaspoon vanilla extract

1　Sift the powdered sugar into a medium bowl.

2　In the bowl of a stand mixer fitted with the whisk attachment, beat the butter on medium-high speed until creamy, about 2 minutes. Add the milk and vanilla and continue beating for another minute.

3　With the mixer running, add the powdered sugar by spoonfuls, scraping down the sides of the bowl as needed. Continue beating until the buttercream is fluffy and holds peaks. It will keep in the refrigerator for up to 1 week. Let it sit at room temperature for at least 4 hours and beat with the paddle attachment on low speed to smooth it again.

CHOCOLATE-COFFEE

Sift 2 tablespoons unsweetened cocoa powder with the powdered sugar in step 1, and use 1 to 2 tablespoons very strong brewed coffee in place of the milk in step 2.

Chocolate Glaze

This chocolate glaze is a healthier version of a ganache or even a chocolate sauce because it is vegan and nearly free of refined sugar. You could also use applesauce in place of the jam for a sugar-free version. It is so simple to make that I use it on many cakes as well as for dipping fruit or spooning over ice cream.

MAKES 1½ CUPS

¾ cup (210 g) Honey-Apricot Jam (page 55) or store-bought apricot jam
¼ cup (80 g) maple syrup
¼ cup (55 g) extra-virgin olive oil
¼ cup (25 g) unsweetened cocoa powder
1 teaspoon vanilla extract
½ teaspoon flaky sea salt

1   Combine all the ingredients in a food processor or blender and mix on high for 2 minutes, until creamy and airy. Transfer to an airtight container and store in the refrigerator for up to 1 week. It will thicken slightly when chilled. You can spread it on a cake as a cream, but if you prefer to use it as a glaze, warm it up slightly, then pour it over.

Coconut-Miso Caramel

This is a very rich and thick caramel. The miso adds an unexpected umami layer that pairs really well with coconut. It is used in the Coconut Layer Cake with Caramel (page 140) and the Apple and Pear Pie with Caramel (page 185). The caramel firms up quite quickly, so reheat it for pouring.

MAKES ABOUT 1 CUP

1 cup (200 g) coconut sugar or light brown sugar
½ cup (115 g) filtered water, at room temperature
1 tablespoon vanilla extract
1 cup (225 g) canned coconut cream
2 tablespoons white miso
2 tablespoons unsalted butter or dairy-free butter

1   Combine the sugar, water, and vanilla in a medium saucepan (preferably with tall sides), and cook over medium-high heat until thick and bubbly, about 4 minutes.

2   Whisk in the coconut cream and miso. Continue cooking, whisking occasionally, until the caramel thickens enough to coat the back of a spoon and a candy thermometer reads 215 to 220 degrees F, which should take 6 to 8 minutes. Stir the caramel occasionally and watch to make sure it doesn't boil over.

3   Pour the caramel into a heatproof bowl. Whisk in the butter until shiny and smooth. The caramel will keep in the refrigerator for up to 1 week. It hardens when chilled, so warm it up in the microwave for a few seconds or in a warm water bath.

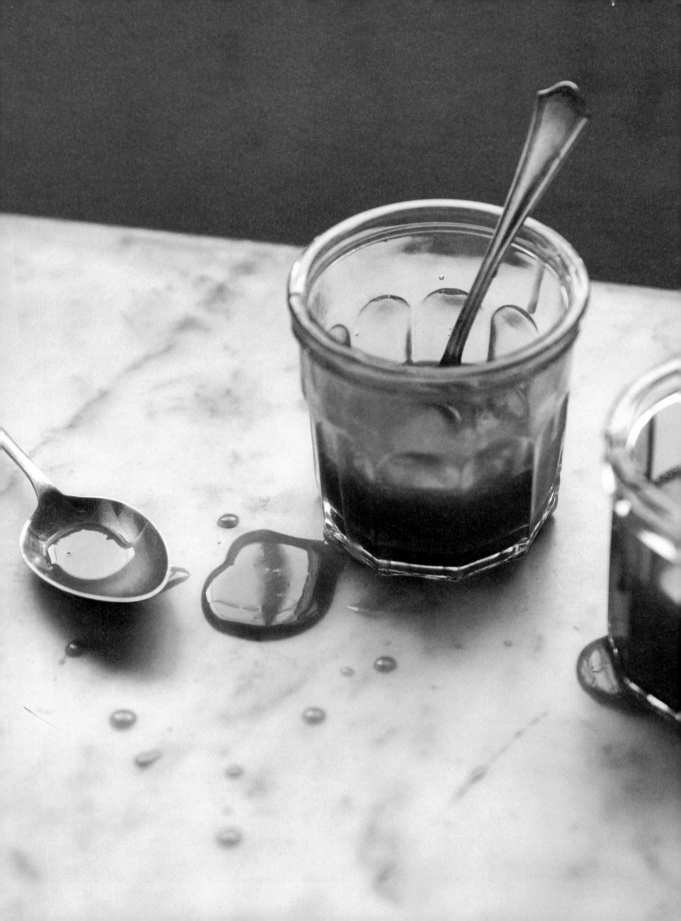

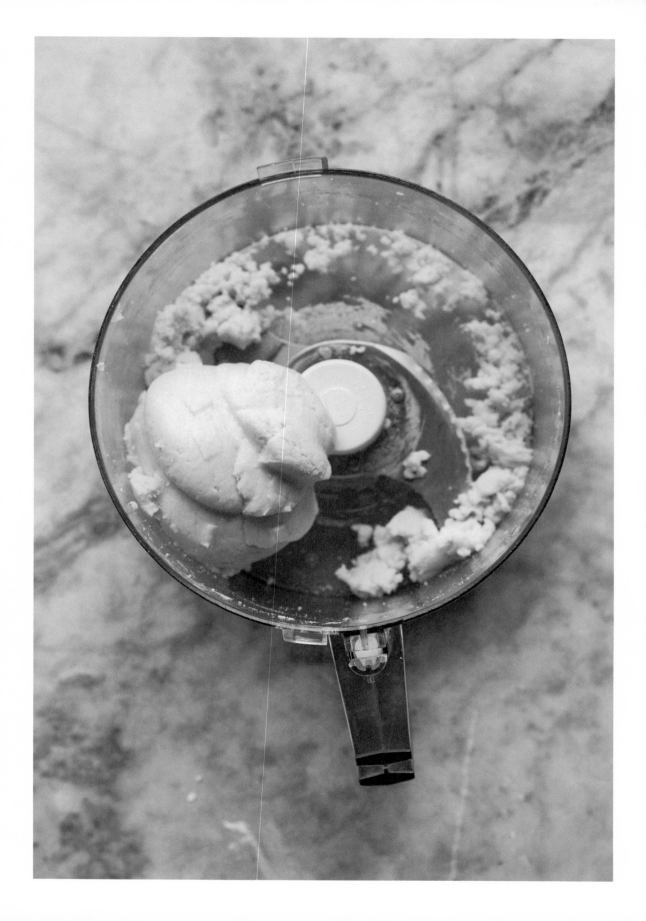

Marzipan

I love making marzipan during the holidays for dotting inside fruit tart fillings or for rich cakes. It is very simple and so much better than store-bought marzipan. You can easily make this vegan by using 1 to 2 tablespoons of aquafaba in place of the egg white.

1½ cups (180 g) powdered sugar
1½ cups (150 g) almond flour
1 large egg white
2 teaspoons almond extract
¼ teaspoon kosher salt

MAKES 1¼ CUPS

1   Combine all the ingredients in a food processor and pulse for a few seconds until it forms a smooth dough. Shape into a log that is 2 inches in diameter, tightly wrap, and refrigerate. The almond paste will keep in the refrigerator for up to 1 month. It hardens when chilled. Make sure it is tightly wrapped at all times so it doesn't dry out.

Streusel

Streusel is one of the straightforward ways to elevate any cake or pastry by adding a layer of crunch. It is a basic topping that works in ratios: one part butter, one part sugar, one part nut flour, and one part whole-grain flour, all by weight. I love adding it to muffins, tarts, or any cake. I usually mix a double batch and freeze half of it for later use.

1 cup (100 g) almond or
  hazelnut flour
¾ cup *minus* 1 teaspoon (100 g)
  superfine brown rice flour or
  light buckwheat flour
½ cup (100 g) light brown sugar
¼ teaspoon kosher salt
7 tablespoons (100 g) cold
  unsalted butter, Cultured
  Cashew-Coconut Butter
  (page 33), or dairy-free butter,
  cut into ½-inch pieces

MAKES 1½ CUPS

1   In a medium bowl, toss together both flours, sugar, and salt. Add the butter and work it into the flour until the mixture is sandy and crumbly. You can use the streusel at this point, refrigerate it for up to 3 days, or freeze it. To freeze, sprinkle it on a baking sheet lined with parchment. Freeze the pan for 15 minutes, then transfer the streusel to a ziplock bag or airtight container and store in the freezer for up to 3 months. There's no need to thaw the streusel before baking: sprinkle it frozen on a cake or tart and bake as directed.

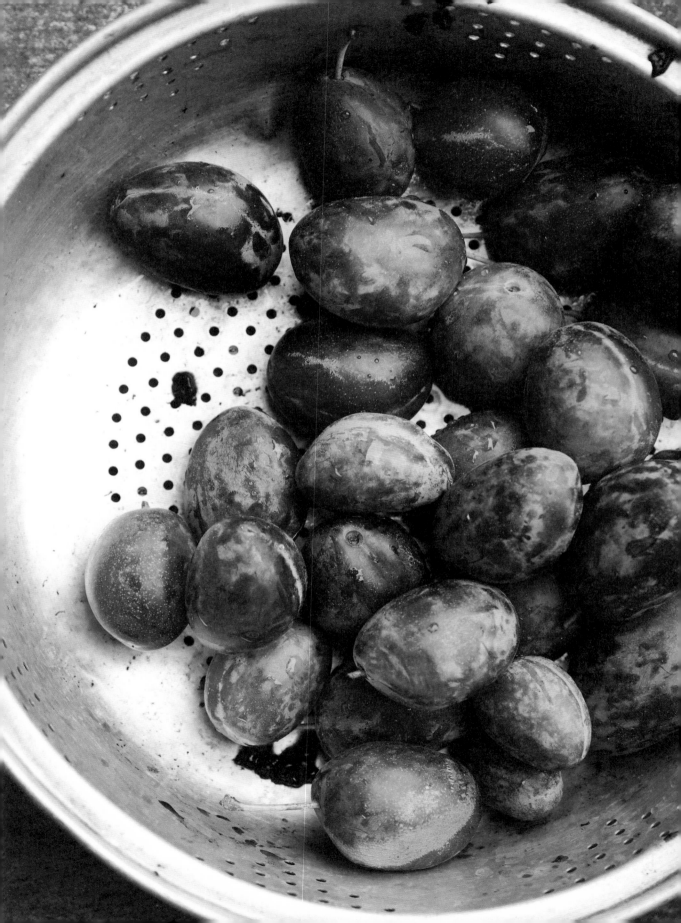

Fruit Jam and Compote

I grew up on toast and jam. My uncle Javi's prolific plum, apple, and pear trees, as well as the wild bramble bushes that tangled all around the sidewalks in our town, supplied my family with endless fresh fruit that eventually turned into compotes and jams. My mom made apricot and plum jam every summer—always using less sugar than traditional recipes called for. My preferred jam texture is just like my mom's, one that is rippled and a bit loose rather than gelled and very set. In general, I don't like using commercial pectin; there is nothing wrong with it, but I prefer to rely on pectin that naturally exists in fruits such as apples and lemons. Macerate the fruit for jamming with sugar in a large bowl. Chop up a lemon or apple core with seeds and skins and wrap them in a muslin bag or cheesecloth to macerate with the fruit for at least 4 hours so their pectin is released into the juice. Then cook the fruit until set.

Jams, not so much compotes, need sugar. It helps thicken the pectin as well as preserve the fruit. You might prefer to use less sugar, in which case you may reduce the amount in a recipe, but remember that you will need enough to reach a set point. Jams are usually set when the sugar syrup reaches 220 degrees F. This is when I do a gel test by spooning some of the jam onto a frozen plate to see how it sets. I don't look for a set gel, because that tells me it will be too hard when it cools completely. Something that ripples but doesn't feel too runny is ideal.

I haven't included instructions for canning as they are easy to look up online, but be sure your jars are sterilized prior to filling them. Fully submerge them in boiling water for 10 minutes or run them through the hottest setting in your dishwasher.

Strawberry-Hibiscus Jam

---

1 tablespoon dried hibiscus
   petals
½ cup (115 g) boiling water
1½ pounds (680 g) strawberries,
   hulled and quartered (if large)
   or halved (if small)
2 cups (400 g) sugar
1 medium lemon

Every early June, I pack the kids in the car with some snacks and rain boots, and we drive north of Seattle to Biringer Farm to pick strawberries. We disperse in the fields and it's quite the competitive endeavor of who picks the most and best-looking strawberries. We head home with our bounty and spend the afternoon processing the fruit—washing, hulling, and then freezing most of it. But I always reserve some to make this jam. The hibiscus adds a touch of tartness that balances the sweetness of the berries well.

MAKES ABOUT 2 CUPS

1   Make a tea with the hibiscus and boiling water. Steep for 10 minutes, then strain into a large bowl. Let the water cool completely. Then stir in the strawberries and sugar.

2   Cut the lemon in half and juice it into the bowl. Chop the entire lemon into large pieces and put the whole thing, including seeds, into a muslin bag, or wrap in a large piece of cheesecloth and tie off the top. Submerge the bag into the strawberry mixture. Cover the bowl with a clean kitchen towel and macerate at room temperature for 4 hours or in the refrigerator overnight.

3   Put two saucers in the freezer at least 20 minutes before cooking the fruit. Transfer the strawberry mixture, including the muslin bag, into a wide pot and bring to a boil over high heat. Skim off any foam or impurities that rise to the surface. Once it reaches a rolling boil, cook for 5 minutes. Then, using a slotted spoon, transfer the strawberries to a clean bowl and continue boiling the syrup until a candy thermometer reads 225 degrees F.

4   Remove a saucer from the freezer and put a small amount of the syrup onto it. Wait a minute to check how it sets. Continue cooking for a few minutes if needed and test again with the other saucer. Once it's ready, remove the pot from the stove and let the syrup cool for about 5 minutes, then stir the strawberries back in. This allows the strawberries to float in the syrup rather than sink. Discard the muslin bag.

5   Ladle the jam into sterilized jars and cool completely. Seal the jars with lids. The jam will last in the refrigerator for 2 to 3 weeks, possibly longer.

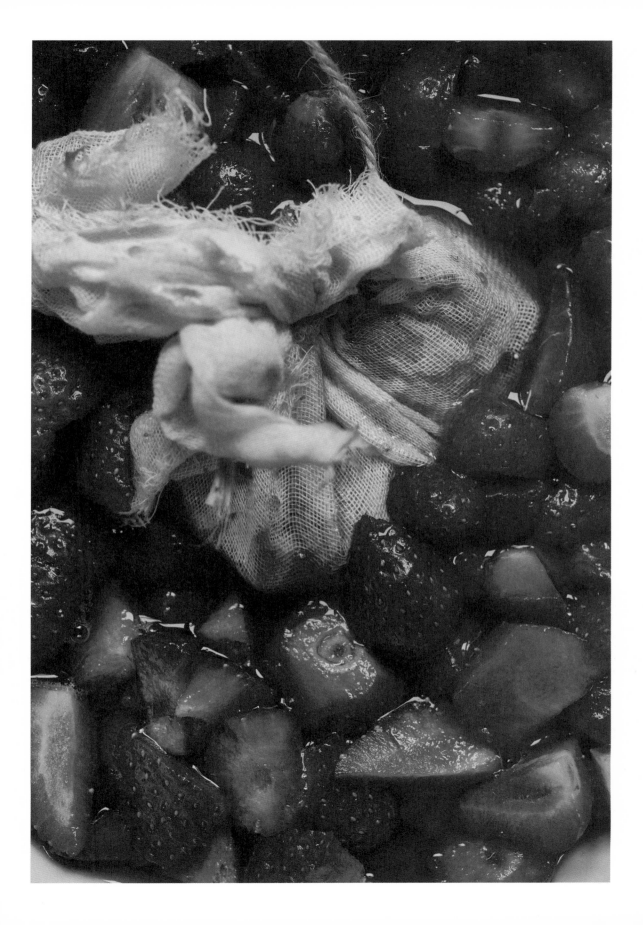

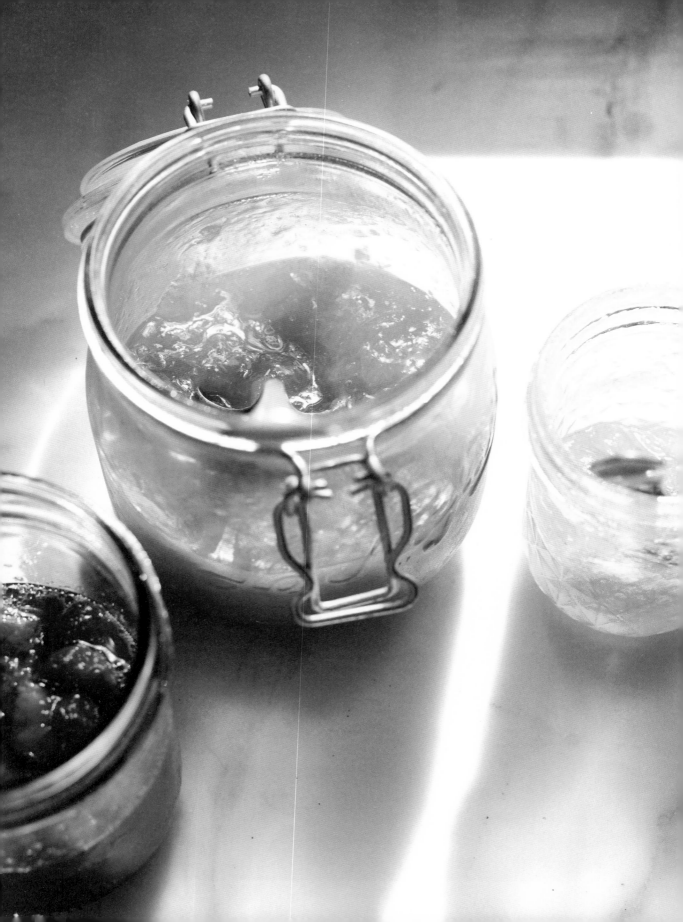

Honey-Apricot Jam

2 pounds (900 g) apricots, halved, pitted, and chopped into ¾-inch pieces
1 cup (200 g) sugar
½ cup (170 g) honey
1 tablespoon freshly grated ginger
1 medium lemon

This is my mom's favorite jam recipe, and I love making it with her when I visit the Basque Country during the summer months. It's adapted from one of Martha Stewart's classic recipes. In general, I like apricots that are very ripe and soft, but this is also a good use for apricots that are on the tart side as they add a nice balance to the sweetness of the honey.

MAKES ABOUT 2 CUPS

1   Toss together the apricots, sugar, honey, and ginger in a large bowl. Cut the lemon in half and juice it into the bowl.

2   Chop the entire lemon into large pieces and put the whole thing, including seeds, into a muslin bag, or wrap in a large piece of cheesecloth and tie off the top. Submerge the bag into the apricot mixture. Cover the bowl with a clean kitchen towel and macerate at room temperature for 4 hours or in the refrigerator overnight.

3   Put two saucers in the freezer at least 20 minutes before cooking the fruit. Transfer the apricot mixture, including the muslin bag, into a wide pot and bring to a boil over high heat. Skim off any foam or impurities that rise to the surface. Once it reaches a rolling boil, cook for 10 minutes, until a candy thermometer reads 225 degrees F.

4   Remove a saucer from the freezer and put a small amount of the jam onto it. Wait a minute to check how it sets. Continue cooking for a few minutes if needed and test again with the other saucer. Once the jam is ready, discard the muslin bag.

5   Ladle the jam into sterilized jars and cool completely. Seal the jars with lids. The jam will last in the refrigerator for 2 to 3 weeks, possibly longer.

Plum-Riesling Compote

The sweetness and acidity of Riesling pairs really well with plums, especially the Italian prune variety, while the vanilla bean adds warmth and balance. This is not a true jam as it doesn't thicken or set quite the same. It is a compote, which cooks fairly quickly, and therefore will be chunky and loose. I love this over ice cream or simply on toast with some cashew cream.

MAKES ABOUT 2 CUPS

2 pounds (900 g) plums, halved, pitted, and cut into ½-inch wedges
1 cup (200 g) sugar
½ cup (115 g) Riesling or other sweet white wine
1 vanilla bean, split lengthwise and seeds scraped
Juice of 1 medium lemon

1   Toss together all the ingredients in a wide pot and bring to a boil over high heat. Skim off any foam or impurities that rise to the surface. Reduce heat to medium-high. Cook until the plums fall apart and the compote thickens, 15 to 20 minutes.

2   Carefully remove the vanilla bean and ladle the compote into sterilized jars. Cool completely and seal the jars with lids. The compote will last in the refrigerator for up to 2 weeks.

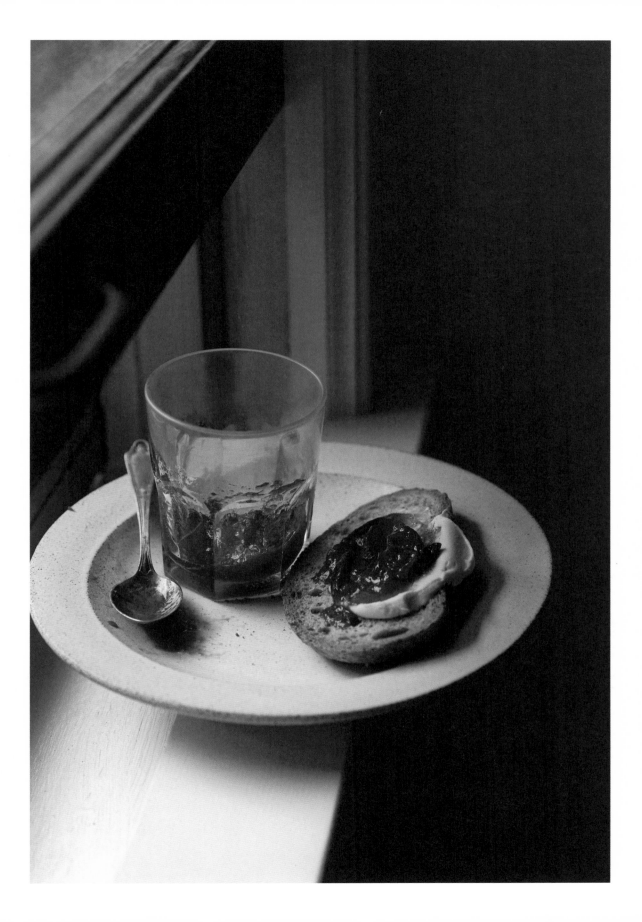

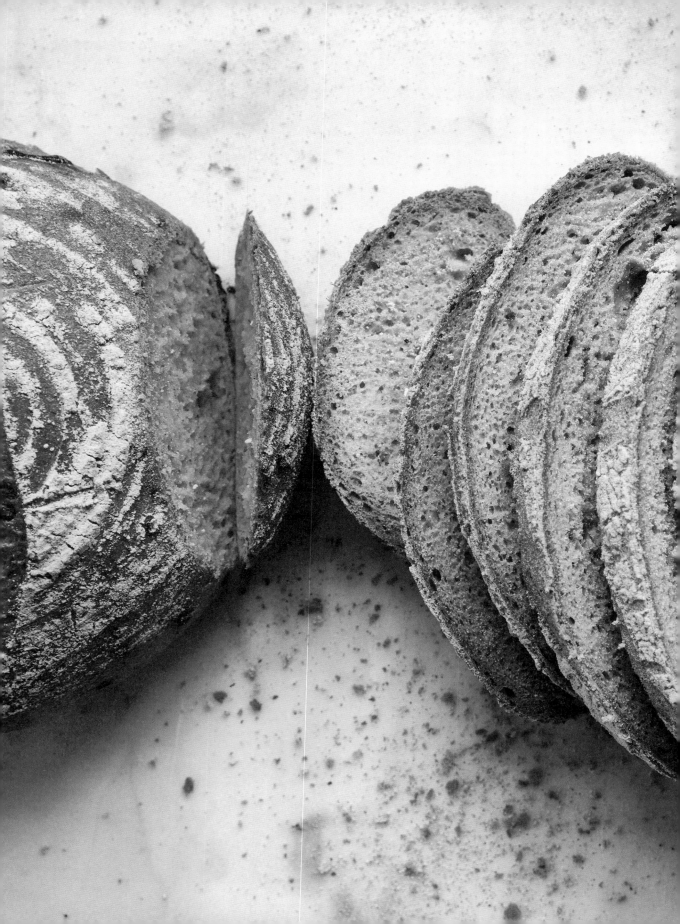

CHAPTER TWO

The Smell of Baking Bread

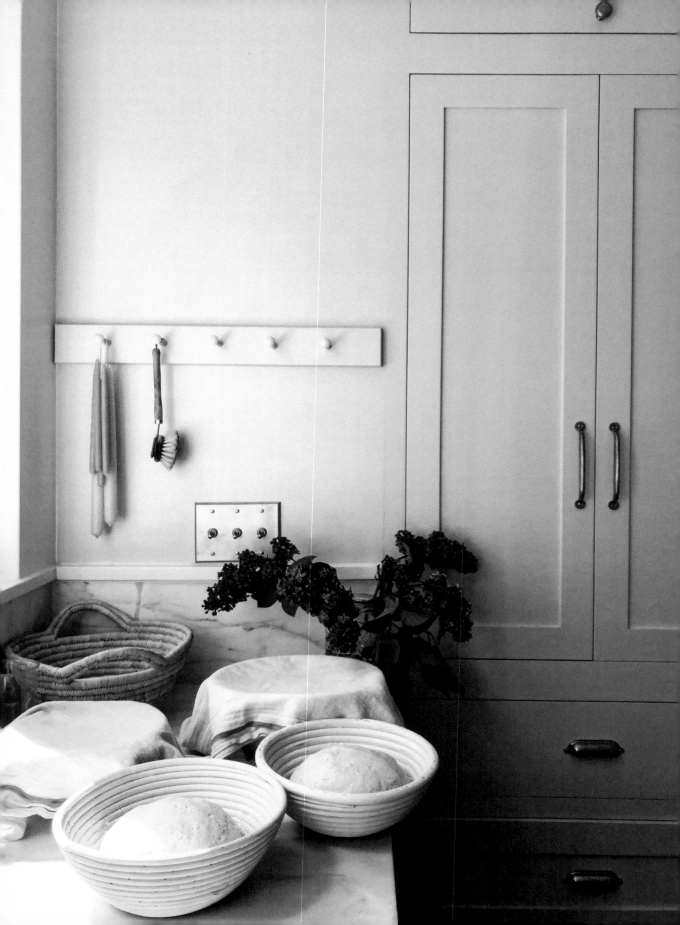

There is an undeniable comfort and warmth that one feels walking into a home where fresh bread is baking. To the lucky among us, baked bread is childhood. It elicits memories of running around the kitchen while someone mixed, kneaded, punched, dusted, and shaped bread. And when you're baking it yourself, it can be a great form of distraction (for me, it's almost like therapy!) to focus attention on this other living organism that is yeast. Baking bread is both science and intuition. It is also about what comes after—about breaking bread together, which is forever a unifying gesture for humankind.

This chapter is filled with an assortment of my favorite bread recipes, all of them yeasted except the Fig and Caramelized Onion Soda Bread (page 87). Many new recipes use sourdough starter, such as All-the-Seeds Sourdough Buckwheat Loaf (page 83), Spiced Sourdough Flatbreads (page 106), or Sourdough English Muffins (page 90). I have also included an updated Sourdough Boule recipe (page 62) with expanded troubleshooting tips. These recipes are straightforward but do take time. If you need to get something on the table within a couple of hours, make the Sandwich Loaf (page 73), Quick Crusty Boule (page 69), or Garlic and Herb Naan (page 105). There are also enriched breads, such as the Olive Oil Brioche (page 81); my personal favorite, the rich Chocolate–Olive Oil Babkas (page 101); and weekend morning crowd-pleasers like the Rhubarb-Cardamom Brioche Rolls (page 99).

Baking and sharing bread is equal parts self-care and love for others.

Sourdough Boules

The recipe for sourdough boules was probably the most sought after one in *Cannelle et Vanille*. As I spent time helping many of you troubleshoot, I learned a lot too! This updated version includes tweaks to the measurements as well as new tips. The most important thing to remember is that all sourdough starters are different, and therefore you must remain flexible and get to know yours. There is trial and error involved.

My current baking schedule goes like this: I mix my sponge at 6 p.m. and it's nice and bubbly by around 10 p.m. I then mix my dough, shape the boules, place them in the bannetons, and transfer them into the refrigerator by about 10:15 p.m. I wake up at 6 a.m. the following morning to preheat the oven, and around 6:40 a.m., the bread goes in. I have fresh bread by about 8 a.m., but no one is allowed to touch it until a couple of hours later.

MAKES 2 BOULES

For the sponge

¾ cup plus 1 tablespoon (245 g) cold sourdough starter (page 25)

1 cup *minus* 1 teaspoon (220 g) filtered water, at room temperature

1 cup plus 2 tablespoons (160 g) superfine brown rice flour, plus more for dusting

For the dough

1¾ cups (210 g) gluten-free oat or light buckwheat flour, plus more for dusting

¾ cup plus 3 tablespoons (120 g) sorghum flour

1 cup (120 g) tapioca starch

¾ cup (120 g) potato starch

2 teaspoons kosher salt

3 cups plus 2 tablespoons (700 g) filtered water, at room temperature

¼ cup (40 g) psyllium husk powder

3 tablespoons (20 g) flaxseed meal

1   To make the sponge, in a medium bowl, mix together the sourdough starter, water, and brown rice flour. Cover the bowl with a clean kitchen towel and proof at room temperature for 3 to 6 hours, until the mixture is bubbly, puffed up, and resembles mousse.

2   To make the dough, once the sponge has fermented, in the bowl of a stand mixer fitted with the dough hook, mix together both flours, both starches, and salt.

3   In a large bowl, whisk the water, psyllium powder, and flaxseed; it will quickly become thick and gel-like. Add this mixture and the sponge to the mixer bowl. Mix on medium speed until the dough comes together and all the flour has been incorporated, about 3 minutes. Alternatively, you can mix the dough by hand in a large bowl, making sure there are no large clumps of unmixed flour.

4   Lightly dust a work surface with brown rice flour. Turn the dough out onto it and cut into 2 equal pieces. Knead each piece, then shape it into a ball, making sure that the seam is sealed. The dough should be moist, with some bounce, and hold its shape.

5   Dust two 8-inch proofing baskets or mixing bowls with brown rice flour. Gently transfer the dough rounds into the baskets with the dough seam facing up. Cover the baskets loosely with clean kitchen towels. Proof the dough at room temperature for 1 to 2 hours or in the refrigerator for 8 to 10 hours. The dough will not double in size or expand much, which makes it hard to visually assess if it's ready to be baked. Give it a try and make adjustments based on the outcome.

6   Approximately 30 minutes before baking the boules, preheat the oven to 500 degrees F and put two 5-quart cast-iron Dutch oven pans inside. Heat them for at least 20 minutes. When ready, invert the proofing basket onto your hand, and gently place the dough into a Dutch oven. Score the top using a lame or sharp knife, sprinkle with a bit of oat flour, and add a couple of ice cubes into each pot beside the dough.

7   Cover the Dutch ovens with lids and bake for 45 minutes. Remove the lids, reduce the oven temperature to 450 degrees F, and bake for another 50 minutes, until the crusts are dark and sound hollow when tapped. The internal temperature should be 210 degrees F.

8   Transfer the boules to a wire rack and cool completely before cutting. This is very important because it allows the crumb to set and not be gummy. If you cut the bread before it is cool, it will collapse and all the air pockets will stick to each other. Be patient. Store the bread in a brown paper bag at room temperature. It is best eaten within 2 days. You can also freeze bread once completely cooled.

CHOCOLATE, WALNUT, AND BUCKWHEAT

Replace the oat flour with buckwheat flour. Add 6 ounces (170 g) coarsely chopped 70 percent chocolate, 1 cup (130 g) coarsely chopped walnuts, 3 tablespoons cacao powder, 3 tablespoons light brown sugar, 1 tablespoon honey, and seeds from 1 vanilla bean at the end of step 2.

FIG, WALNUT, AND CUMIN

Soak 3 ounces (90 g) dried figs in boiling water for 1 hour. Drain well and coarsely chop. At the end of step 2, add them in with ½ cup (65 g) coarsely chopped walnuts and 1 tablespoon cumin seeds. If any figs or walnuts stay on the surface after shaping, I like to gently push them inside the dough so they don't burn during baking.

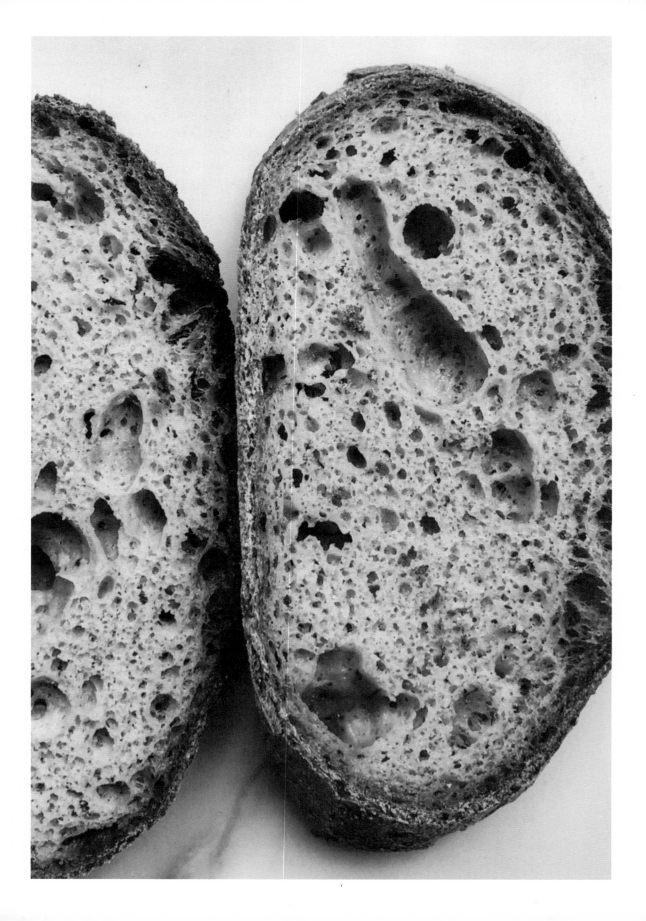

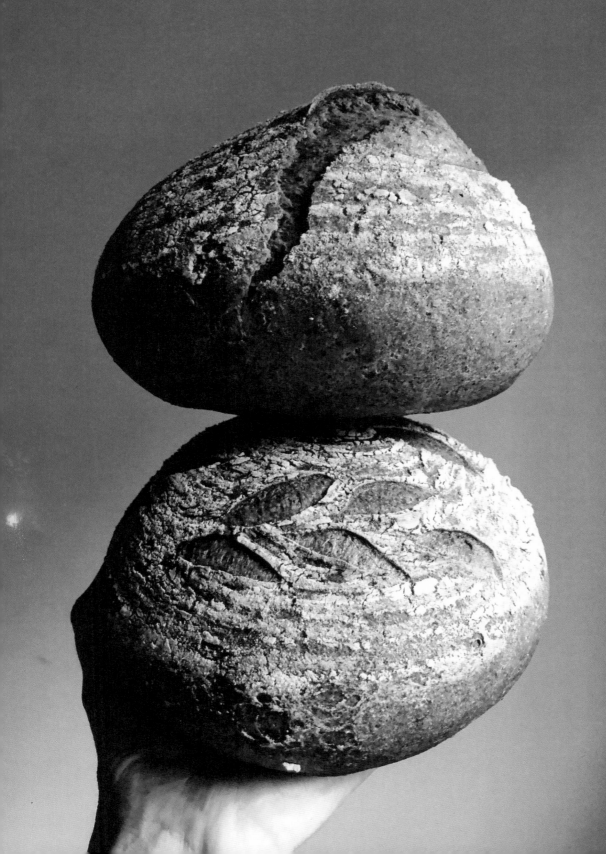

Sourdough Boule Trouble-shooting Tips

Lack of Rise

If your crumb is not aerated and open, make sure that your starter is refreshed and activated. You might have to discard some of the starter and refresh it with flour and water. If your crumb is open but you wish your boule looked taller, make sure you seal the seams really well and your boule is perfectly rounded when it goes into the proofing basket. Use proofing baskets that are narrow and deep (mine are 8 inches in diameter). This will give it the appearance of a traditional tall and rounded sourdough loaf because the shape in which the dough goes into the oven is essentially the shape it will come out.

Overproofing

This is probably the number one issue with gluten-free breads, and it is caused by the lack of elastic proteins like gluten. If your bread is overproofed, you will clearly see it as the crumb and crust detach, and many times the crumb collapses onto itself, creating a gummy interior. There are two variables to play with if this happens.

- Reduce the amount of sourdough starter. If your starter is very active, you might not need as much in your dough. Begin by reducing the amount by 10 percent and see if that helps, which it usually does.

- Reduce the fermentation time. Proofing for less time can help, especially if the room temperature has increased.

Gummy Crumb

The crumb in these boules is moist, especially the first few hours after baking. But if you feel like it's gummier than usual, it could be caused by any of the following:

- Using psyllium or flaxseed that is flaky or coarse. Make sure you are using high-quality finely milled psyllium husk powder and flaxseed meal.

- Using coarse stone-ground flour. If your flour is not superfine, use 10 percent less water.

- Not enough fermentation. If the dough hasn't fully proofed, the crumb won't aerate and becomes gummy.

- Overproofing. Similarly, if your dough is overproofed and the crumb has collapsed onto itself, it will also become gummy.

Burnt Exterior

The boules are meant to be dark and crispy, but if the bottom of yours is too dark, raise the oven rack one level and place parchment paper beneath your dough.

Cracked Crust

If you ferment your dough in the fridge and cover it only with a towel, the surface can dry out, which can cause the crust to crack during baking. If this is the case for you, cover the bannetons with plastic wrap tightly secured with rubber bands. Also, don't skip adding the ice cubes into the Dutch oven if you have issues with cracking. The steam created will keep the dough moist.

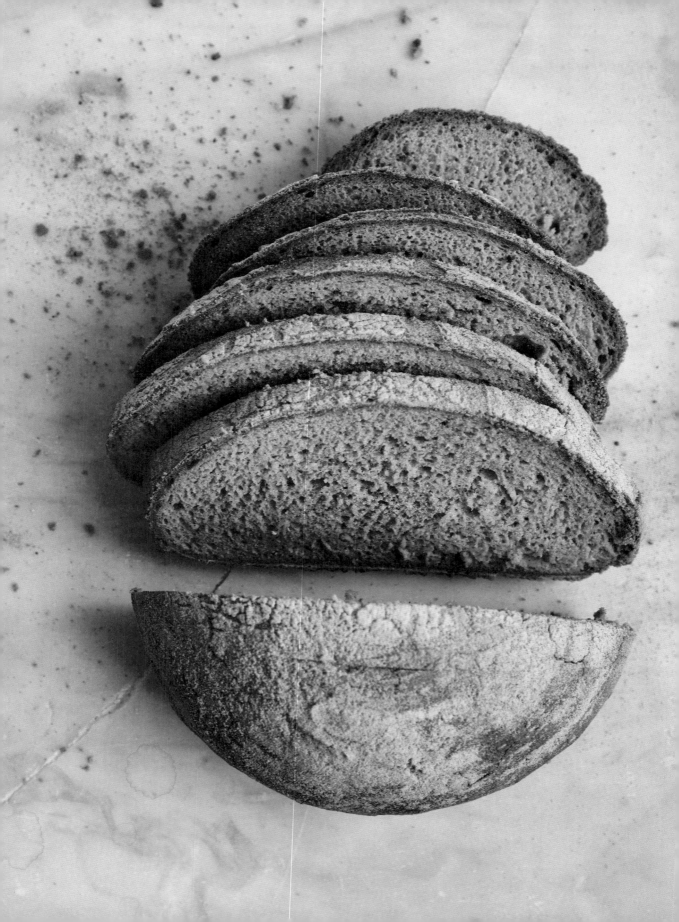

Quick Crusty Boule

2 cups (455 g) filtered water, heated to 105 degrees F
2 teaspoons (8 g) active dry yeast
2 tablespoons (20 g) psyllium husk powder
4 teaspoons (10 g) flaxseed meal
1 tablespoon apple cider vinegar
¾ cup (105 g) sorghum flour
¾ cup (105 g) superfine brown rice flour
⅔ cup (90 g) light buckwheat flour, plus more for dusting
⅔ cup (80 g) tapioca starch
½ cup (80 g) potato starch
1½ teaspoons kosher salt

I love sourdough boules, but sometimes you just need to speed things up. This boule made with baker's yeast is quick to assemble and bake, allowing you to have fresh crusty bread in just a couple of hours. It is also very versatile—you can add herbs, cheese, and other savory additions to create more texture and flavor. See some of my suggested flavor combinations on page 70.

MAKES 1 BOULE

1 In a medium bowl, whisk together the water and yeast. Proof until the yeast bubbles and a thin layer of foam forms on top, about 10 minutes. Whisk in the psyllium powder, flaxseed, and vinegar. Let the mixture gel for 5 minutes.

2 In the bowl of a stand mixer fitted with the dough hook, combine the three flours, both starches, and salt. Add the psyllium gel and mix on medium speed until the dough is smooth, about 3 minutes. Alternatively, you can mix the dough by hand in a large bowl.

3 Turn the dough out onto a work surface and shape it into a ball. Dust a proofing basket with buckwheat flour, place the dough seam side up inside, cover with a clean kitchen towel, and proof for 30 minutes, or until doubled.

4 Meanwhile, put a cast-iron Dutch oven in the oven and preheat to 450 degrees F. When the dough is ready, place it in the Dutch oven and score the top with a sharp knife or lame.

5 Cover the pot with its lid and bake for 45 minutes. Remove the lid and continue baking for another 45 minutes. Transfer the bread to a wire rack and let it cool for at least 1 hour before slicing. Store the bread wrapped in parchment paper for 2 days. It can also be tightly wrapped and frozen whole or sliced for up to 3 months. ⟶

CARAMELIZED ONION AND FENNEL WITH TURMERIC

Heat a medium sauté pan over medium heat. Add 1 tablespoon olive oil; ½ medium red onion, sliced; 1 tablespoon cumin seeds; 1 teaspoon fennel seeds; and ¼ teaspoon kosher salt. Stir and cook for 5 minutes, or until the onions are softened and slightly caramelized. Remove from the heat and cool to room temperature. Add them along with 1 teaspoon ground turmeric to the mixer bowl in step 2. If any onion pieces are at the surface after shaping, gently press them into the dough so they don't burn during baking.

ROSEMARY-OLIVE

Add ¾ cup (100 g) chopped olives, 1 tablespoon olive oil, and 1 tablespoon chopped fresh rosemary (or 2 teaspoons dried) to the mixer bowl in step 2.

GRUYÈRE-THYME

Add 3 ounces (90 g) grated Gruyère and 1 tablespoon fresh thyme leaves to the mixer bowl in step 2.

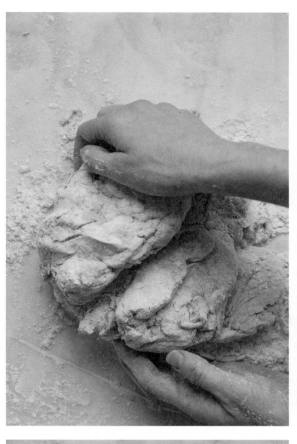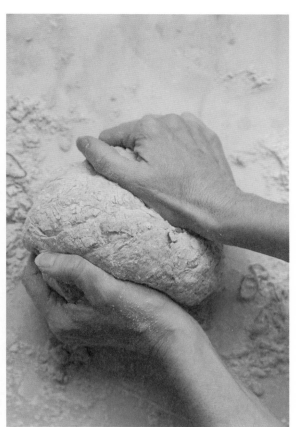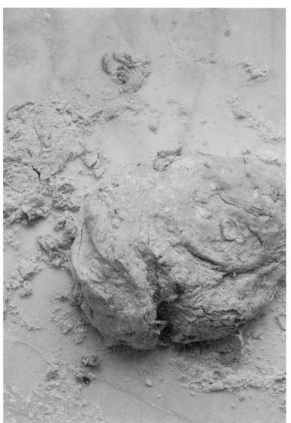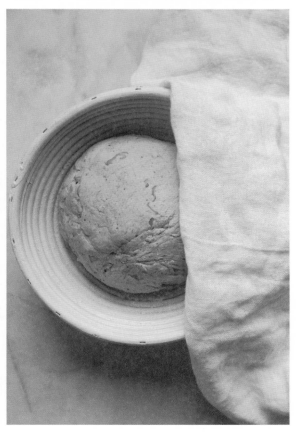

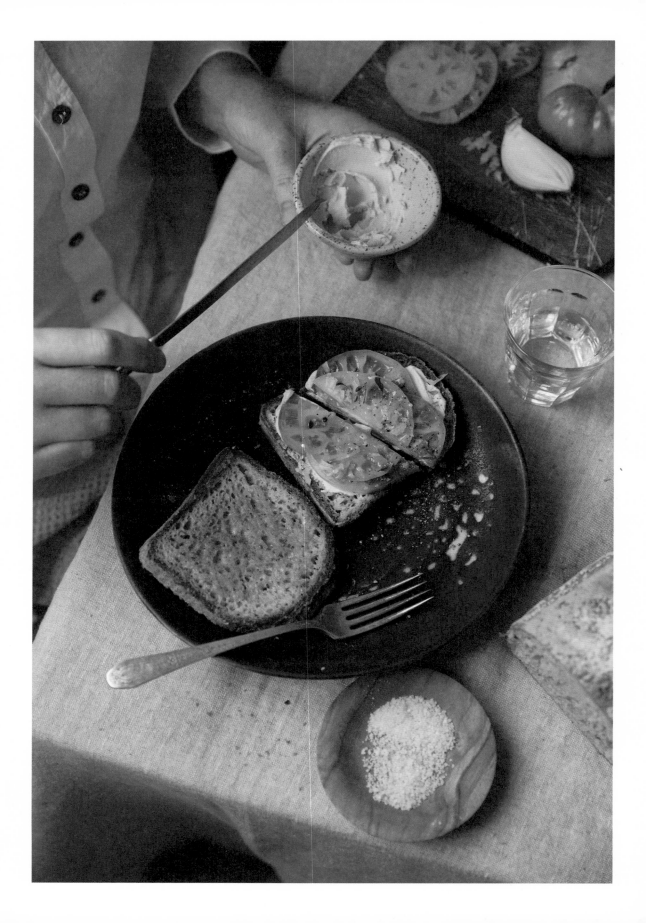

Sandwich Loaf

2¾ cups (620 g) filtered water, heated to 105 degrees F
1 tablespoon (12 g) active dry yeast
2 teaspoons sugar or honey
2½ tablespoons (25 g) psyllium husk powder
1 tablespoon (7 g) flaxseed meal
1 tablespoon apple cider vinegar
1½ cups (210 g) superfine brown rice flour, plus more for dusting
1 cup (140 g) sorghum flour
1 cup (120 g) tapioca starch
2 teaspoons kosher salt
Extra-virgin olive oil, for greasing

This bread has a moist, open crumb and a thin, crunchy crust. It slices like sturdy bread, leaving crumbs all over your cutting board. However, if you prefer a sandwich loaf that has a slightly softer crust, replace half of the total water with milk. Make this recipe as is or load it with herbs, nuts, and other additions. See some of my favorite variations on page 74.

MAKES 1 LOAF

1   In a medium bowl, whisk together the water, yeast, and sugar. Proof until the yeast bubbles and a thin layer of foam forms on top, about 10 minutes. Whisk in the psyllium powder, flaxseed, and vinegar and let it gel for 5 minutes.

2   In the bowl of a stand mixer fitted with the dough hook, combine both flours, tapioca starch, and salt. Add the psyllium gel and mix on medium speed for 2 minutes, or until the dough comes together. It should be a little sticky yet bouncy. Alternatively, you can mix the dough by hand in a large bowl.

3   Preheat the oven to 425 degrees F. Grease the inside of an 8½-by-4½-inch loaf pan with olive oil and dust with brown rice flour.

4   Dust a work surface with brown rice flour. Turn the dough out onto it and knead a couple of times, shaping the dough into a log about 8 inches long. Gently transfer the dough to the prepared pan. Cover with a clean kitchen towel or plastic wrap and proof for 30 minutes, or until nearly doubled.

5   Bake the bread for 1 hour. Carefully remove the bread from the pan and set it back in the oven directly on a rack. Bake for another 30 minutes.

6   Transfer the bread to a wire rack and cool completely before cutting into it, about 1 hour. It needs to set in the center as the steam evaporates, otherwise the crumb will be gummy. The bread keeps best wrapped in a clean kitchen towel or parchment paper for 2 days. ⟶

SESAME-CURRANT-HAZELNUT

Add 1 cup (130 g) coarsely chopped and toasted hazelnuts, 1 cup (130 g) dried currants, and ½ cup (60 g) black sesame seeds to the mixer bowl in step 2. Sprinkle some sesame seeds inside the loaf pan in step 3, then after the dough proofs, spray the top with a bit of water and sprinkle more seeds over the dough before baking. If there are any currants at the surface of the dough, tuck them in so they do not burn during baking.

CARROT-SUNFLOWER SEED

Add 1 cup (120 g) shredded fresh carrot, ½ cup (75 g) toasted sunflower seeds, and 1 tablespoon cumin seeds to the mixer bowl in step 2.

CINNAMON-RAISIN

Soak 1¼ cups (120 g) raisins in boiling water for 10 minutes, then drain. Add the drained raisins and 1 tablespoon ground cinnamon to the mixer bowl in step 2.

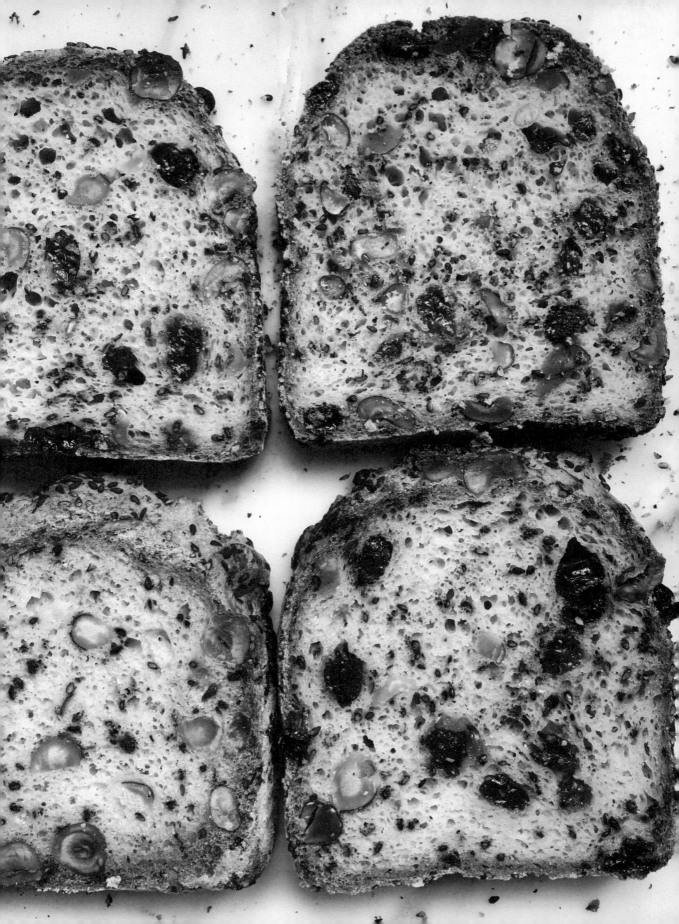

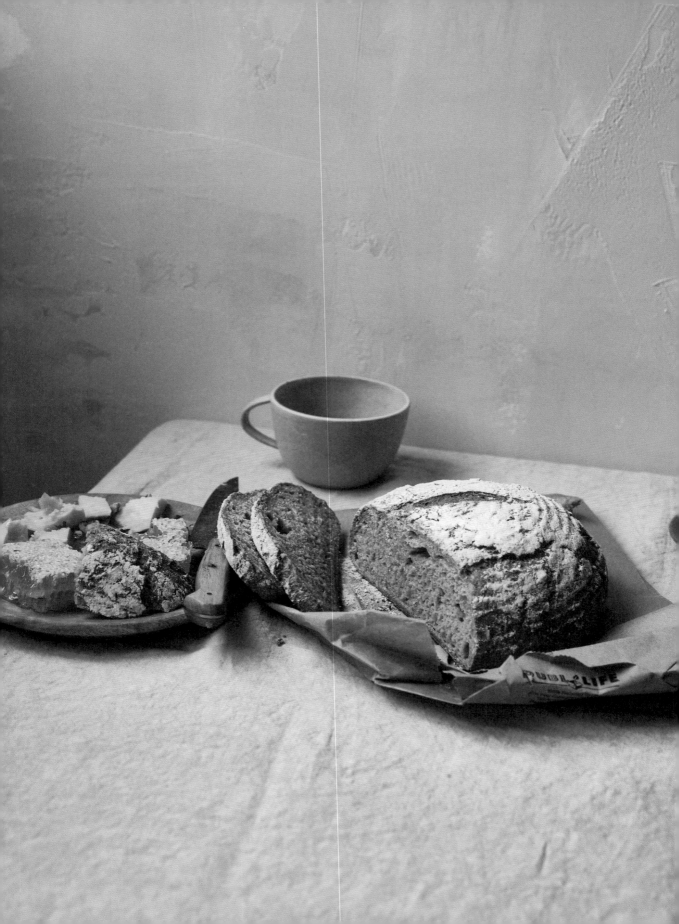

Oat Milk and Honey Bread

2 cups (450 g) oat milk or whole
    milk, heated to 105 degrees F
3 tablespoons honey
2 teaspoons (8 g) active dry yeast
¼ cup (55 g) apple cider vinegar
3 tablespoons (30 g) psyllium
    husk powder
1 cup (140 g) sorghum flour
1 cup (100 g) gluten-free oat
    flour, plus more for dusting
1 cup (120 g) tapioca starch
1 cup (75 g) gluten-free rolled
    oats, plus more for topping
1½ teaspoons kosher salt

This bread smells just as you imagine it would when you hear the words "oats, honey, and milk." The loaf is perfect for sandwiches fresh out of the oven, and for making French toast with day-old slices. If you prefer, you can bake the bread in a traditional 1-pound loaf pan instead of a Dutch oven. After mixing, shape it into a log, place in a greased loaf pan dusted with oat flour, and proof the dough for 30 to 40 minutes. Bake for 30 minutes, then gently remove from the pan and bake for another 30 minutes directly on an oven rack.

MAKES 1 LOAF

1   In a large bowl, whisk together the milk, honey, and yeast. Proof until the yeast bubbles and a thin layer of foam forms on top, about 10 minutes. Whisk in the vinegar and psyllium powder and let it gel for 5 minutes.

2   In the bowl of a stand mixer fitted with the dough hook, combine both flours, tapioca starch, oats, and salt. Add the psyllium gel and mix on medium speed until the dough comes together, about 2 minutes. It will feel sticky but don't worry, it will smooth out with a bit of flour. Alternatively, you can mix the dough by hand in a large bowl.

3   Dust a work surface with oat flour. Scrape the dough onto the surface and shape it into a ball, dusting with more flour if needed. Dust a proofing basket with oat flour and place the dough in it. Cover with a clean kitchen towel and let the dough proof for 30 to 40 minutes, or until nearly doubled.

4   Meanwhile, put a cast-iron Dutch oven in the oven and preheat to 450 degrees F. When the dough is ready, invert it onto your hand and gently place it inside the heated Dutch oven. Score the top with a sharp knife or lame.

5   Cover the pot with its lid and bake for 30 minutes. Remove the lid, reduce the oven temperature to 400 degrees F, and continue baking for another 30 minutes, until golden brown. The crust will be thin and crispy and the interior moist. Transfer the dough to a wire rack and cool completely before cutting, at least 1 hour. It's very important to allow all the steam to evaporate and the crumb to set. Store the bread at room temperature wrapped in parchment paper or a brown paper bag for 2 days.

Roasted Concord Grape Bread

1½ cups plus 3 tablespoons
  (375 g) filtered water, heated
  to 105 degrees F
2 teaspoons (8 g) active dry yeast
1 teaspoon honey
1 tablespoon (10 g) psyllium
  husk powder
1 tablespoon (7 g) flaxseed meal
1 tablespoon apple cider vinegar
1 cup (140 g) sorghum flour
¾ cup (90 g) tapioca starch
½ cup (70 g) superfine brown rice
  flour, plus more for dusting
1½ teaspoons kosher salt
5 ounces (140 g) Concord grapes
2 tablespoons extra-virgin olive
  oil, plus more for drizzling
¼ to ½ teaspoon flaky sea salt
2 tablespoons za'atar (optional)

When I was a child, we spent our August days camping in Spain's La Rioja region, which is known for its wine. I remember the silence on the plains and the blanket of dry warmth that enveloped us. We visited orchards, picked blackberries in the wild open fields, and ferociously stuffed our mouths with muscat grapes. We turned them into jelly occasionally but hardly ever were they roasted. It was years later that I was introduced to the pleasure of roasted grapes on bread. This recipe is somewhere between a focaccia and a boule. It's wonderful on its own but also pairs well with a slice of aged cheese, such as cheddar or Idiazabal.

MAKES 1 LOAF

1 In a medium bowl, whisk together the water, yeast, and honey. Proof until the yeast bubbles and a thin layer of foam forms on top, about 10 minutes. Whisk in the psyllium powder, flaxseed, and vinegar and let it gel for 5 minutes.

2 In a large bowl, mix the sorghum flour, tapioca starch, brown rice flour, and kosher salt. Add the psyllium gel and stir with a wooden spoon until it comes together into a lumpy dough. Dust a work surface with brown rice flour, turn out the dough, and knead it until smooth. Shape it into a round boule.

3 Preheat the oven to 400 degrees F. Position a rack in the bottom third of the oven. Line a baking sheet with parchment paper.

4 Place the dough on the baking sheet and gently press down with your fingertips until it is about 8 inches wide and 1½ inches thick. Scatter the grapes on top, lightly pressing on them. Dust the bread with a bit of brown rice flour (this is to give the surface a rustic look). Cover the dough with a clean kitchen towel and proof for 30 to 40 minutes, until puffed up and nearly doubled.

5 Drizzle the dough with the olive oil and sea salt. Bake for 40 to 45 minutes, until golden brown and the grapes are caramelized. Some grapes might burn slightly, which I don't mind. While the bread is still hot, drizzle a bit more olive oil on top and sprinkle the za'atar all over. Let the bread cool completely before cutting into it. It is best eaten the same day.

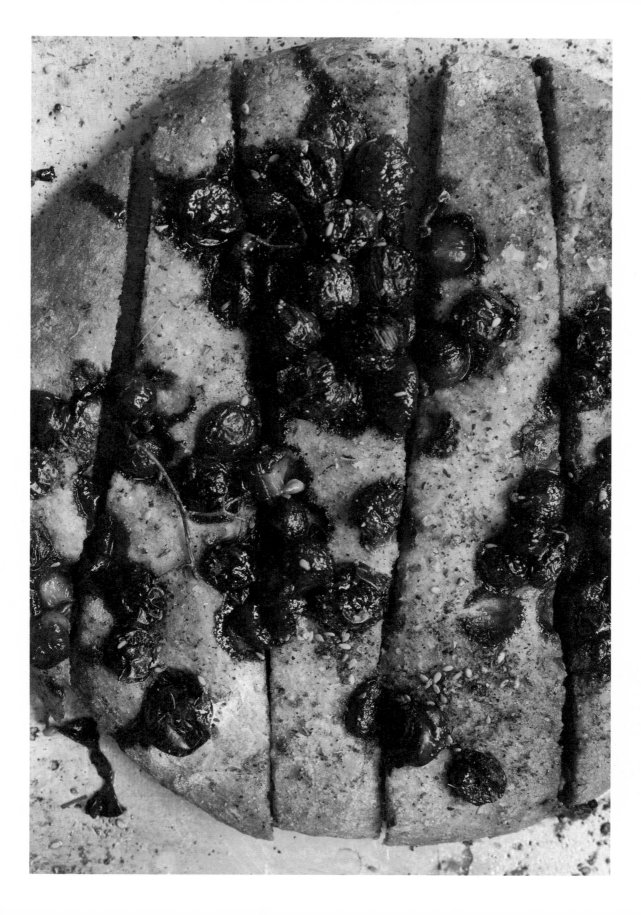

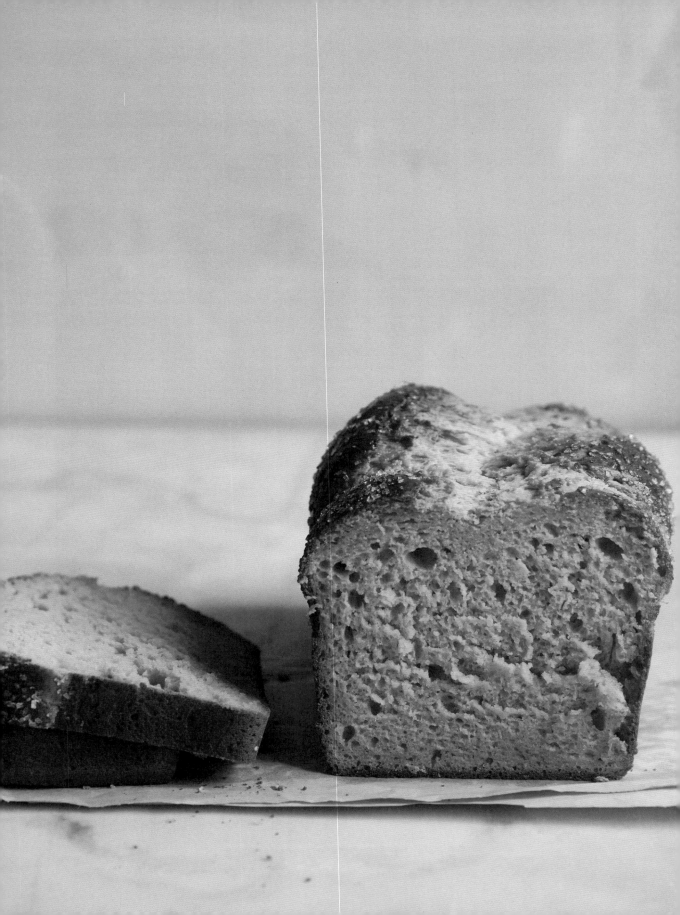

Olive Oil Brioche

1¼ cups (300 g) whole milk or oat milk, heated to 100 degrees F
1 tablespoon (12 g) active dry yeast
3 tablespoons (30 g) psyllium husk powder
1 cup (160 g) potato starch
1 cup (120 g) tapioca starch, plus more for dusting
1 cup (140 g) sweet white rice flour
½ cup (70 g) superfine brown rice flour
½ cup (100 g) sugar
1½ teaspoons kosher salt
Finely grated zest of 1 medium orange
Finely grated zest of 1 medium lemon
¼ cup (55 g) extra-virgin olive oil, plus more for greasing
4 large eggs, divided
Sparkling sugar (optional)

Brioche always brings up memories of my childhood: the smell of the enriched dough fermenting overnight, spreading buttercream on brioche rolls to make *bollos de mantequilla*, and the sight of my grandmother standing alone in the dimly lit old pastry kitchen late into the evening. My version includes olive oil rather than butter. I use this recipe as a base for rolls and other enriched breads. See page 82 for a chocolate brioche and a savory bun variation.

MAKES 1 LOAF

1   In a medium bowl, whisk together the milk and yeast. Proof until the yeast bubbles and a thin layer of foam forms on top, about 10 minutes. Whisk in the psyllium powder and let it gel for 5 minutes.

2   In the bowl of a stand mixer fitted with the dough hook, combine both starches, both flours, sugar, salt, orange and lemon zests, and the psyllium gel. Turn the mixer on medium speed, adding the olive oil and 3 of the eggs, one at a time. Mix the dough for 2 minutes, or until it comes together and is lump free. It will be sticky and feel like thick cake batter.

3   Grease a large bowl with olive oil. Scrape the dough into it and shape into a ball as much as possible. Turn the dough around to coat it. At this point, it won't feel as sticky and you will be able to round it a bit more. Cover the bowl with a clean kitchen towel and ferment for 45 minutes, or until nearly doubled.

4   Grease the inside of an 8½-by-4½-inch loaf pan with olive oil. Lightly dust a work surface with tapioca starch and turn the dough out onto it. Gently press down the dough to deflate it a bit. It should feel airy. Cut it into 6 equal pieces, then roll each piece into a ball. Tightly pack the pieces of dough inside the loaf pan so they are pressing against each other. Cover with a towel and proof for 45 minutes, or until nearly doubled.

5   Halfway through proofing, preheat the oven to 375 degrees F. Whisk the remaining egg in a small bowl and brush the dough with it. Sprinkle the top with sparkling sugar. $\longrightarrow$

6 Bake the brioche for 40 minutes, or until golden brown. Let it cool in the pan for 15 minutes, then invert it onto a wire rack and cool completely before slicing. It is best eaten the same day, but any leftover slices make great French toast or Almond Bostock with Apricots (page 97).

CHOCOLATE

Knead 4 ounces (115 g) coarsely chopped bittersweet chocolate into the dough at the end of step 2, then proceed with the recipe as directed.

SAVORY BRIOCHE BUNS

Cut the sugar amount in half. Follow steps 1 through 4 as directed, but divide the dough into 12 equal pieces (each about 100 g) instead of 6. Shape the dough into balls and place them on a parchment-lined 9-by-13-inch baking sheet, leaving about ½ inch between. Cover with a towel and proof for 20 to 30 minutes, or until doubled and the dough balls touch each other. Brush all exposed sides with a lightly beaten egg and sprinkle with sesame seeds. Bake at 375 degrees F for 25 to 30 minutes, until golden brown.

All-the-Seeds Sourdough Buckwheat Loaf

This is a tall, hearty, dense, and texture-rich loaf. I refer to it as the "Summer of Love" bread because it reminds me of the rustic, hippie breads in old cookbooks and what I imagine people in communes were baking back in the seventies. It is full of all kinds of seeds and is wonderful topped with a simple jam and butter, or with something savory like hummus and roasted vegetables. You can use all the seeds called for or simply a combination of whatever is in your pantry.

MAKES 1 LOAF

For the sponge
⅔ cup (200 g) cold sourdough starter (page 25)
⅔ cup (90 g) light buckwheat flour
½ cup (115 g) filtered water, at room temperature

For the dough
Extra-virgin olive oil, for greasing
½ cup (75 g) raw sesame seeds, plus more for sprinkling
¼ cup (30 g) poppy seeds, plus more for sprinkling
2¼ cups (500 g) filtered water, room temperature
3 tablespoons (30 g) psyllium husk powder
1¾ cups (245 g) light buckwheat flour, plus more for dusting
½ cup (60 g) tapioca starch
4 ounces (115 g) dried apricots, chopped
½ cup (75 g) raw pumpkin seeds
½ cup (75 g) raw sunflower seeds
¼ cup (30 g) chia seeds
¼ cup (30 g) flaxseeds
1 tablespoon honey
1 tablespoon unsweetened cocoa powder
2 teaspoons whole coriander seeds
2 teaspoons kosher salt

1 To make the sponge, in a medium bowl, whisk together the sourdough starter, brown rice flour, and water until smooth. It should be the consistency of a pourable thick cream. Cover the bowl with a clean kitchen towel and proof at room temperature for 4 to 6 hours, until the mixture is bubbly and resembles mousse.

2 To make the dough, lightly grease the inside of an 8½-by-4½-inch loaf pan with olive oil and sprinkle some sesame and poppy seeds all around.

3 In a medium bowl, whisk together the water and psyllium powder and let it gel for 5 minutes.

4 In the bowl of a stand mixer fitted with the dough hook, combine the sourdough sponge, psyllium gel, and all remaining ingredients. Mix on medium speed until the dough comes together, about 2 minutes. It will be very sticky, like thick cake batter. Spoon the dough into the prepared pan and smooth the top. Cover with a clean kitchen towel and proof for 3 to 4 hours. The dough won't rise much as it ferments. I recommend the first time you make it, you bake the dough after 3 hours of proofing and then reassess for next time if you needed to go longer or shorter. Alternatively, you can ferment the dough in the refrigerator overnight, then bake it straight from the fridge.

5 Preheat the oven to 450 degrees F. Bake the bread for 45 minutes, then reduce the oven temperature to 400 degrees F. Gently remove the loaf from the pan, put it directly on an oven rack, and bake for another 30 minutes. Let the bread cool on a wire rack for at least 1 hour before cutting. The bread keeps best wrapped in parchment paper at room temperature for up to 3 days.

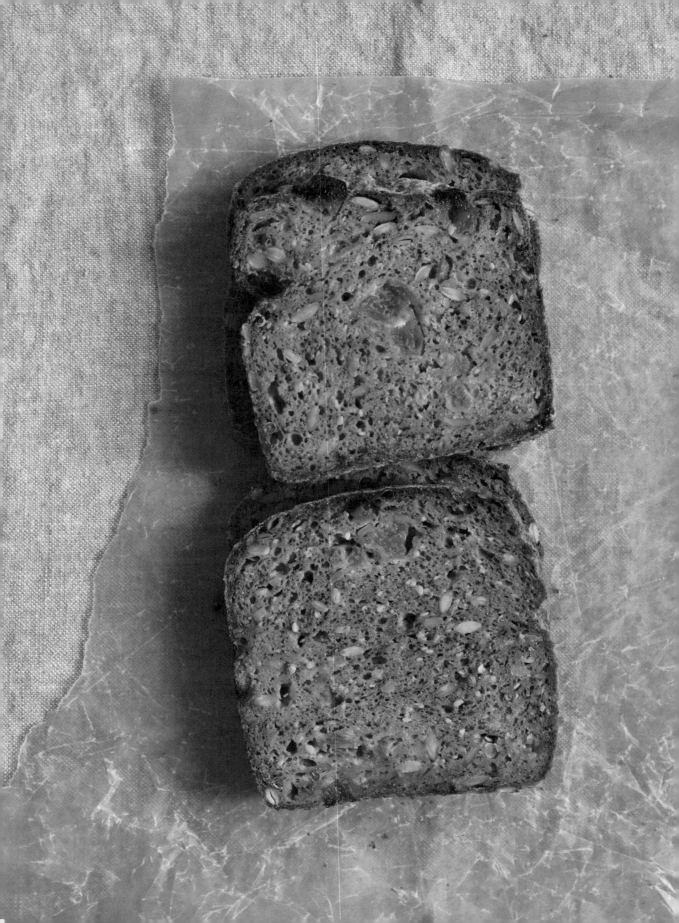

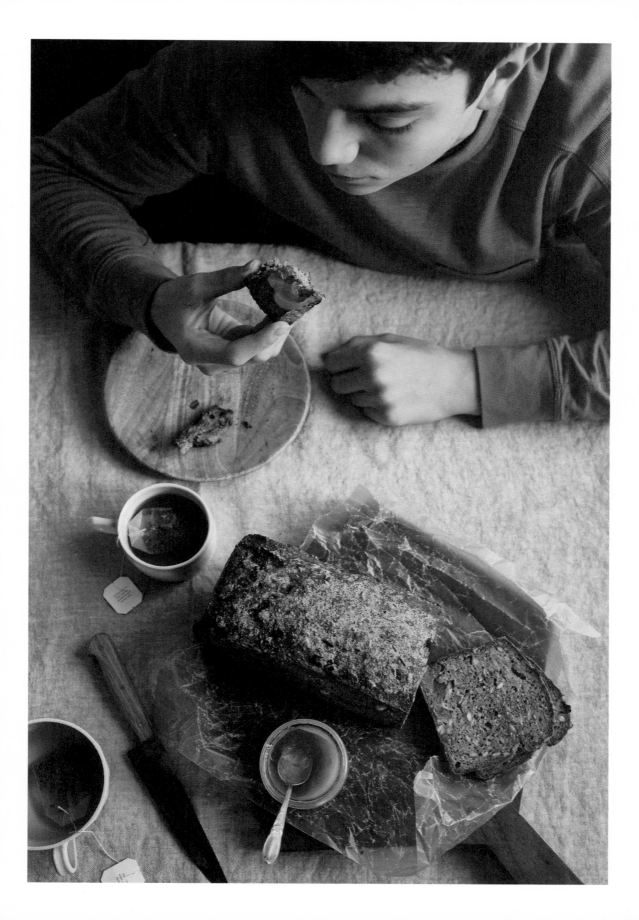

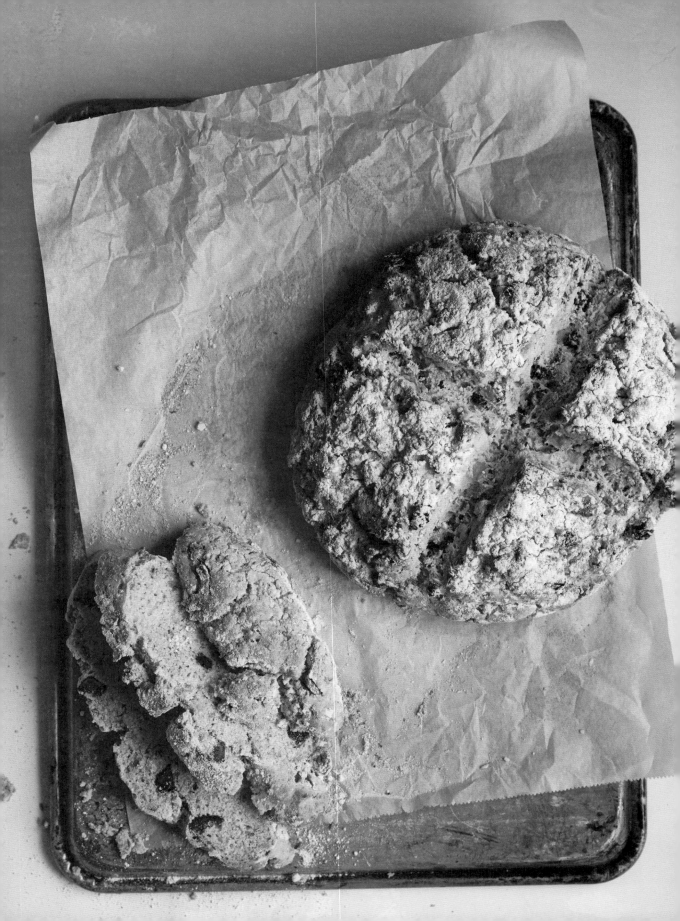

Fig and Caramelized Onion Soda Bread

This bread leavened simply with baking soda is like a giant savory scone. The trick is to not overmix the dough, keeping it loose and lumpy so it gets the rough exterior texture. Do not let the dough sit on the counter for long—make sure your oven is preheated so you can bake the bread as soon as it comes together.

MAKES 1 LOAF

3 ounces (90 g) dried figs (about 8) or currants (no soaking required)

1 tablespoon extra-virgin olive oil

½ medium yellow onion, cut into ¼-inch dice

1¼ teaspoons kosher salt, divided

1 teaspoon whole caraway seeds (optional)

1½ cups (210 g) light buckwheat flour or sorghum flour

1 cup (120 g) gluten-free oat flour, plus more for dusting

½ cup (80 g) potato starch

½ cup (60 g) tapioca starch

¼ cup (50 g) sugar

2 tablespoons (20 g) psyllium husk powder

2½ teaspoons baking powder

½ teaspoon baking soda

2 large eggs, lightly beaten

1¼ cups (300 g) oat milk

3 tablespoons apple cider vinegar

1   Preheat the oven to 450 degrees F. Line a baking sheet with parchment paper and dust it with oat flour.

2   Put the figs in a small bowl, cover with boiling water, and soak for 15 minutes. Drain and coarsely chop them.

3   Meanwhile, heat a small sauté pan over medium heat, then add the olive oil, onion, and ¼ teaspoon of the salt. Reduce the heat to medium-low and cook, stirring occasionally, until caramelized, about 10 minutes. Add the caraway seeds, cook for another 30 seconds, and transfer the mixture to a plate to cool.

4   In a large bowl, whisk together both flours, both starches, sugar, psyllium powder, baking powder, baking soda, and the remaining 1 teaspoon salt. Add the chopped figs and caramelized onions and stir.

5   In a small bowl, whisk together the eggs, milk, and vinegar. Pour this over the dry ingredients and, using a fork, whisk until it comes together in a lumpy dough. You want to be sure almost all the flour is incorporated, but do not overmix. It's OK if it's loose. I don't touch the dough with my hands or knead it in the bowl.

6   Invert the bowl over the prepared pan and let the dough fall onto the flour. Dust your hands with more oat flour and bring the dough together, shaping it into a circle about 7 inches wide and 2½ inches thick. Top with a light dusting of flour. Make two ½-inch-deep crisscross cuts on top.

7   Bake for 15 minutes, then reduce the oven temperature to 400 degrees F and bake for another 15 minutes, until golden brown. Let the bread cool for 15 minutes before cutting. It's best eaten immediately as it dries out quickly.

Chewy Bagels

2¼ cups plus 2 tablespoons
(525 g) filtered water, heated
to 105 degrees F
2 teaspoons (8 g) active dry yeast
1 tablespoon plus 1 teaspoon
sugar, divided
2 tablespoons (20 g) psyllium
husk powder
1 tablespoon (7 g) flaxseed meal
1 teaspoon apple cider vinegar
1 cup (140 g) superfine brown
rice flour
1 cup (140 g) sorghum flour
¾ cup (90 g) gluten-free oat flour
¾ cup (90 g) tapioca starch
1½ teaspoons kosher salt
Sesame, poppy, or caraway
seeds, for topping (optional)

I didn't grow up with bagels. I never tasted one until I was a teenager and visited the US for the first time, but from the first bite, I was hooked. To me, a bagel is not simply any bread that has a donut shape. It must have a tender crumb with a thin, chewy crust that comes from boiling them before baking. The trick to a smooth skin is to shape them very well into even balls. You can dust your work surface with a bit of sorghum flour while rolling them, but don't use too much as you need friction to create that perfect smooth exterior.

MAKES 8 BAGELS

1 In a medium bowl, whisk together the water, yeast, and 1 teaspoon of the sugar. Proof until the yeast bubbles and a thin layer of foam forms on top, about 10 minutes. Whisk in the psyllium powder, flaxseed, and vinegar, and let the mixture gel for 5 minutes.

2 In the bowl of a stand mixer fitted with the dough hook, combine the three flours, tapioca starch, and salt. Add the psyllium gel and mix on medium speed for 2 minutes, until the dough comes together and is smooth. Alternatively, you can mix the dough by hand in a large bowl.

3 Turn the dough out onto a work surface. Using a bench scraper or knife, cut the dough into 8 equal pieces (each about 130 g). Shape each piece into a ball, then use the end of a wooden spoon or your thumb (lightly floured to avoid sticking) to press a hole through the center of the dough, gently expanding it to about 1½ inches in diameter. Repeat with all of the dough pieces.

4 Line two baking sheets with parchment paper. Place the bagels on them, cover with a clean kitchen towel or plastic wrap, and proof at room temperature for 45 minutes, until nearly doubled. You can cook the bagels at this point, but refrigerating them develops their flavor. Cover and transfer the pans to the fridge and proof overnight or up to 24 hours. Make sure the bagels are well covered so their skin doesn't dry out. I personally prefer plastic wrap, but a towel should protect the dough well enough.

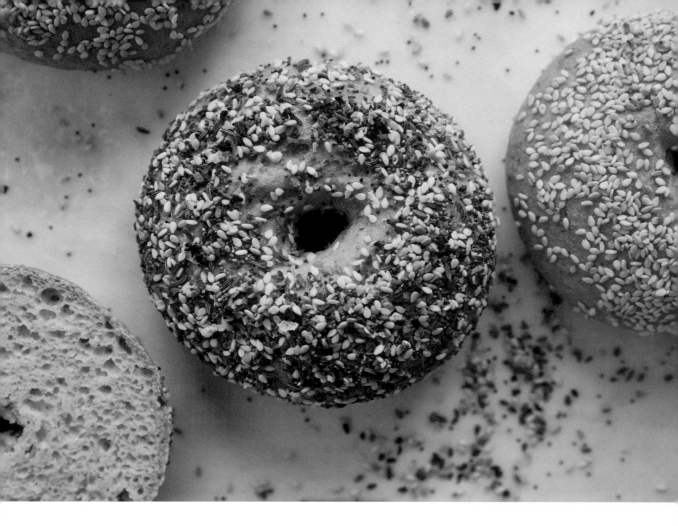

5   Preheat the oven to 450 degrees F. Fill a large pot with 3 inches of water and the remaining 1 tablespoon sugar. Bring to a boil over high heat, then reduce to maintain a simmer.

6   Remove the bagels from the refrigerator, gently lower them into the simmering water, and cook for 20 to 30 seconds on each side. Some of the skin might crack a little and that is OK. Boil no more than 4 bagels at a time. Remove them with a slotted spoon or spatula and place them back on the baking sheets. Sprinkle them with the seeds or any other toppings. Bake for 25 to 30 minutes, or until golden brown. Cool completely before cutting to prevent a gummy crumb. The bagels are best eaten the same day, but they freeze well, tightly wrapped, for up to 3 months.

Sourdough English Muffins

These English muffins are made with a mixture of baker's yeast and sourdough discard, meaning the starter doesn't need to be activated. The leavening is mostly done by the baker's yeast and baking powder, which also provides a sweet flavor, while the sourdough adds tang. Some English muffin recipes resemble traditional crumpets; for those, you need special molds. However, the dough in this recipe is cut using a round cutter, then fermented and baked without a mold.

MAKES SIX 3-INCH ENGLISH MUFFINS

1 cup (225 g) filtered water, heated to 105 degrees F
2 teaspoons (8 g) active dry yeast
1 teaspoon sugar
2 tablespoons apple cider vinegar
1 tablespoon (10 g) psyllium husk powder
1 tablespoon (7 g) flaxseed meal
½ cup (70 g) superfine brown rice flour, plus more for dusting
½ cup (70 g) sorghum flour
¼ cup (30 g) tapioca starch
2½ teaspoons baking powder
1½ teaspoons kosher salt
½ cup (150 g) cold sourdough starter (page 25)
Cornmeal, for dusting
Unsalted butter or dairy-free butter, for frying

1 In a medium bowl, whisk together the water, yeast, and sugar. Proof until the yeast bubbles and a thin layer of foam forms on top, about 10 minutes. Whisk in the vinegar, psyllium powder, and flaxseed and let it gel for 5 minutes.

2 In a large bowl, whisk together both flours, tapioca starch, baking powder, and salt. Add the psyllium gel and sourdough starter. Mix the dough with a wooden spoon and knead by hand until it comes together and is lump-free. The dough should feel airy and bouncy and shouldn't be terribly sticky.

3 Dust a baking sheet with cornmeal and a work surface with brown rice flour. Turn the dough out onto the surface and shape it into a rectangle that is ½ to ¾ inch thick. Using a 3-inch cookie cutter, cut 6 circles of dough and place them on the prepared pan. Reroll the dough if needed. Cover the pan with a clean kitchen towel and proof the dough for 60 to 90 minutes. The English muffins won't double in size, but they will feel springy to the touch and very light when you lift them.

4 When the dough is ready, preheat the oven to 350 degrees F. Preheat a cast-iron griddle over medium-low heat. Add about ½ teaspoon of butter per English muffin and cook for 3 to 5 minutes, until golden brown. Check that the bottom doesn't burn, then flip and cook for another 3 to 5 minutes on the other side.

5 Return the English muffins to the baking sheet and bake for 15 to 20 minutes, until baked thoroughly inside. Let them cool on the pan completely before slicing. They are best eaten the same day but can be tightly wrapped and frozen for up to 3 months.

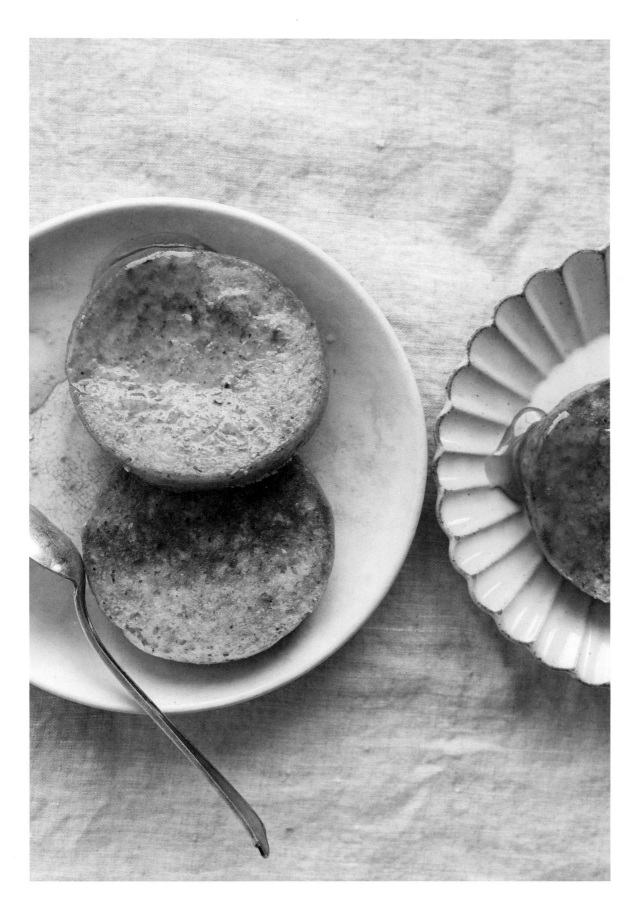

Crusty Baguettes

---

2 cups plus 2 tablespoons (475 g) filtered water, heated to 105 degrees F, divided

1 cup (140 g) sorghum flour, plus more for dusting

2 teaspoons (8 g) active dry yeast

2 tablespoons (20 g) psyllium husk powder

1 tablespoon apple cider vinegar

1 tablespoon (7 g) flaxseed meal

1½ cups (240 g) potato starch

¾ cup (90 g) tapioca starch

1 tablespoon sugar

1½ teaspoons kosher salt

Cornmeal, for dusting

A baguette is not only a distinct bread shape. When I think of a baguette, I think of a thin, crispy crust, an airy interior with distinct pockets, light but with a bit of chew. It is best consumed the day it is baked. When I was growing up, we would pick up a baguette at the bakery early in the morning and sometimes another in the afternoon. It takes practice to perfect the technique of shaping and scoring baguettes. I highly recommend watching tutorial videos online and then practice, practice, practice to get a feel for your dough.

MAKES 2 BAGUETTES

1   Whisk 1 cup of the water, sorghum flour, and yeast in a medium mixing bowl, and proof for 1 hour, or until the mixture puffs up. Whisk in the remaining 1 cup plus 2 tablespoons (250 g) water, psyllium powder, vinegar, and flaxseed. Let the mixture gel for 5 minutes.

2   In the bowl of a stand mixer fitted with the dough hook, combine both starches, sugar, salt, and the yeast mixture. Mix on medium speed for 2 minutes, until the dough comes together and is smooth. Alternatively, you can mix the dough by hand in a large bowl. Add a small amount of water if the dough feels dry.

3   Transfer the dough to a work surface. Using a bench scraper or sharp knife, cut the dough into two equal pieces (each approximately 500 g). You can dust the surface with a bit of sorghum flour, but don't use too much as you will need friction to help shape the baguettes. Shape each piece into a ball, then roll into a 15- to 16-inch log. Use your palms to taper the ends of the dough to resemble the shape of a traditional baguette.

4   Dust a baking sheet with cornmeal or sorghum flour. Place the baguettes on top, cover with a clean kitchen towel or plastic wrap, and proof at room temperature for 30 to 40 minutes.

5   While the dough is proofing, preheat the oven to 450 degrees F. Position one rack in the middle of the oven and another at the bottom. Put a metal or ceramic tray on the bottom rack. Boil 1 cup of water.

6   Spritz the baguettes with room temperature water and lightly dust the tops with sorghum flour. Using a sharp knife or lame, make five ¼-inch-deep slashes on the top of each baguette, each score overlapping slightly with the previous one. Place the baguettes in the oven and pour the boiling water into the bottom tray. Or, if you are using the oven's steam function, release steam at the 1-, 6-, and 12-minute marks. Bake for 35 to 40 minutes, until the baguettes are crusty and deep golden brown. Check that the bottoms are crispy and sound hollow when tapped. It's OK if parts have cracked; you might also get protruding air bubbles.

7   Transfer the baguettes to a wire rack and cool for at least 30 minutes and ideally 1 hour before cutting. It's important to let the internal steam release so the crumb can set and the crust can soften slightly. The baguettes will keep at room temperature wrapped in parchment paper for 2 days but are best eaten the same day.

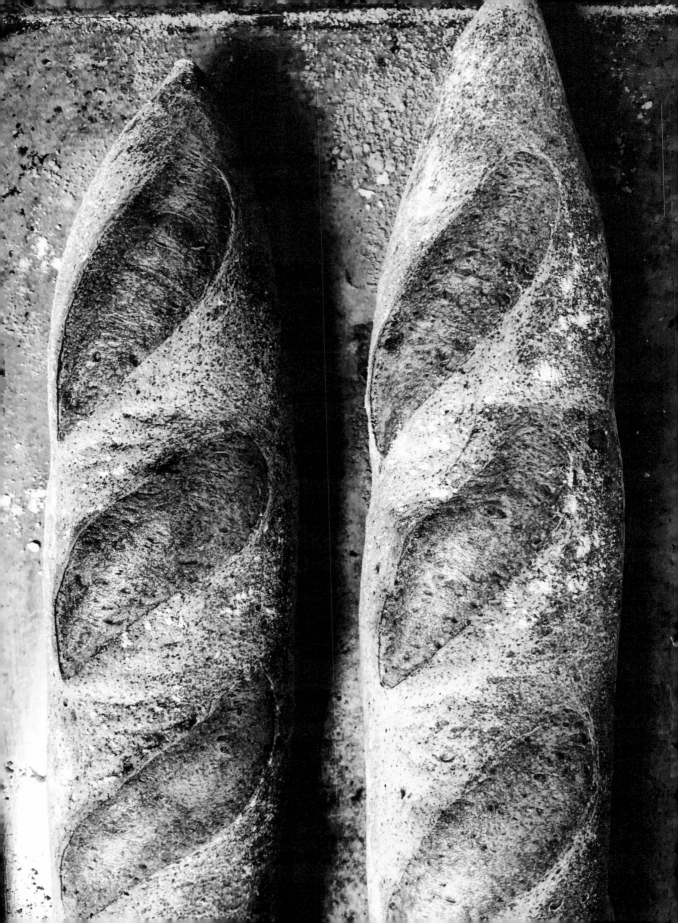

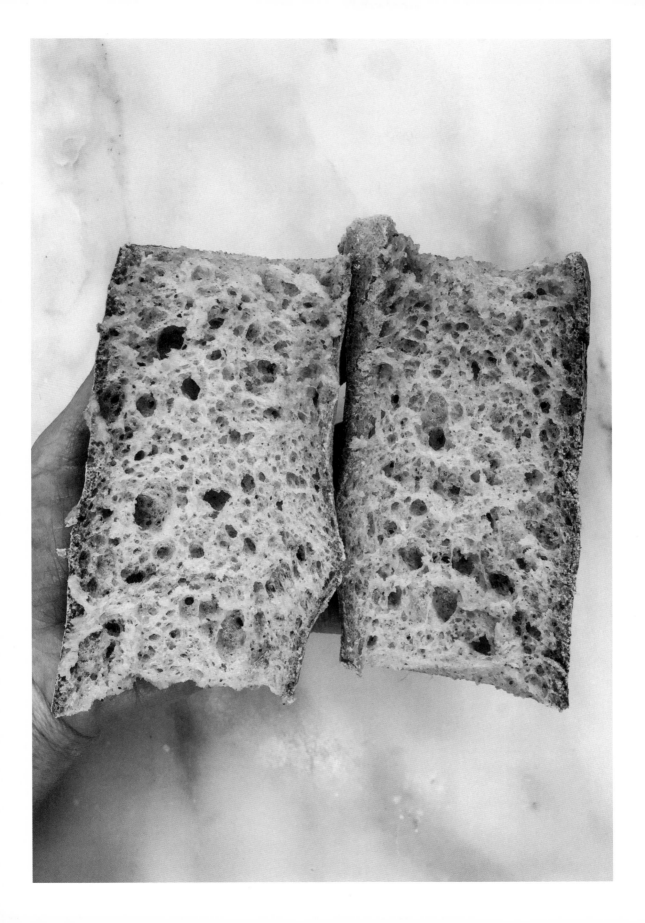

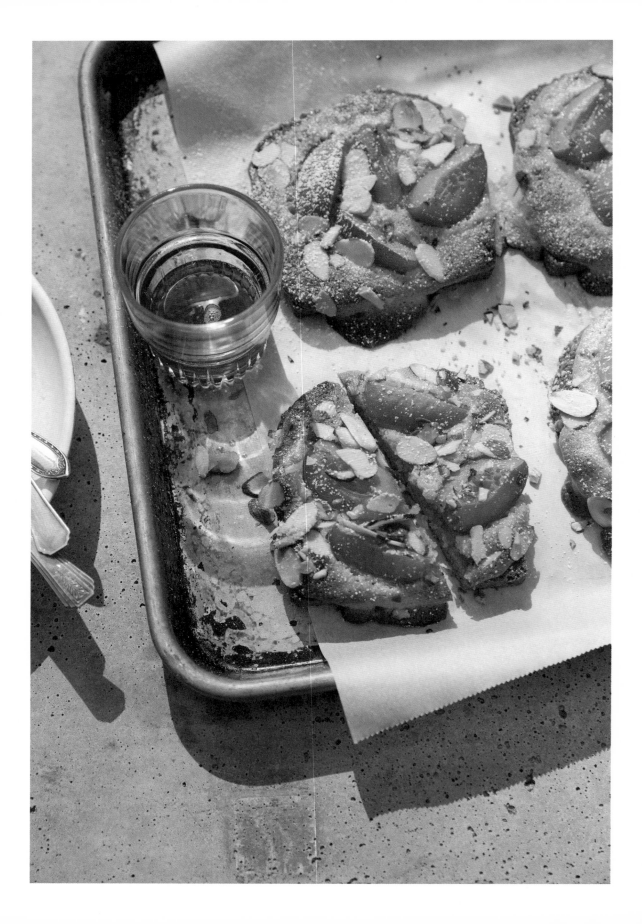

Almond Bostock with Apricots

3 tablespoons maple syrup
2 tablespoons water
6 (½-inch) slices Olive Oil
  Brioche (page 81)
1½ cups Basic Frangipane
  (page 38)
3 medium apricots, halved,
  pitted, and cut into wedges
½ cup (75 g) raw sliced almonds
Powdered sugar, for dusting

Bostock is an enriched French toast. Instead of using milk and eggs, the bread slices are soaked in syrup, slathered with frangipane, and baked until golden brown. This means it is a great option for brunch, but it also serves as a great dessert when cut into small pieces and topped with whipped cream. In place of the apricots, try it with sliced pears, apples, bananas, or peaches.

MAKES 6 SERVINGS

1 Preheat the oven to 400 degrees F. In a small bowl, whisk together the maple syrup and water.

2 Lay the brioche slices on a baking sheet. Brush the tops generously with the maple syrup mixture. Gently spread ¼ cup of the frangipane over the top of each brioche, being careful not to rip the crumb too much. Lay the apricot wedges on top, pressing them into the frangipane. Top with the sliced almonds.

3 Bake the bostock for 20 to 22 minutes, until golden brown. Dust with powdered sugar and serve warm.

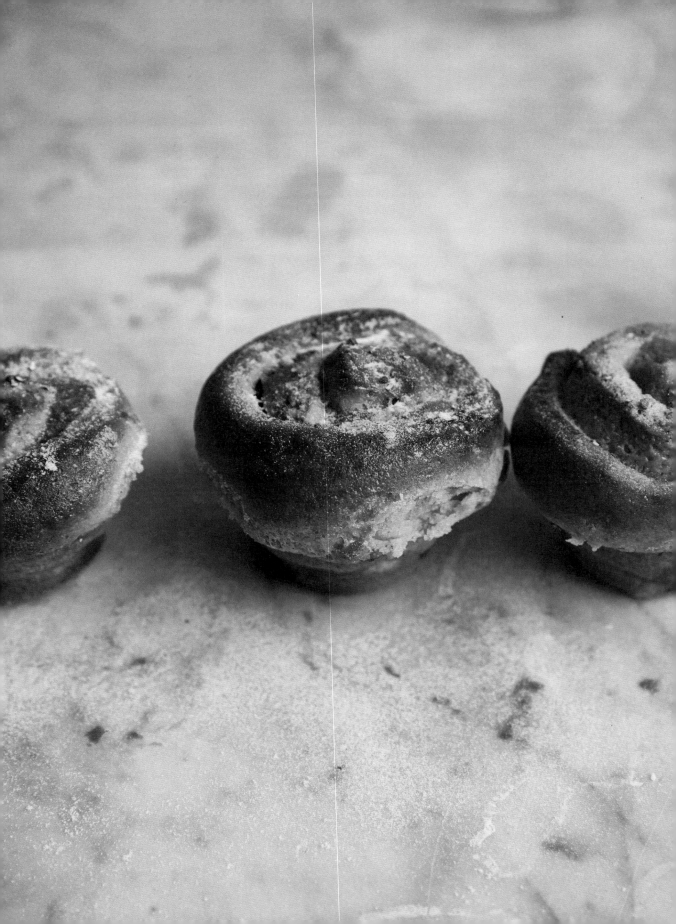

Rhubarb-Cardamom Brioche Rolls

The Olive Oil Brioche serves as the ideal base for making these rolls with rhubarb compote. You can also use any other fruit compote or jam you enjoy, or turn these into traditional cinnamon rolls with a buttery cinnamon-sugar filling. A note about rhubarb color: Use stalks that are red throughout for rosy effect since green stalks will turn slightly brown. Even though it will taste perfectly fine, it won't achieve the same beautiful color.

MAKES 12 ROLLS

For the compote
30 whole cardamom pods, divided
8 ounces (225 g) rhubarb (about 3 medium stalks), cut into ¼-inch-thick slices
½ cup (100 g) sugar
¼ cup (55 g) freshly squeezed orange juice

For the rolls
1 recipe Olive Oil Brioche dough (page 81)
Extra-virgin olive oil, for greasing
Tapioca starch, for dusting
2 tablespoons sugar

1 To make the compote, begin by cracking the cardamom pods open with the back of a knife. Discard the pods and pulverize the seeds in a mortar and pestle or a clean coffee grinder. You should have 1 heaping tablespoon. You will use 1 teaspoon for the compote; reserve the remainder for the rolls.

2 Combine the rhubarb, sugar, orange juice, and 1 teaspoon cardamom in a small saucepan and cook over medium heat until the rhubarb breaks down and the sauce thickens, 7 to 10 minutes. Remove from the heat and let the compote cool completely. If it is too chunky, you can mash or puree it. It can be made up to 2 days in advance.

3 To make the rolls, prepare the brioche dough as directed in steps 1 and 2 on page 81, adding 1½ teaspoons of the reserved ground cardamom with the dry ingredients. Proof the dough in a large bowl greased with olive oil and covered with a clean kitchen towel for 30 minutes, then transfer the bowl to the refrigerator for at least 4 hours and up to 8 hours. Chilling the dough makes it easier to roll and shape.

4 Lightly dust a work surface with tapioca starch. Turn the dough out onto it, pat it down, and form it into a square. Roll the brioche dough into a rectangle, approximately 13 by 16 inches. Move the dough around as you are rolling and continue dusting the bottom as needed to prevent sticking. You might need to work quickly if it's warm in your kitchen, but work gently.

5 Spread the compote evenly over the dough. Starting from the long side, gently roll up the dough, being careful not to rip it. Position it seam side down and cut the dough into 12 equal pieces. ⟶

6   Preheat the oven to 375 degrees F. Grease a muffin pan with olive oil and place a dough piece into each cavity, cut side up. Loosely cover the pan with a clean kitchen towel and proof for 20 to 30 minutes.

7   In a small bowl, whisk together the sugar and remaining ½ teaspoon ground cardamom and sprinkle it over the rolls. Bake for 30 minutes, or until golden brown. Let the rolls cool in the pan for 10 minutes, then transfer them to a plate. They are best eaten the same day.

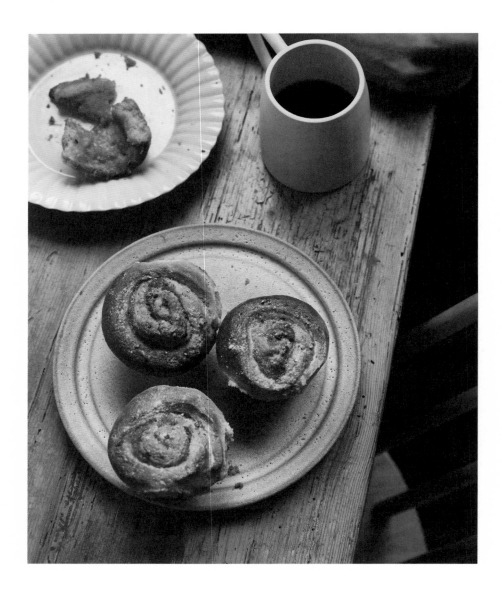

Chocolate–Olive Oil Babkas

Chocolate babka is one of my favorite enriched breads—brioche-style dough that is filled with chocolate and twisted for a beautiful effect. This might look like a complicated recipe, but it's surprisingly straightforward. You just need time. Plan to let the dough rest for a few hours, which will allow you to manipulate it without it falling apart. Don't worry if the shape is not flawless as that's part of the beauty of the babka, the uneven texture.

For the dough

1¼ cups (300 g) whole milk or oat milk, heated to 105 degrees F

2 teaspoons (8 g) active dry yeast

3 tablespoons (30 g) psyllium husk powder

1 cup (160 g) potato starch

1 cup (120 g) tapioca starch

1 cup (140 g) sweet white rice flour

½ cup (70 g) sorghum flour, plus more for dusting

½ cup (100 g) sugar

1½ teaspoons kosher salt

Zest of 1 medium orange

3 large eggs

¼ cup (55 g) extra-virgin olive oil, plus more for greasing

For the chocolate filling

¼ cup (55 g) heavy cream or canned full-fat coconut milk

2 tablespoons maple syrup

¼ teaspoon kosher salt

5 ounces (145 g) 70 percent chocolate, very finely chopped, divided

For the glaze

¼ cup (55 g) freshly squeezed orange juice

1 tablespoon maple syrup

MAKES 2 BABKAS

1 To make the dough, in a medium bowl, whisk together the milk and yeast. Proof until the yeast bubbles and a thin layer of foam forms on top, about 10 minutes. Whisk in the psyllium powder and let it gel for 5 minutes.

2 In the bowl of a stand mixer fitted with the dough hook, combine both starches, both flours, sugar, salt, orange zest, and psyllium gel. Mix on medium-high speed until the dough begins to come together. Add the eggs and olive oil, then mix for 2 minutes, or until the dough comes together and is smooth. It should be moist but hold its shape. Add a bit more milk if the dough feels dry.

3 Shape the dough into a ball. Grease a large bowl with olive oil, place the dough in the bowl, and move it around to coat. Cover the bowl with a clean kitchen towel, proof for 45 minutes at room temperature, then refrigerate for least 4 hours or up to 8 hours. The dough will have nearly doubled and hardened slightly.

4 Make the chocolate filling right before you will roll out the dough. Combine the heavy cream, maple syrup, and salt in a small saucepan and bring to a simmer over medium heat. Put 3 ounces (85 g) of the chopped chocolate in a small bowl and pour the hot cream over it. Let it sit undisturbed for 1 minute, then stir until smooth. Set aside.

5 Line two 8½-by-4½-inch loaf pans with a strip of parchment paper, letting some hang over the sides. $\longrightarrow$

6 Lightly dust a work surface with sorghum flour and remove the dough from the refrigerator. Flatten the dough with your hands and shape it into a square. Roll it out into a rectangle that is about 18 by 15 inches and a little less than ¼ inch thick. Roll gently so the dough doesn't tear, and move it around if it starts to stick to the surface. It might not be a perfect rectangle, but try to get it as close as possible. Trim off the edges.

7 Spread the chocolate filling all over the dough. Scatter the remaining 2 ounces (60 g) chopped chocolate on top. Starting from the long side, tightly roll the dough into a log and position it seam side down.

8 Use a sharp knife to cut the log in half crosswise, then cut each half lengthwise. Twist the first two halves together and gently place into one of the prepared pans. Repeat with the remaining halves. The babka might tear slightly in parts and that's OK—it will come together when baking.

9 Cover the pans with a clean kitchen towel, and proof for 45 minutes to 1 hour, or until doubled in size.

10 Preheat the oven to 375 degrees F. Bake the babkas for 40 to 45 minutes, until golden brown.

11 Meanwhile, make the glaze by heating the maple syrup and orange juice in a small saucepan over medium heat until it comes to a simmer.

12 Remove the babkas from the oven and immediately brush the glaze all over the tops. Let the babkas cool in the pans for 20 minutes, then use the parchment to lift them out. They are best eaten the same day.

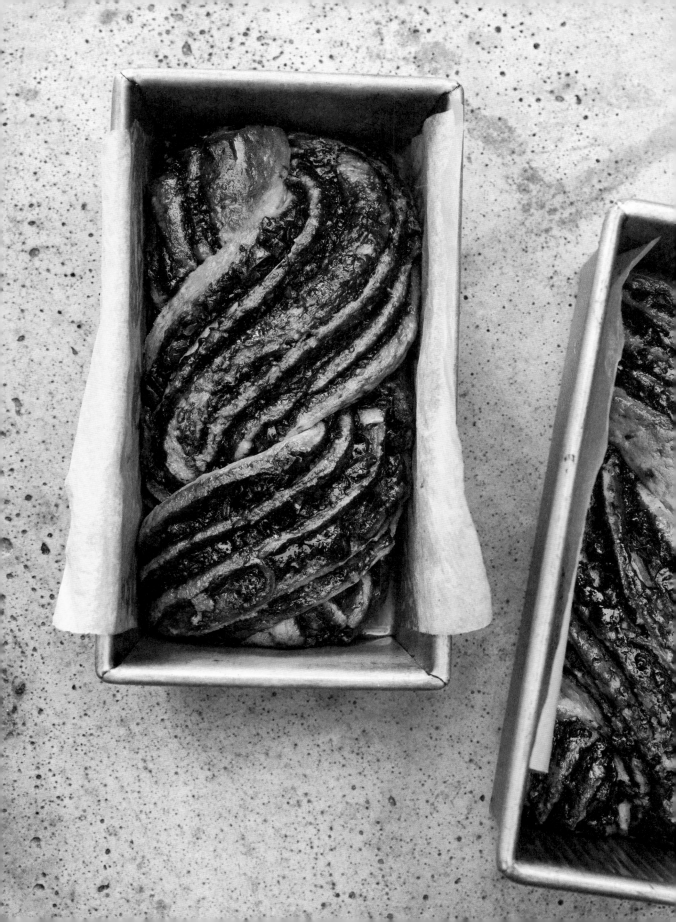

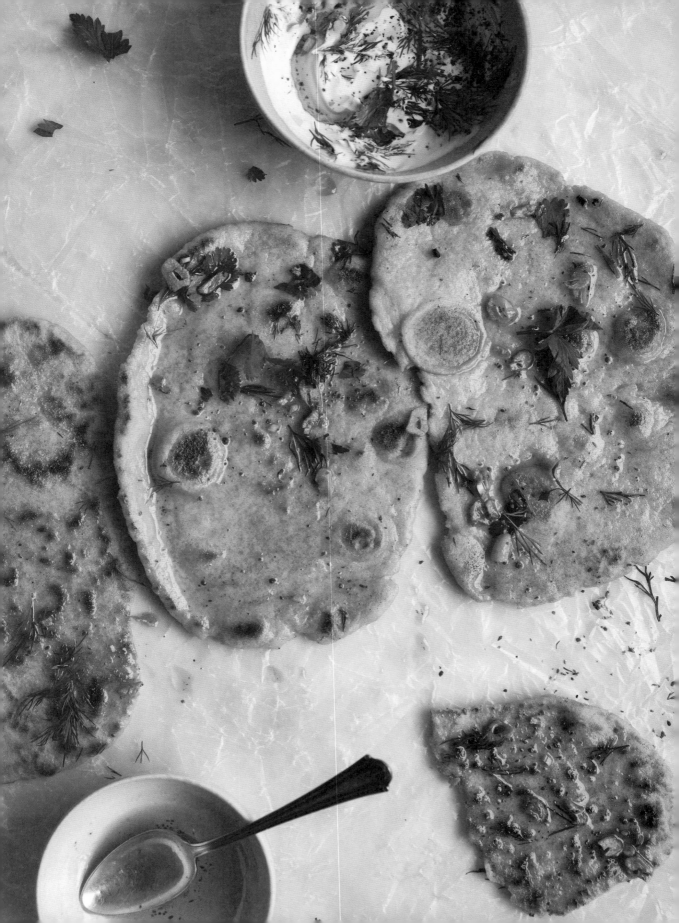

Garlic and Herb Naan

1¼ cups plus 1 tablespoon (315 g) filtered water, heated to 105 degrees F

1 tablespoon sugar

2 teaspoons (8 g) active dry yeast

2 tablespoons (20 g) psyllium husk powder

1 cup (140 g) sorghum flour, plus more for dusting

1 cup (120 g) light buckwheat flour

½ cup (80 g) potato starch

⅓ cup (80 g) full-fat buttermilk or Cashew-Coconut Yogurt (page 30)

½ cup (110 g) plus 3 tablespoons extra-virgin olive oil, divided

1 teaspoon kosher salt

2 medium cloves garlic, finely chopped

¼ to ½ teaspoon red pepper flakes

¼ cup chopped fresh herbs (parsley, chives, oregano)

Naan is a leavened flatbread original, mainly, to western and southern Asia, although there are similar versions all over the world. It often accompanies stews and dips. It is very tender and pliable, which also makes it suitable as a sandwich wrap. You can use whole-milk or dairy-free yogurt in place of the buttermilk or Cultured Cashew-Coconut Yogurt, but if you do, add a tablespoon of water to thin it out to a buttermilk consistency.

MAKES 10 NAAN

1 In a medium bowl, whisk together water, sugar, and yeast and proof for 10 minutes, until bubbly. Whisk in the psyllium powder and let it gel for 5 minutes.

2 In the bowl of a stand mixer fitted with the dough hook, combine both flours, potato starch, buttermilk, 3 tablespoons of the olive oil, salt, and psyllium gel. Mix on medium speed until a smooth dough forms, about 2 minutes. Shape the dough into a ball inside the bowl. Cover with a clean kitchen towel and let it ferment for 40 minutes, or until nearly doubled.

3 Meanwhile, gently heat the remaining ½ cup (110 g) olive oil, garlic, and red pepper flakes in a small sauté pan over medium-low heat, until the garlic begins to color, 2 to 3 minutes. Remove from the heat and set aside.

4 Preheat a cast-iron griddle or grill pan over medium heat. Transfer the dough to a work surface and cut it into 10 equal pieces (each about 80 g). Work with one piece at a time, covering the rest with a towel. Shape each piece into a ball and flatten it. Generously dust each side with sorghum flour and roll the dough ⅛ inch thick. The naan will be free-form and rustic, so don't worry too much about shape. Gently round the edges with your palm if they begin to crack.

5 Lightly brush one side of the naan with the infused olive oil and place it on the preheated griddle. Brush the top with more oil. Cook for 2 to 3 minutes, until small bubbles appear and the bottom is golden brown. Flip over and cook for another 2 to 3 minutes, until golden brown. Transfer to a plate and sprinkle with some herbs. Continue cooking the rest of the dough. Naan is best eaten right away. They can also be tightly wrapped and frozen for up to 3 months.

Spiced Sourdough Flatbreads

I love how versatile this recipe is. Top the flatbreads with a variety of spices, herbs, and seeds, such as za'atar, paprika, sesame or poppy seeds, oregano, thyme, sumac, cumin, turmeric, and more. You can serve flatbread alongside soups, salads, and dips; turn it into Crispy Potato, Leek, and Kale Focaccia Pie (page 204); or use it as a base for your favorite pizza.

MAKES 2 FLATBREADS OR PIZZAS OR 1 FOCACCIA

For the sponge
½ cup (150 g) cold sourdough starter (page 25)
½ cup (70 g) superfine brown rice flour
⅓ cup (75 g) filtered water, at room temperature

For the dough
1¼ cups (280 g) filtered water, at room temperature
1 tablespoon (10 g) psyllium husk powder
1 tablespoon (7 g) flaxseed meal
1 cup (140 g) sorghum flour, plus more for dusting
1 cup (120 g) tapioca starch
1 tablespoon extra-virgin olive oil, plus more for brushing and greasing
1½ teaspoons kosher salt, plus more for topping
Sesame seeds, freshly ground black pepper, sumac, dried herbs, or any other seeds, for topping

1   To make the sponge, whisk together the sourdough starter, brown rice flour, and water in a medium bowl until smooth. Cover the bowl with a clean kitchen towel and proof at room temperature for 3 to 6 hours, until the mixture is bubbly and resembles mousse.

2   To make the dough, in another medium bowl, whisk together the water, psyllium powder, and flaxseed and let it gel for 5 minutes.

3   In the bowl of a stand mixer fitted with the dough hook, combine the fermented sponge, psyllium gel, sorghum flour, tapioca starch, olive oil, and salt, and mix on medium speed until the dough is smooth, about 2 minutes.

4   Dust a work surface with sorghum flour and turn the dough out onto it. Cut the dough in half and shape each piece into a ball. Transfer the dough to a baking sheet. Cover the dough with a clean kitchen towel and let them proof for 1 to 2 hours, until they begin to expand. At this point, you can tightly wrap and refrigerate the dough for up to 24 hours.

5   When you are ready to bake the flatbreads, preheat the oven to 450 degrees F and lightly grease two baking sheets with olive oil. Roll each piece of dough to ¼ inch thick and place each on its own baking sheet. Top with salt, pepper, seeds, herbs, or other desired toppings. Bake for 25 minutes, until golden brown.

PIZZA CRUST

Prepare the dough as directed in steps 1 through 4 on page 106. Preheat a pizza stone in a 450-degree-F oven for 20 minutes. The pizza stone helps bake the underside of the crust nicely. Lightly dust a work surface with brown rice flour and roll the dough ¼ inch thick. If you will bake the dough directly on the pizza stone, use a pizza peel dusted with cornmeal to help you transfer it. If you don't have a pizza peel, you can also place the dough on a baking sheet drizzled with olive oil and dusted with cornmeal. Add the desired pizza toppings and place the pizza or pan directly on the stone. Bake for 25 minutes, until the bottom of the pizza is golden brown, the toppings are cooked, and any cheese is melted.

FOCACCIA

Prepare the dough as directed in steps 1 through 4 on page 106, but don't cut it in half. Preheat the oven to 450 degrees F. Drizzle olive oil on a 9-by-13-inch baking sheet. Gently stretch the dough with your fingers to fill the pan as much as possible, but be careful not to tear it. Spritz the top with warm water and drizzle with 3 tablespoons of olive oil and a pinch of salt, black pepper, rosemary, and other desired toppings. Bake for 25 to 30 minutes, until golden brown.

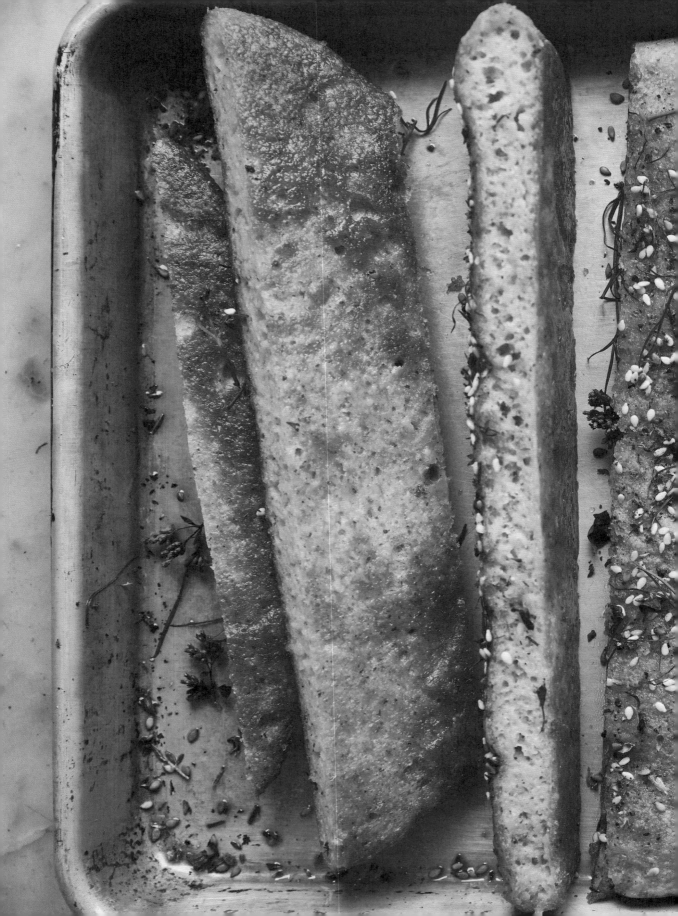

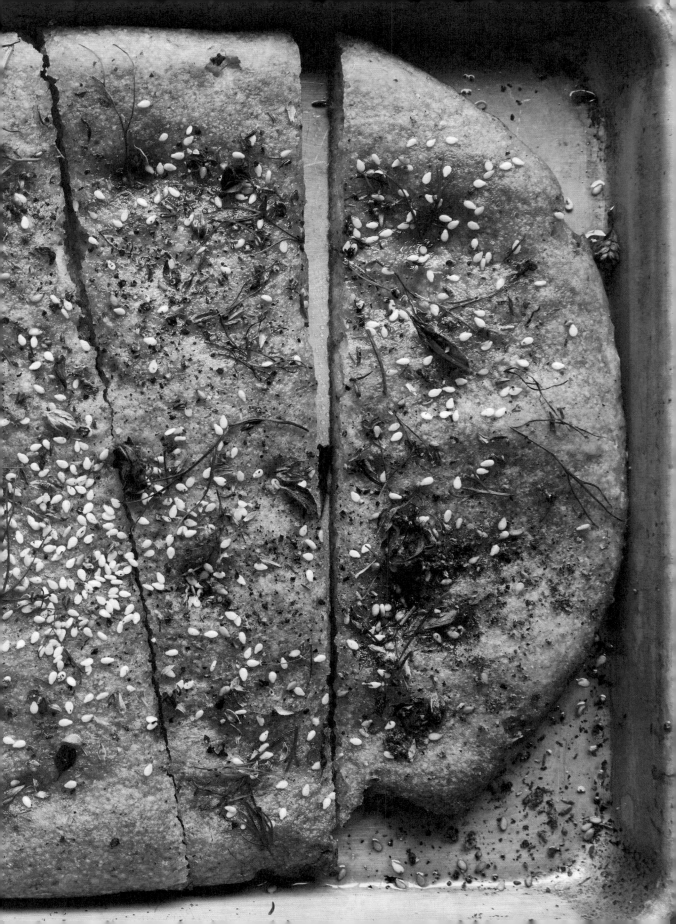

Herby Sourdough Crackers

I love serving these crackers in large uneven pieces alongside hummus or chunky salads. The trick is to roll them as thinly as possible so they become crispy and even develop some air pockets. If you prefer to have perfect squares or rectangles instead of shards, you can lightly score the dough before baking (don't cut all the way through)—the crackers should easily snap apart once cool.

MAKES 2 BAKING SHEETS OF CRACKERS

For the sponge

½ cup (150 g) cold sourdough starter (page 25)

½ cup *minus* 1 tablespoon (60 g) light buckwheat flour

⅓ cup (75 g) filtered water, at room temperature

For the dough

½ cup (70 g) sorghum flour

½ cup (60 g) tapioca starch

¼ cup (55 g) extra-virgin olive oil

¼ cup (55 g) filtered water, at room temperature

2 tablespoons (15 g) flaxseed meal

1 tablespoon (10 g) psyllium husk powder

1 teaspoon kosher salt

3 tablespoons finely chopped fresh herbs (chives, tarragon, cilantro, parsley, oregano, rosemary)

1 large egg, lightly beaten, or 2 tablespoons extra-virgin olive oil, for brushing

Sesame seeds, poppy seeds, cumin seeds, dried thyme, dried rosemary, or other herbs, for topping

1   To make the sponge, whisk together the sourdough starter, buckwheat flour, and water in a large bowl until smooth. Cover the bowl with a clean kitchen towel and proof at room temperature for 3 to 6 hours, until the mixture is bubbly and resembles mousse.

2   Once the sponge has fermented, preheat the oven to 400 degrees F.

3   To make the dough, add the sorghum flour, tapioca starch, olive oil, water, flaxseed, psyllium powder, and salt to the bowl with the sponge. Stir together with a wooden spoon, then mix with your hands until you have a smooth dough. Add another teaspoon of water if the dough feels dry. It should be firm but moist and smooth, similar to fresh pasta dough.

4   Divide the dough into two equal pieces. Roll each piece between two sheets of parchment paper until it is paper thin (about ¹⁄₁₆ inch). The thinner the dough, the crispier the crackers will be. As the dough rolls and stretches, it might get stuck to the parchment, so gently lift it up, set it back down, and continue rolling. If there are any thin pieces that stick out at the edges, trim and use them to fill an empty corner. This will help the dough bake evenly in the oven.

5   Peel off the top piece of parchment paper. Slide the sheets of dough with parchment underneath onto two baking sheets. Lightly brush the tops with the beaten egg, and sprinkle with seeds, herbs, or other desired toppings. Bake for 15 to 20 minutes, until golden brown. If your oven doesn't heat very evenly, rotate the pans halfway through. Gently slide the parchment from the pan onto a work surface to cool completely. Once cooled, break the sheets into large pieces. Store the crackers in an airtight container for up to 5 days.

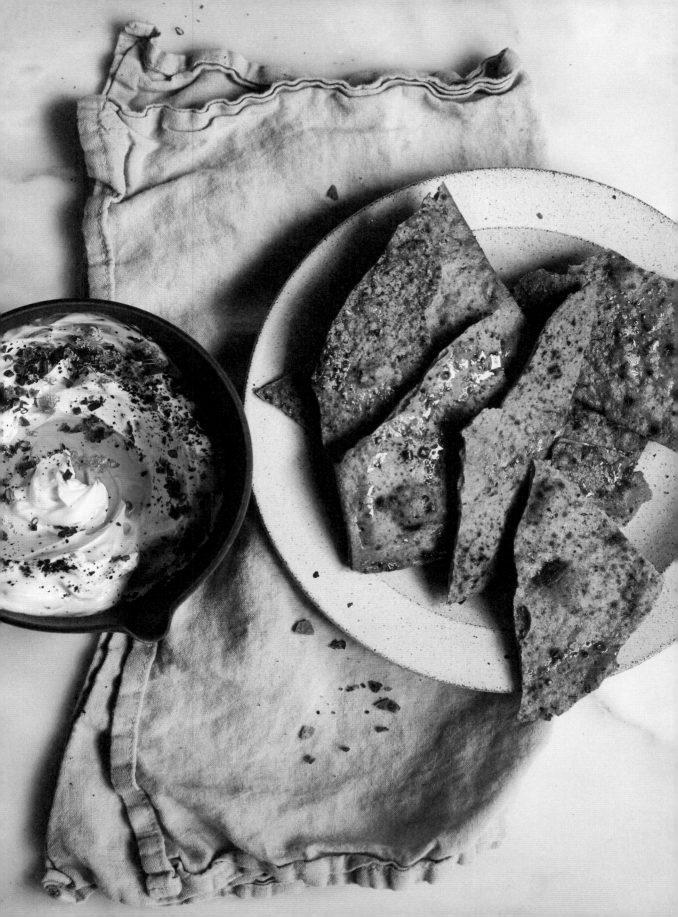

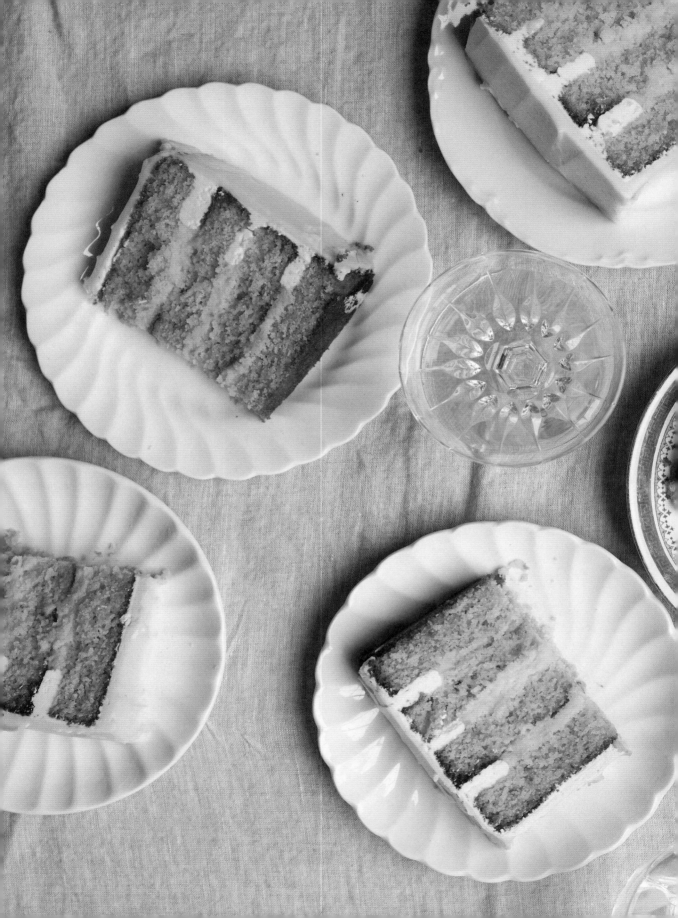

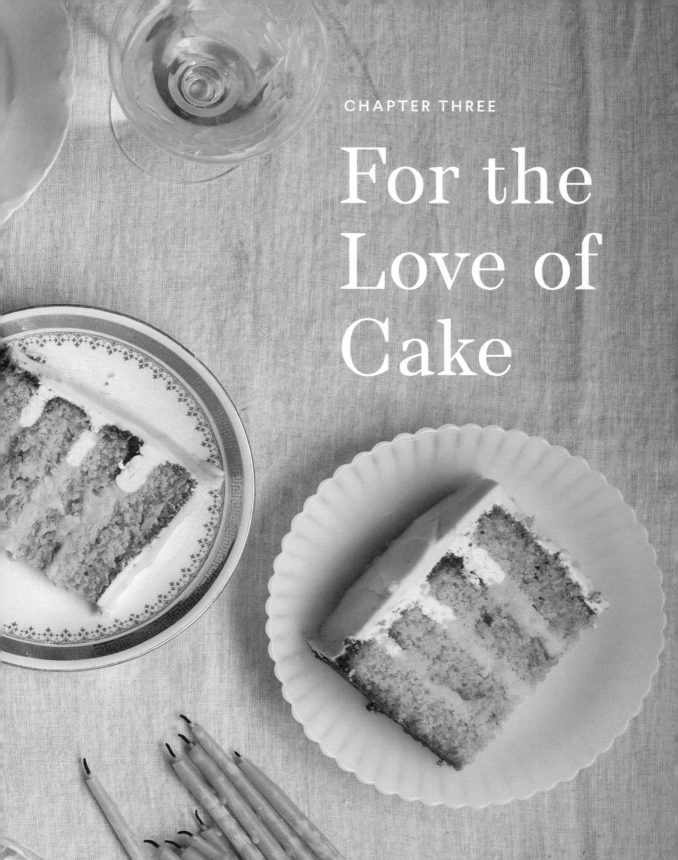

CHAPTER THREE

For the Love of Cake

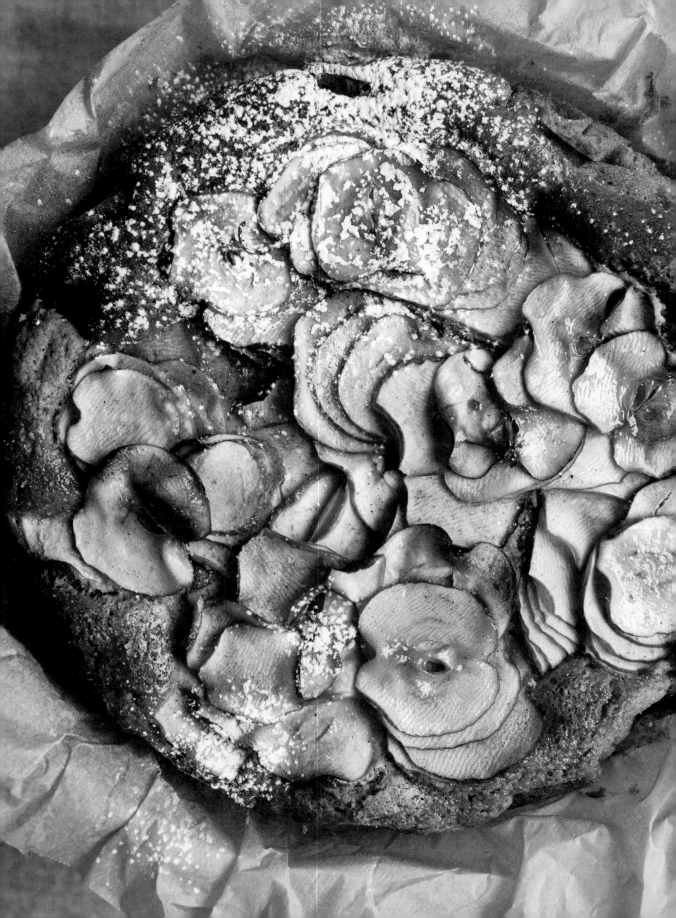

My mother loves cake. As the legend goes in my family, she went into labor right after indulging in an enormous slice of *tarta San Marcos*—heavily drunken sponge cake with an egg-yolk custard filling and mounds of whipped cream. It was the dead of winter after all, and by that point in her pregnancy, she was given everything she craved. She ate the cake with a cup of *café con leche* after a big lunch at the pastry shop with the rest of the family to celebrate my aunt Aran's birthday. She claims she knew I would be born once she finished that slice. Soon after, she was rushed to the hospital in Bilbao and I was.

Ever since I can remember, I have been baking cakes. The first one I made, at age ten or eleven, was the yogurt and olive oil cake I've included in this chapter. My mother hardly ever followed a recipe, and in this case she simply used a yogurt container to measure all the ingredients. The first time she taught me how to make it, though, she wrote the recipe down on a piece of paper that I kept for years but have since lost. I began making variations with sliced fruit and spices, and I bought myself different baking pans with the little money I earned in my younger years.

As you read through the cake recipes here, you will notice that none of them are overtly sweet or elaborate. I adore simple cakes. Cakes that you can have on your counter as a snack in the afternoon or serve to anyone who stops by to say hello. Cakes that you mix in one bowl and bake, such as the Chocolate Sourdough Cake (page 147); One-Bowl Apple, Yogurt, and Maple Cake (page 130); or Fig, Honey, and Lemon Tea Cakes (page 124). In general, I have always been more interested in textures and how flavors interconnect than in more decorative affairs, but one must have a couple of go-to cakes for special occasions and to wow guests. For that, try the Lemon Curd and Honey Celebration Cake (page 150), Coconut Layer Cake with Caramel (page 140), or Raspberry-Rhubarb Cream Sponge (page 135).

Cake makes people happy . . . especially my mother.

Glazed Lemon, Yogurt, and Olive Oil Pound Cake

This is the basic snack cake of my childhood. I would come home from school to find it displayed on an old red melamine tray cooling on the outdoor balcony. It is very lemony and moist with a simple glaze. You can add orange zest or poppy seeds to it if you'd like.

MAKES 1 LOAF

1 Preheat the oven to 350 degrees F. Grease the inside of an 8½-by-4½-inch loaf pan with a little bit of olive oil.

2 To make the cake, in a large bowl, rub together the sugar and lemon zest until fragrant. This helps release the natural lemon oil. Whisk in the remaining ingredients until the batter is smooth. Pour the batter into the prepared pan and bake for 45 to 50 minutes, until a toothpick inserted in the center comes out clean. Let the cake cool in the pan for 15 minutes, then invert onto a wire rack. Let the cake cool completely if you want the glaze to stay thick on top of the cake. If the cake is warm, the glaze will melt and run off.

3 To make the glaze, in a medium bowl, whisk together the powdered sugar and lemon juice until smooth and lump free. As you begin to whisk, it might seem too thick, but as the sugar absorbs the juice, the glaze will thin out. The glaze should be pourable but not too runny.

4 Put a tray or baking sheet under the wire rack and pour the glaze all over the cake, letting it run over the edges. Wait a few minutes for the glaze to set. Sprinkle the top with the pistachios, then serve. The cake will keep at room temperature for 3 days. If you refrigerate it, the glaze will soften.

For the cake
1 cup (200 g) sugar
1 tablespoon finely grated lemon zest (from 2 to 3 medium lemons)
1 cup (140 g) superfine brown rice flour
1 cup (100 g) almond flour, any lumps broken up
3 large eggs
½ cup (115 g) whole-milk yogurt or Cashew-Coconut Yogurt (page 30)
½ cup (110 g) extra-virgin olive oil, plus more for greasing
1 tablespoon vanilla extract
1 tablespoon baking powder
½ teaspoon kosher salt

For the glaze
2 cups (240 g) powdered sugar
2 to 3 tablespoons freshly squeezed lemon juice
2 tablespoons finely chopped pistachios, for topping

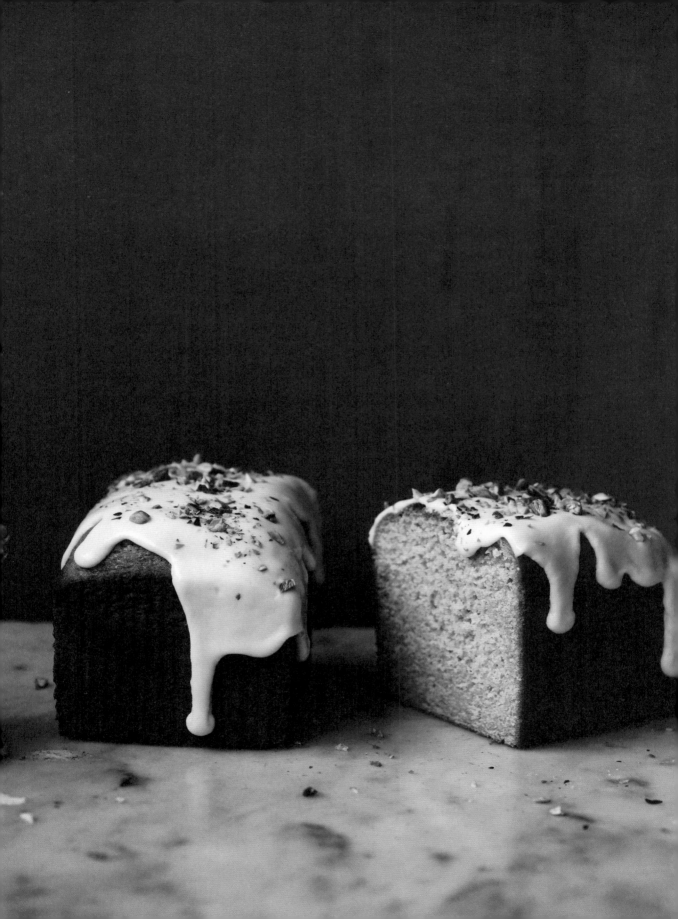

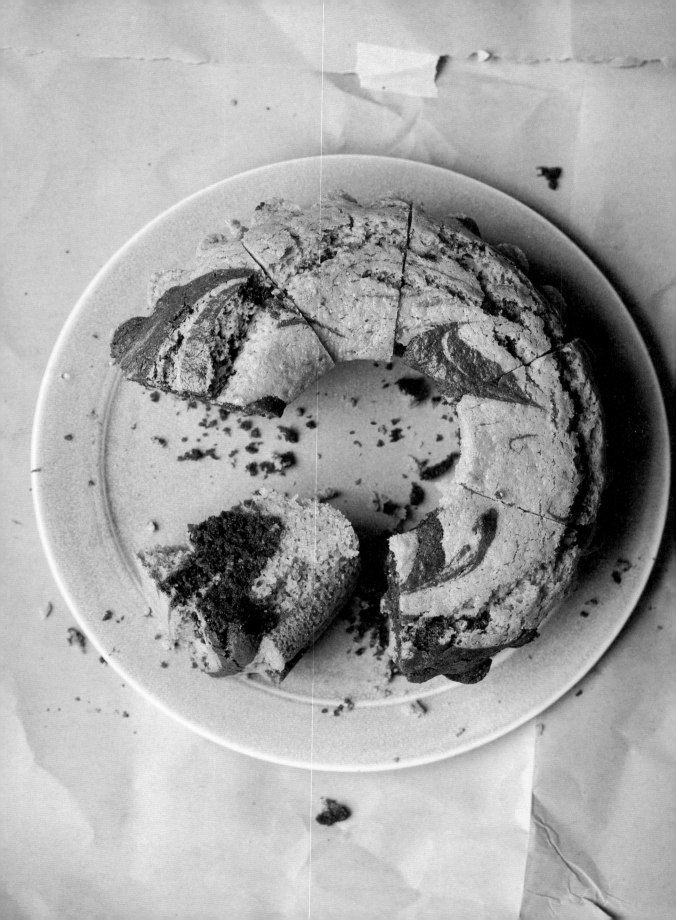

Chocolate-Tahini Buckwheat Marble Cake

1 cup (140 g) light buckwheat
  flour or superfine brown
  rice flour
1 cup (100 g) almond flour
¾ cup (150 g) sugar
1½ teaspoons baking powder
½ teaspoon baking soda
½ teaspoon kosher salt
½ cup (115 g) melted virgin
  coconut oil or extra-virgin olive
  oil, plus more for greasing
½ cup (115 g) well-stirred tahini
½ cup (115 g) whole milk, oat
  milk, or canned full-fat
  coconut milk
2 large eggs
1 tablespoon freshly squeezed
  lemon juice
1 tablespoon vanilla extract
2 tablespoons unsweetened
  cocoa powder
Chocolate Glaze (page 46),
  optional

During my university years and before I had dreams of becoming a pastry chef, my friend Estibaliz Goicoechea and I used to bake a recipe of *marmorkuchen* we found in an old German cooking magazine. Estibaliz had studied in a German school and she introduced me to the Northern European baking tradition. I still have that tear sheet at my parents' home in the old recipe notebook I kept. During exams, Estibaliz and I baked together to calm our anxiety and minds. That recipe was full of butter, too much sugar, and gluten. The old tin Bundt pan needed to be coated with bread crumbs so the heavy cake wouldn't stick. This cake is an adaptation of that *marmorkuchen* but uses tahini and almonds for a portion of the fat and buckwheat flour for added earthiness. Use light buckwheat flour (see page 7) here as darker buckwheat flour will not provide a distinct swirl with the chocolate layer.

MAKES 1 BUNDT CAKE

1 Preheat the oven to 350 degrees F. Grease the inside of a 9-cup Bundt pan with coconut oil.

2 In a large bowl, whisk together both flours, sugar, baking powder, baking soda, and salt. Add the coconut oil, tahini, milk, eggs, lemon juice, and vanilla. Whisk vigorously until the batter is smooth. Transfer half of the batter to a separate bowl and whisk in the cocoa powder.

3 Alternate spooning the two batters into the pan until all of it has been used. To marble the cake, run the tip of a knife or a toothpick through the batters to create swirls, but try not to overdo it or you won't get distinct marbling in the baked cake.

4 Bake for 35 to 40 minutes, until a toothpick inserted in the center comes out clean. Let the cake cool in the pan for 15 minutes, then invert it onto a wire rack. If you will glaze the cake, let it cool completely. Put the wire rack on a tray lined with parchment paper and pour the chocolate glaze over the top. The cake will keep tightly wrapped in the refrigerator for 3 days.

Date-Sweetened Banana Bread with Chocolate and Walnuts

4 ounces (120 g) plump pitted Medjool dates (about 8)

⅓ cup (120 g) maple syrup

4 ripe medium bananas, divided

3 large eggs

½ cup (110 g) extra-virgin olive oil, plus more for greasing

1 tablespoon vanilla extract

1 tablespoon finely grated fresh ginger

¾ cup (105 g) light buckwheat flour

1 cup (100 g) almond flour

3 ounces (85 g) 70 percent chocolate, coarsely chopped

¾ cup (90 g) raw walnuts or pecans, coarsely chopped

3 tablespoons raw sesame seeds, plus more for topping

1 teaspoon ground cinnamon

1 teaspoon baking powder

½ teaspoon ground nutmeg

½ teaspoon baking soda

½ teaspoon kosher salt

This banana bread is free of refined sugar, relying on bananas, dates, and maple syrup for sweetness, and it's heavily spiced with fresh ginger, cinnamon, and nutmeg. The chocolate, walnuts, and sesame seeds add texture and richness. Your kitchen will smell amazing when you bake this, and I warn you, the bread won't last long on your kitchen counter. A quick tip: if your dates are a bit dry, soak them in boiling water for 15 minutes, then squeeze them dry before blending with the bananas.

MAKES 1 LOAF

1   Preheat the oven to 350 degrees F. Grease the inside of an 8½-by-4½-inch loaf pan with olive oil, then line it with a piece of parchment paper large enough to hang over the sides. This will help you lift the bread out of the pan after baking.

2   In a food processor, pulse the dates until roughly chopped. Add the maple syrup and 3 of the bananas and puree to a creamy and smooth paste. It's OK if there are some date chunks, but it should be as smooth and creamy as possible. Add the eggs, olive oil, vanilla, and ginger and pulse a few times until well blended.

3   In a large bowl, stir together both flours, chocolate, walnuts, sesame seeds, cinnamon, baking powder, nutmeg, baking soda, and salt. Add the date puree and, using a spatula, mix until the all the ingredients are well incorporated.

4   Pour the batter into the pan. Cut the remaining banana in half lengthwise and place the halves on top of the batter. Sprinkle some sesame seeds on top. Bake for 55 to 60 minutes, until a toothpick inserted in the center comes out clean. Let the bread cool in the pan for 15 minutes, then invert onto a wire rack or platter. Store the bread wrapped in the refrigerator for up to 3 days.

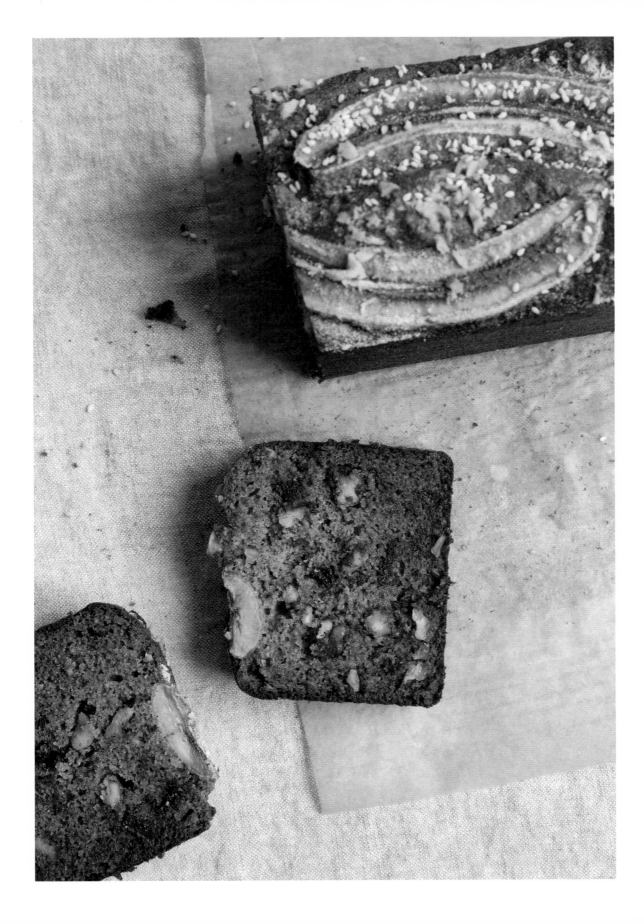

Coriander-Cornmeal Cake with Honey-Candied Lemon

You might be surprised to see coriander seeds in a cake, but they are a wonderful addition with their floral, bright, and citrus flavor profile. Just like in savory cooking, they are a perfect match for lemons and, consequently, a perfect match for honey.

MAKES ONE 8-INCH CAKE

4 teaspoons coriander seeds, divided
4 to 5 medium lemons, divided
1 cup (200 g) sugar
¾ cup (170 g) very soft unsalted butter or dairy-free butter, plus more for greasing
3 large eggs, at room temperature
¾ cup (105 g) superfine brown rice flour
½ cup (60 g) tapioca starch
½ cup (60 g) fine cornmeal
2 teaspoons baking powder
½ teaspoon kosher salt
½ cup (180 g) honey

1 Preheat the oven to 350 degrees F. Grease the inside of an 8-inch cake pan with butter and place a circle of parchment paper on the bottom.

2 Toast the coriander seeds in a small sauté pan over medium-high heat until fragrant, about 3 minutes. Reserve 1 teaspoon of the seeds and grind the rest into a fine powder in a spice grinder or with a mortar and pestle.

3 Finely grate lemon zest from 2 of the lemons until you have about 2 teaspoons. Put it in a large bowl. Cut the zested lemons in half and juice them into a separate bowl. You will need ½ cup of juice total, so juice additional lemons as needed. Set the juice aside.

4 Add the sugar to the bowl with the zest and rub it between your fingers to release the lemon oils from the zest. Add the soft butter and whisk until the mixture is creamy and smooth. Add the eggs, one at a time, whisking after each addition. Whisk in ¼ cup of the lemon juice.

5 In a small bowl, stir together the brown rice flour, tapioca starch, cornmeal, baking powder, salt, and finely ground coriander. Add to the wet ingredients and whisk to combine. Pour the batter into the prepared pan and bake for 45 minutes, until a toothpick inserted in the center comes out clean. Let the cake cool in the pan for 30 minutes.

6 While the cake is cooling, thinly slice 2 of the remaining lemons. Combine the honey and remaining ¼ cup lemon juice in a large shallow 10- to 12-inch sauté pan. Bring the liquid to a light simmer over medium heat, then add the lemon slices in a single layer. Cook them over medium heat, flipping occasionally, until the slices are soft and caramelized, about 12 minutes. They should be soft and jammy with some caramelized edges.

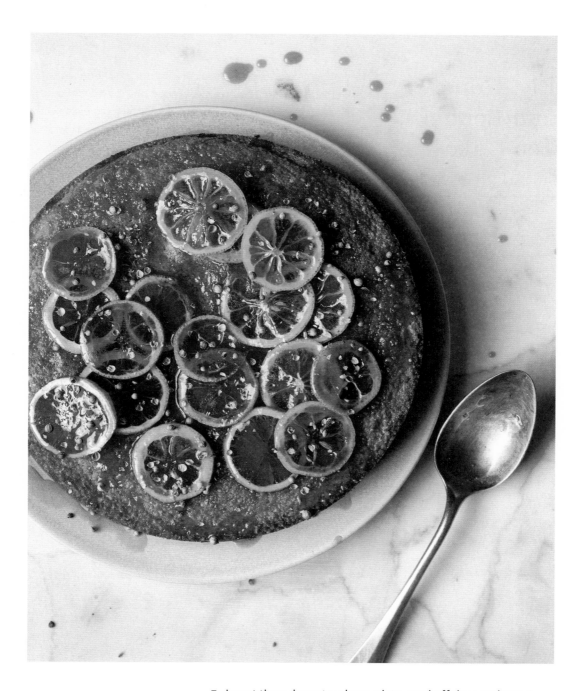

7   Invert the cake onto a large plate, peel off the parchment, and spoon the lemons and honey all over the top, letting the syrup run down the sides. Sprinkle the toasted whole coriander seeds on top. The cake will keep tightly wrapped in the refrigerator for up to 3 days.

Fig, Honey, and Lemon Tea Cakes

These little cakes are perfect to serve in the afternoon with a cup of tea or coffee. They are sweetened only by the figs and a bit of honey. If figs are out of season, try topping the cakes with sliced peaches, nectarines, apricots, pears, or berries. I use a friand mold, but you can bake them in a standard muffin pan.

MAKES 12 TEA CAKES

1¼ cups (125 g) almond flour

¾ cup (75 g) gluten-free oat flour

2 tablespoons tapioca starch

2 tablespoons finely chopped fresh rosemary

1½ teaspoons baking powder

½ teaspoon kosher salt

2 large eggs, lightly beaten

½ cup (115 g) unsalted butter, dairy-free butter, or virgin coconut oil, melted, plus more for greasing

5 tablespoons honey

3 tablespoons freshly squeezed lemon juice

1 teaspoon finely grated lemon zest

6 fresh figs, stemmed and halved

1   Preheat the oven to 350 degrees F. Grease the inside of a 12-muffin pan with melted butter.

2   In a large bowl, whisk together all the ingredients except for the figs. Pour the batter into the muffin cups, filling them only halfway. Let the batter sit for 5 minutes. This will activate the baking powder and thicken the batter so when the figs are added, they don't sink. Top each muffin with half a fig.

3   Bake for 20 to 22 minutes, until the cakes are golden brown, puffed, and a toothpick inserted in the center comes out clean. Let the cakes cool in the pan for 15 minutes, then invert onto a plate. The cakes will keep in an airtight container at room temperature for 2 days.

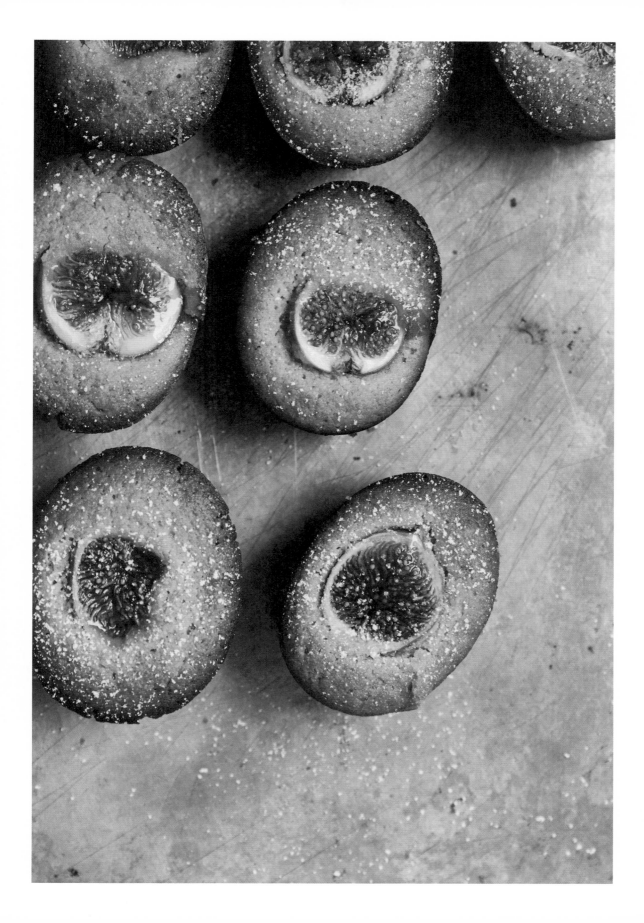

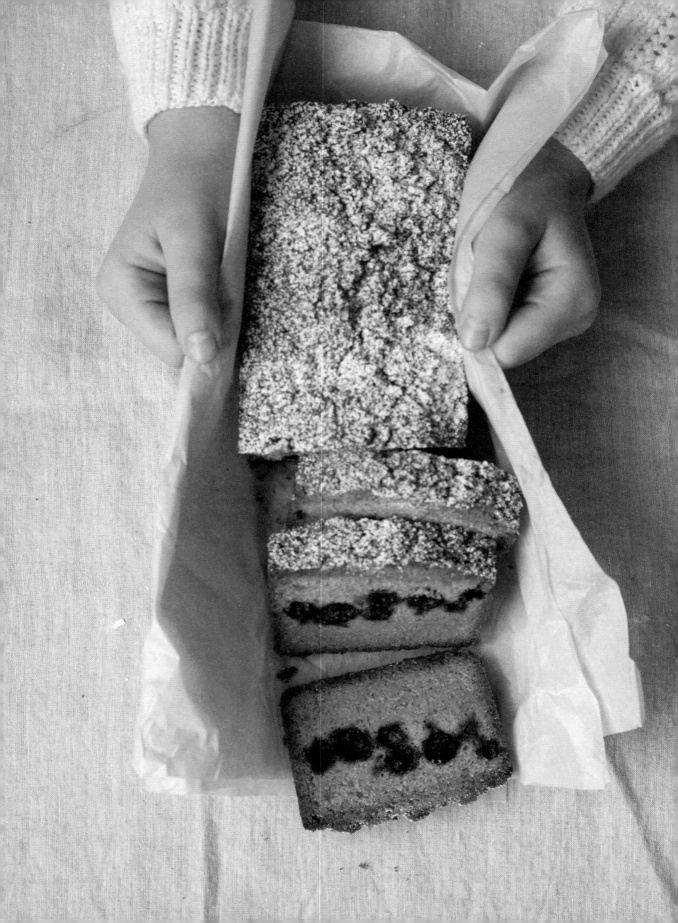

Blueberry Crumb Coffee Cake

2 cups (225 g) blueberries
¼ cup (30 g) plus 1 tablespoon tapioca starch, divided
1 teaspoon ground cinnamon
½ teaspoon ground ginger
¾ cup (150 g) light brown sugar
2 teaspoons finely grated lemon zest
1 cup (225 g) unsalted butter or dairy-free butter, at room temperature, plus more for greasing
1 tablespoon vanilla extract
3 large eggs, at room temperature
1 cup (140 g) sorghum flour
¾ cup (75 g) almond flour
2½ teaspoons baking powder
½ teaspoon kosher salt
½ cup Streusel (page 49)

This blueberry cake is a mix between a pound cake and a traditional coffee cake. It is heavy and rich and even better the next day, after all the flavors have mingled. A couple of tips: First, if you use frozen blueberries, thaw them first. If they release too much liquid, drain some off, as it can make the cake soggy. Second, make sure you use a 1-pound loaf pan, as the batter will fill it almost all the way to the top. You could also bake the cake in an 8-inch square pan.

MAKES 1 LOAF

1 Preheat the oven to 350 degrees F. Position a rack in the lower third of the oven. Grease the inside of an 8½-by-4½-inch loaf pan with butter, then line with a piece of parchment paper large enough to hang over the sides. This will help you lift the cake out of the pan after baking.

2 In a medium bowl, toss together the blueberries, 1 tablespoon of the tapioca starch, cinnamon, and ginger. Set aside.

3 In the bowl of a stand mixer, combine the brown sugar and lemon zest and rub them between your fingers until sandy and fragrant. Add the butter and vanilla. Attach the bowl to the mixer fitted with the paddle attachment and beat on medium speed until creamy and light, about 2 minutes. Scrape the paddle and sides of the bowl well. Add the eggs, one at a time, beating between additions.

4 In a small bowl, stir together both flours, remaining ¼ cup (30 g) tapioca starch, baking powder, and salt. Add the dry ingredients to the mixer bowl and beat on medium speed until you have a creamy, smooth batter, about 1 minute. Spread half of the batter evenly inside the prepared pan. Top with the blueberries. Spread the remaining batter on top, then sprinkle with the streusel.

5 Bake for 60 to 70 minutes, until the cake is golden brown and a toothpick inserted in the center comes out clean. Check the cake near the end of baking, and if the top begins to darken too much, cover it with foil. Let the cake cool in the pan for 20 minutes, then lift it out onto a wire rack. Store the cake tightly wrapped at room temperature for up to 3 days.

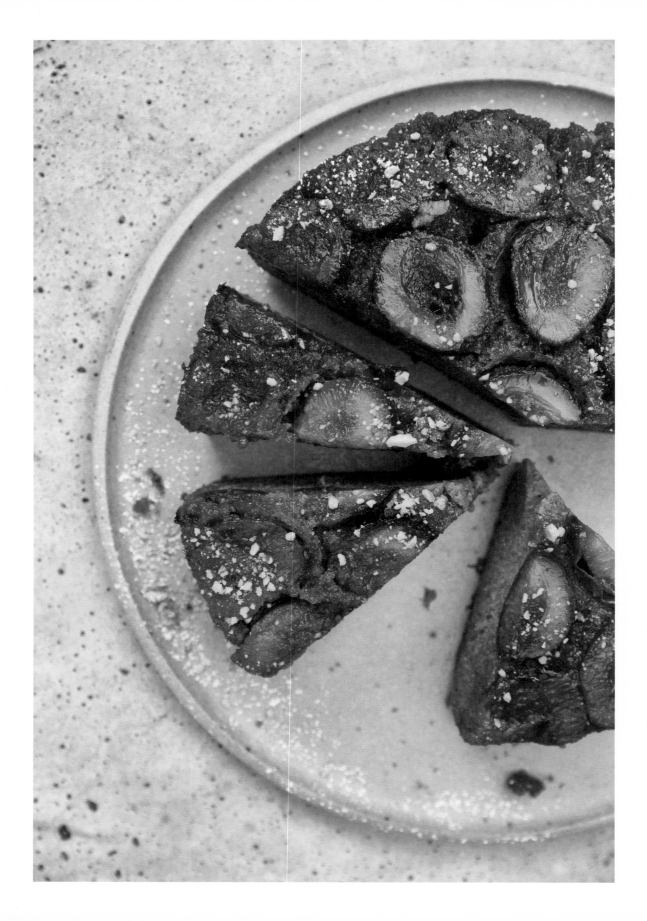

Plum and Toasted Miso Upside-Down Cake

The combination of toasted miso, brown sugar, and buckwheat gives this cake umami-butterscotch notes. The cake is so rich that every bite appears loaded with butter, however it is completely dairy-free. You can use any plums you'd like, but make sure they are ripe yet firm or they might fall apart during baking. This is also delicious made with cherries or pears.

MAKES ONE 9-INCH CAKE

⅔ cup (130 g) sugar

1¼ pounds (680 g) Italian prune plums or other medium plum, halved and pitted

3 tablespoons white miso

⅓ cup (85 g) whole milk or oat milk

1 cup (200 g) light brown sugar

3 large eggs

½ cup (110 g) sunflower oil or extra-virgin olive oil

2 teaspoons vanilla extract

1 cup (140 g) light buckwheat flour or sorghum flour

½ cup (50 g) almond flour

½ teaspoon baking soda

¼ teaspoon kosher salt

Heavy cream, whipped, for serving

1 Preheat the oven to 350 degrees F.

2 Heat a medium stainless steel sauté pan over medium-high heat. Sprinkle half of the sugar evenly around the pan. As the sugar melts, sprinkle the other half all over the pan and cook until all the sugar turns a deep caramel color. If it isn't melting evenly, stir the sugar with a wooden spoon to incorporate any coarse areas into the melting ones. Scrape all the caramel into a 9-inch cake pan. Swirl the pan around so the entire bottom is covered with caramel. The pan will get hot, so be careful when you touch it. Set the sauté pan aside as you will need it again.

3 Carefully arrange the plums in a circular pattern over the caramel. Set aside.

4 Spread the miso thinly on the sauté pan. Have the milk close by because you will need it right away. Cook the miso over medium-high heat until it begins to stick to the pan, stirring it around with a wooden spoon to toast it, 1 to 2 minutes. It will turn dark and smoky. Immediately pour in the milk and whisk it around to break down the miso just as you would to make a roux. It will thicken and become a dark paste. Scrape it into a medium bowl and let it cool for 5 minutes.

5 Whisk the brown sugar, eggs, oil, and vanilla into the miso paste until smooth. Then whisk in both flours, baking soda, and salt until you have a smooth batter. Pour it over the plums.

6 Bake for 50 to 55 minutes, or until a toothpick inserted in the center comes out clean. Let the cake cool in the pan for 15 minutes. Run a knife close to the edge of the pan to release the cake, then invert it onto a plate. Serve the cake warm or at room temperature with a bit of whipped cream. It will keep tightly wrapped in the refrigerator for up to 3 days.

One-Bowl Apple, Yogurt, and Maple Cake

1 tablespoon sugar
¾ teaspoon ground cinnamon, divided
1 cup (100 g) almond flour
¾ cup (105 g) superfine brown rice flour
¼ cup (30 g) tapioca starch
1½ teaspoons baking powder
½ teaspoon baking soda
½ teaspoon kosher salt
2 large eggs
¾ cup (240 g) maple syrup
¾ cup (170 g) unsweetened whole-milk or dairy-free yogurt
⅓ cup (75 g) extra-virgin olive oil
1 tablespoon vanilla extract
2 medium or 4 small juicy but firm apples, such as Honeycrisp or Gala
Warm apricot jam or powdered sugar, for topping

Here is one of the simplest cakes you can make. Add all the ingredients to a large bowl, whisk away, and top with thinly sliced apples. It comes together in an instant and it's always a crowd-pleaser. The cake is sweetened with maple syrup and spiced only with a touch of cinnamon. It also works great with other fruits, such as pears, peaches, apricots, or plums. Add more spices to the batter if you really want to play with flavors, such as orange zest, finely chopped candied ginger, or cardamom.

MAKES ONE 9-INCH CAKE

1   Preheat the oven to 350 degrees F. Line a 9-inch cake pan with parchment paper, letting some hang over the sides. In a small bowl, stir together the sugar and ¼ teaspoon of the cinnamon. Set aside.

2   In a large bowl, whisk together both flours, tapioca starch, baking powder, baking soda, salt, and the remaining ½ teaspoon cinnamon. Whisk in the eggs, maple syrup, yogurt, olive oil, and vanilla until you have a smooth batter. Pour it into the prepared pan.

3   Using a mandoline, thinly slice the apples lengthwise. If you don't have a mandoline, cut the apples with a very sharp knife as thinly as possible. If the slices are too thick, they will not bake through. Remove any seeds, stem, or tough bottoms, then layer the apple slices over the batter. I like to arrange them in a rustic way, without following a pattern, but you can follow a concentric form. Sprinkle the apples with the reserved cinnamon-sugar.

4   Bake for 45 to 50 minutes, until a toothpick inserted in the center comes out clean. Let the cake cool in the pan for 20 minutes, then use the parchment to lift it out. Brush the top with a bit of warm apricot jam or dust with powdered sugar. The cake will keep tightly wrapped at room temperature for 3 days.

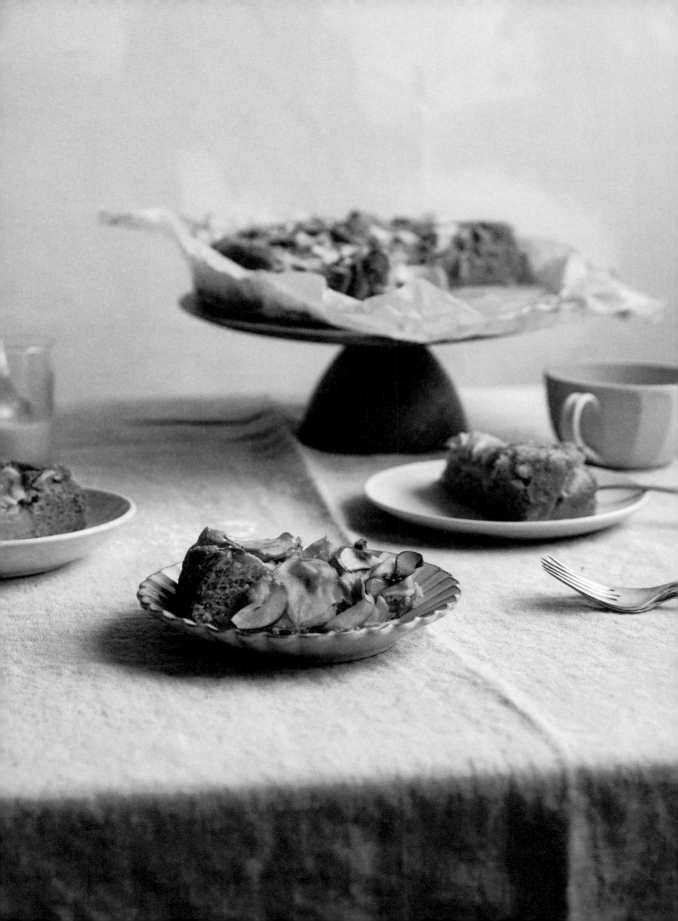

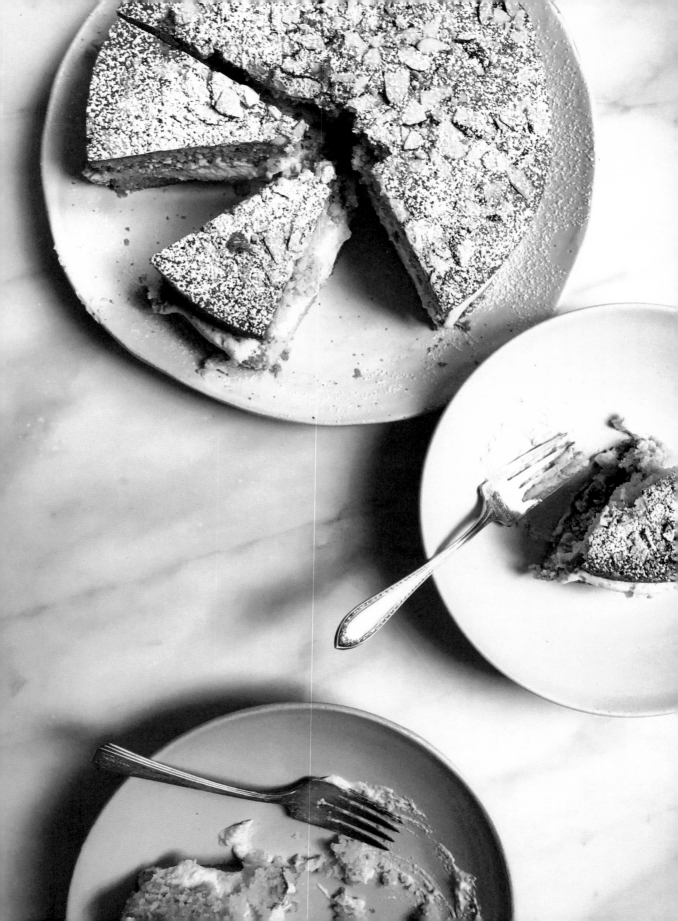

Orange-Flower Water and Saffron Cake

Orange-flower water, or *agua de azahar*, as it is called in Spanish, reminds me of my grandfather, who kept a small bottle of the precious extract in a drawer next to his workbench at the old pastry shop. He would reminisce about the streets of Seville during orange blossom season and the syrup-soaked cakes he tasted there. He used orange-flower water to flavor the brioche doughs. You can find orange-flower water in specialty and Middle Eastern markets. A little goes a long way.

MAKES ONE 8-INCH LAYER CAKE

½ cup (115 g) whole milk or
    oat milk
⅛ teaspoon saffron threads
¾ cup (150 g) sugar
2 tablespoons finely grated
    orange zest
2 large eggs
½ cup (110 g) extra-virgin olive
    oil, plus more for greasing
3 tablespoons freshly squeezed
    orange juice
1 tablespoon orange-flower water
1 cup (140 g) superfine brown
    rice flour
1 cup (100 g) almond flour
1½ teaspoons baking powder
¾ teaspoon kosher salt
½ teaspoon baking soda
¼ cup (35 g) raw sliced almonds
1 recipe Whipped Cashew-
    Coconut Cream (page 39),
    or 1 cup (225 g) heavy cream,
    whipped
Powdered sugar, for dusting

1　Preheat the oven to 350 degrees F. Grease the inside of an 8-inch cake pan with olive oil and line the bottom with a circle of parchment paper.

2　Combine the milk and saffron in a small saucepan and warm over low heat for 2 minutes, or until the saffron begins to stain the milk. Do not boil. Remove the pot from the heat and let steep for 5 minutes.

3　In a large bowl, combine the sugar and orange zest. Rub the mixture between your fingers so the zest releases its natural oils and becomes fragrant. Whisk in the milk, eggs, olive oil, orange juice, and orange-flower water.

4　In a small bowl, whisk together both flours, baking powder, salt, and baking soda. Add to the wet ingredients and whisk until well incorporated. Pour the batter into the prepared pan and top with the sliced almonds.

5　Bake for 40 to 45 minutes, or until golden brown and a toothpick inserted in the center comes out clean. Let the cake cool in the pan for 20 minutes, then invert onto a wire rack and peel off the parchment. Let the cake cool completely before cutting.

6　Place the cake on a cake stand or a platter. Using a serrated knife, cut the cake in half crosswise. I press one hand on the top center of the cake and cut with the other hand as I turn the cake, which helps with cutting even layers. The cake is delicate, so be gentle.

7　Spread the cashew-coconut cream over the bottom cake layer. Place the top layer on the cream and dust the cake with powdered sugar. Store the cake in the refrigerator for up to 2 days.

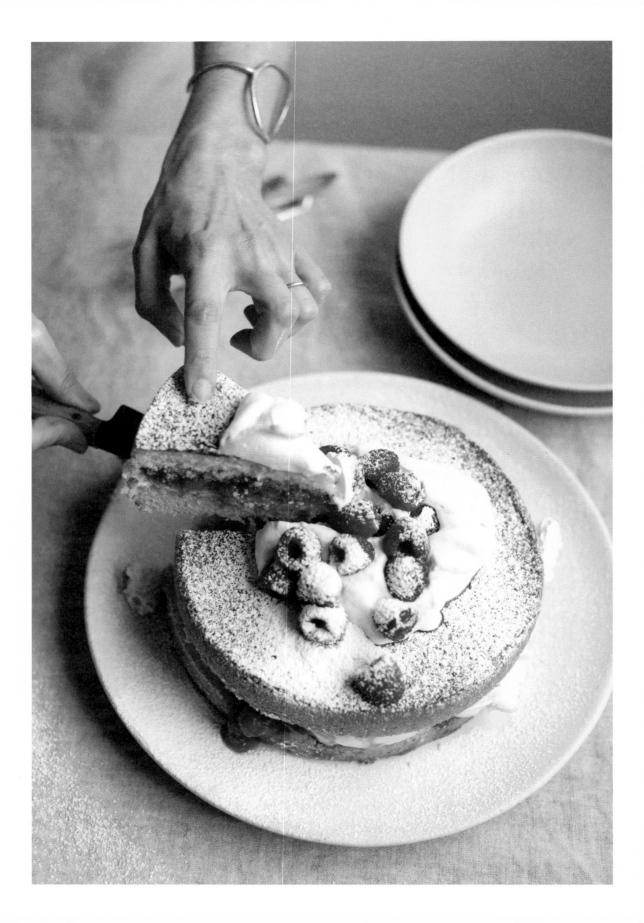

Raspberry-Rhubarb Cream Sponge

For the compote
8 ounces (225 g) fresh
    raspberries
8 ounces (225 g) rhubarb (about
    3 medium stalks), cut into
    ½-inch slices
⅓ cup (130 g) honey
2 tablespoons freshly squeezed
    orange juice
1 teaspoon vanilla extract

For the sponge
3 large eggs
1 cup (200 g) sugar
1 teaspoon vanilla extract
1 cup (100 g) almond flour
¾ cup plus 1 tablespoon (130 g)
    potato starch
1½ teaspoons baking powder
¼ teaspoon kosher salt
½ cup plus 2 tablespoons (140 g)
    unsalted butter or dairy-free
    butter, melted and cooled to
    room temperature, plus more
    for greasing
1 cup (225 g) chilled heavy cream
    or coconut cream
Fresh berries, for garnish
Powdered sugar, for dusting

Itziar Arriola, a distant family relative, migrated to London in the 1960s. She married a Sicilian man and they started a family there. She worked at a traditional English tea house and he was a maître d'. When I was twelve, my parents sent me to live with them for the summer so I could immerse myself in the English language. But more than the language, I learned about the English tradition of cakes (along with where to find the best Sicilian charcuteries in the city). This recipe is an homage to that time and traditional Victoria sponge cakes with a simple raspberry-rhubarb filling, but you may use any other fresh fruit or jam you prefer. The sponge layers can be baked a day in advance, but the cake should not be assembled until right before serving as it doesn't hold well.

MAKES ONE 8-INCH LAYER CAKE

1   To make the compote, combine the raspberries, rhubarb, honey, orange juice, and vanilla in a small saucepan and cook over medium-high heat for 8 to 10 minutes, until you have a loose jam-like consistency. Transfer the compote to a bowl or glass jar and cool completely. You should have about 2 cups. It will keep in the refrigerator for up to 1 week.

2   Preheat the oven to 350 degrees F. Grease the inside of two 8-inch cake pans with melted butter. Line the bottoms with a circle of parchment paper in each.

3   To make the sponge, in the bowl of a stand mixer fitted with the whisk attachment, combine the eggs, sugar, and vanilla. (Note: Don't let eggs and sugar sit without whisking for long or the eggs can burn.) Whip on high speed for 5 minutes, until the eggs are very thick, pale, and have tripled in volume.

4   In a medium bowl, whisk together the almond flour, potato starch, baking powder, and salt, making sure there are no lumps. Reduce the mixer speed to medium and add heaping tablespoons of the dry ingredients to the eggs. Once you have added all the flour, pour in the melted butter in a steady stream. Increase the mixer speed to high and whip for 1 minute. $\longrightarrow$

5   Divide the batter equally into the prepared pans. Bake for 25 to 30 minutes, until the top feels springy when touched and a toothpick inserted in the center comes out clean. Let the cakes cool in the pans for 30 minutes. Run the tip of a small knife all around the pan edges, then invert the cakes onto a wire rack, peel off the parchments, and cool completely. The cakes can be made 1 day in advance and stored tightly wrapped in the refrigerator.

6   In the clean bowl of the stand mixer with whisk attachment, whip the cream on high speed until thick, about 1 minute.

7   Place one cake layer on a platter or cake stand. Spread about 1 cup of the compote all over it (serve the rest on the side). Spread about three-quarters of the whipped cream over the compote, then carefully place the second cake layer on top. Dollop with the remaining cream and decorate with fresh fruit and a dusting of powdered sugar. Serve immediately—the cake is best eaten the same day.

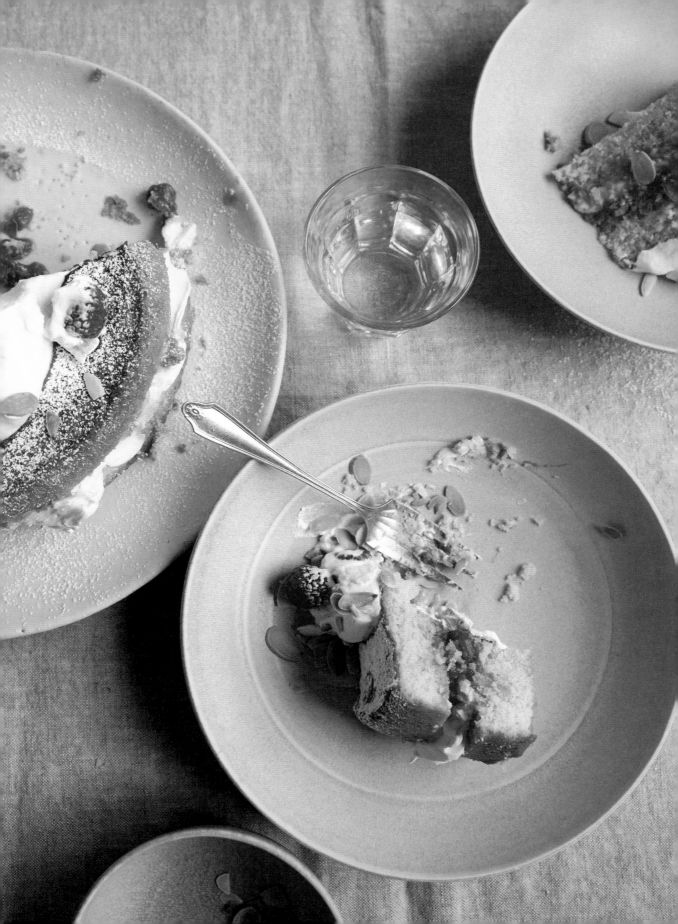

Berry Meringue Roll

Unsalted butter or nonstick
   spray, for greasing
5 large egg whites
1 cup plus 2 tablespoons (225 g)
   superfine or castor sugar
1 tablespoon cornstarch or
   tapioca starch
1 teaspoon freshly squeezed
   lemon juice
¼ cup (35 g) raw sliced almonds
2 cups (450 g) crème fraîche,
   whipped, or 1 recipe Whipped
   Cashew-Coconut Cream
   (page 39)
Finely grated zest of 1 medium
   lemon
6 ounces fresh strawberries,
   tayberries, raspberries, or
   currants

This cake is made with a layer of meringue that is baked, then filled with cream and berries and rolled into a log. As the cake sits, the meringue softens; the result is crunchy edges with a very creamy interior. The meringue is quite sweet, so the Whipped Coconut-Cashew Cream or crème fraîche make for a perfect tangy filling. If you cannot find superfine or castor sugar in your supermarket, make it yourself by pulverizing granulated white sugar in a blender or food processor until it is very powdery and fine.

MAKES 8 SERVINGS

1 Preheat the oven to 400 degrees F. Grease a 13-by-17-inch baking sheet with butter or spray. Line with parchment and grease it as well.

2 In the bowl of a stand mixer fitted with the whisk attachment, whip the egg whites on medium-high speed until they begin to foam and thicken, 1 to 2 minutes. Reduce the mixer speed to medium-low and add the sugar, 1 tablespoon at a time, waiting a few seconds between additions to make sure it is well incorporated. Once all the sugar has been added, increase the speed to medium-high again and whip until the whites are glossy and form soft peaks.

3 Gently fold in the cornstarch and lemon juice, then spread the meringue evenly on the prepared pan. Sprinkle the sliced almonds all over the top.

4 Bake for 7 to 8 minutes, until the meringue begins to turn slightly golden, then reduce the oven temperature to 325 degrees F and bake for another 8 minutes, until the top feels set, the edges begin to pull away from the pan, and the almonds are golden brown. The meringue might puff up in the oven and that's OK—it will deflate.

5 Lay a piece of parchment paper on a work surface and carefully flip the meringue onto it so the almonds are on the bottom. Peel off the parchment and cool for at least 20 minutes before filling.

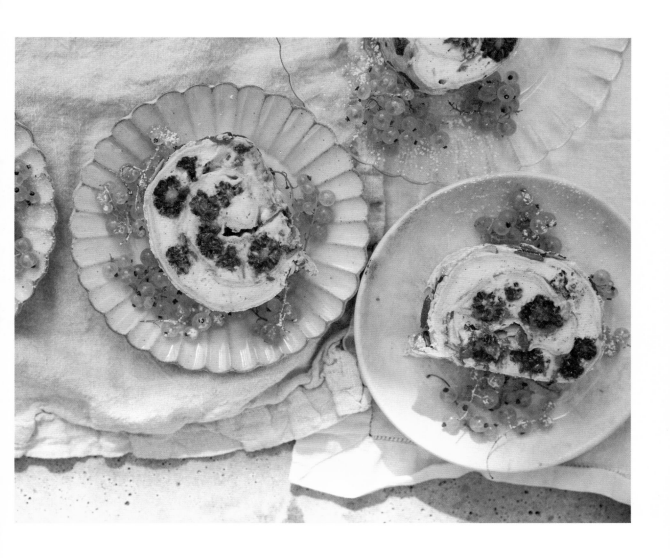

6   Using a whisk, whip the crème fraîche with the lemon zest, then spread it all over the meringue and scatter the berries on top. Starting from the short end, roll up the meringue tightly, using the parchment paper to help. Place the log on a platter and refrigerate for at least 2 hours so the flavors mix well and the cream sets. Slice and serve. The cake will keep tightly wrapped in the refrigerator for up to 2 days.

Coconut Layer Cake with Caramel

2 cups (150 g) unsweetened
  finely grated coconut
1 cup (140 g) superfine brown
  rice flour
1 cup (100 g) almond flour
¾ cup (120 g) potato starch
½ cup (60 g) tapioca starch
2½ teaspoons baking powder
1 teaspoon baking soda
1 teaspoon kosher salt
4 large eggs, at room temperature
1½ cups (300 g) coconut sugar
  or light brown sugar
1 cup (225 g) melted virgin
  coconut oil, plus more for
  greasing
1 cup (225 g) canned full-fat
  coconut milk
¼ cup (55 g) freshly squeezed
  lemon juice
1 teaspoon finely grated
  lemon zest
3 teaspoons coconut extract,
  divided
3 cups Swiss Buttercream
  (page 42)
1 recipe Coconut-Miso Caramel
  (page 46)
1½ cups (135 g) toasted
  unsweetened coconut flakes

This tower of a cake is a showstopper that is deceptively simple to put together. I took the classic coconut layer cake and made it a little bit more wholesome and extra coconutty. The cake layers are crumbly and delicate, so I recommend refrigerating the cake for a few hours before cutting it in half. Be sure your caramel is liquid before drizzling it on the cake layers—you might have to warm it up in the microwave or over a water bath if it has set. The cake firms up quite a bit when refrigerated, so let it come to temperature for at least 30 minutes before serving.

MAKES ONE 8-INCH FOUR-LAYER CAKE

1   Preheat the oven to 350 degrees F. Grease the inside of two 8-inch-wide by 2-inch-deep cake pans with coconut oil. Place a circle of parchment paper in the bottom of each pan.

2   In a large bowl, whisk together the grated coconut, both flours, both starches, baking powder, baking soda, and salt.

3   In another large bowl, whisk together the eggs, coconut sugar, coconut oil, coconut milk, lemon juice and zest, and 1 teaspoon of the coconut extract. Pour the wet ingredients over the dry and whisk until the batter is smooth.

4   Divide the batter equally into the prepared pans and bake for 30 to 35 minutes, until golden brown and a toothpick inserted in the centers comes out clean. Let the cakes cool completely in the pans, then invert onto a wire rack and peel off the parchments. You can make the cakes 3 days in advance and keep them tightly wrapped in the refrigerator.

5   Make sure the cakes are completely cooled before cutting or they can fall apart. Using a serrated knife, cut each cake in half crosswise. I press one hand on the top center of the cake and cut with the other hand as I turn the cake, which helps with cutting even layers. This cake is crumbly, which is what makes it so tender, so work carefully.

6   Fold the remaining 2 teaspoons coconut extract into the buttercream.

7   Place one cake layer on a cake stand. Spread 1 to 2 tablespoons of the caramel around on top in a very thin layer. Wait until it soaks into the cake, then cover the top with a thin layer of buttercream. Place another cake layer over the buttercream and gently press down so it adheres well to the buttercream. Repeat this sequence with the remaining cake layers.

8   Once you have stacked the fourth cake layer on top, spread a very thin layer of buttercream over the top and sides of the entire cake. Scrape off as much as possible. This will be your crumb coat. I like to use a bench scraper to even out the tall sides. You should be able to see some of the cake through the buttercream. Refrigerate the cake for at least 15 minutes to firm up the buttercream. You can keep the cake in the refrigerator for up to 24 hours at this point and finish icing the following day.

9   If you like the look of a naked cake, simply pile the coconut flakes on the top and serve. Otherwise, spread another, thicker layer of buttercream over the top and sides of the entire cake. You can smooth out the buttercream or use your spatula to create some texture. Cover all sides with the coconut flakes and drizzle the cake with the remaining caramel before serving. The cake will keep in the refrigerator for up to 3 days.

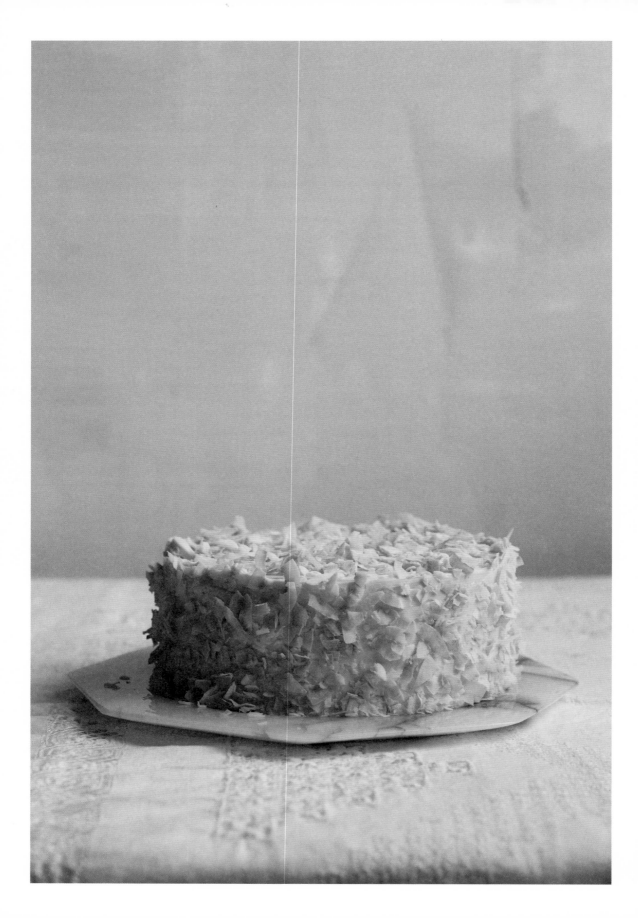

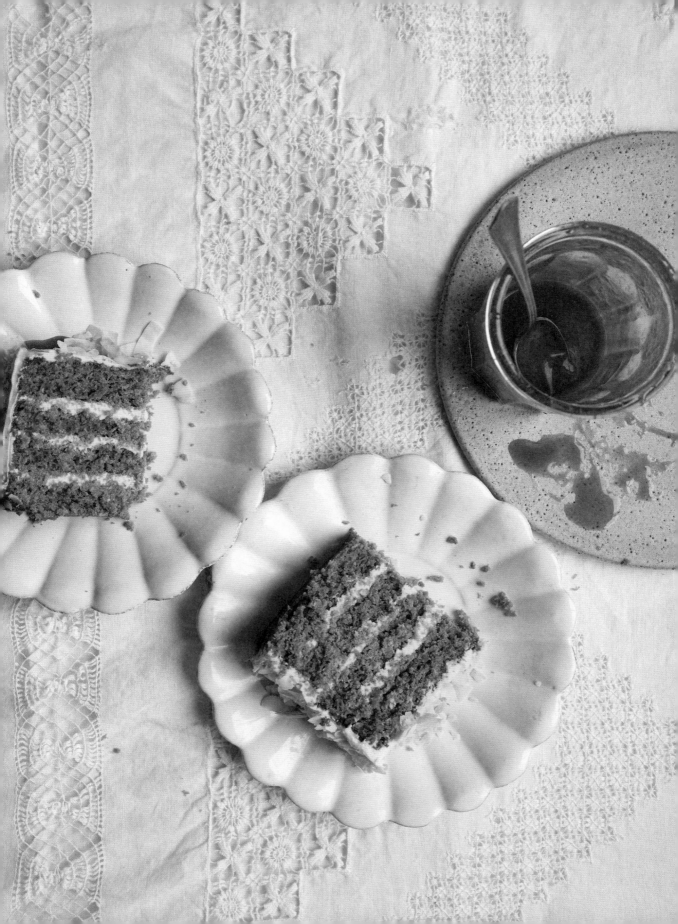

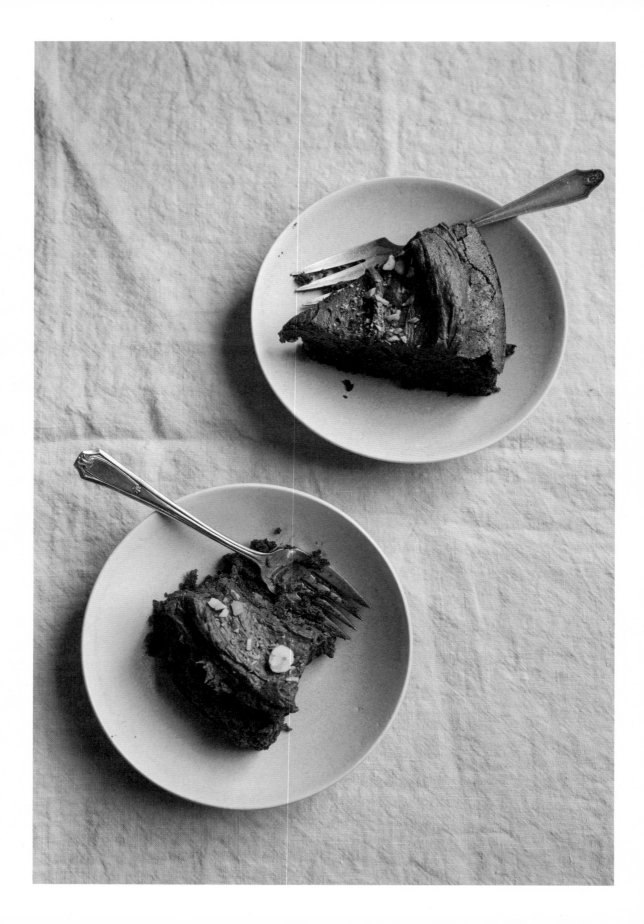

Chocolate-Hazelnut Torte with Chocolate-Coffee Buttercream

I like to serve this cake next to some shots of espresso in the dark afternoons of the winter months. It's one of my favorites. The cake is rich, with a gooey interior and crunchy exterior—the pieces of hazelnut add texture to each bite. You can certainly serve this cake naked, but the buttercream adds another delectable level of richness.

MAKES ONE 9-INCH CAKE

1 Preheat the oven to 325 degrees F. Grease the inside of a 9-inch cake pan with olive oil and cover the bottom with a circle of parchment paper.

2 Spread the hazelnuts on a baking sheet and roast for 15 to 18 minutes, until golden brown and fragrant. Let them cool slightly on the pan, then transfer them to a thick kitchen towel. Rub the towel and hazelnuts together to loosen their skins. Once they are mostly peeled (it's OK if they still have some skin), transfer them to a food processor and cool completely. Increase the oven temperature to 350 degrees F.

3 Once the hazelnuts are cool, add ½ cup (100 g) of the sugar, buckwheat flour, and salt to the food processor and pulse until the hazelnuts turn into a fine powder. Be careful not to overprocess or they will turn into butter.

4 Fill a saucepan one-quarter full with water and bring to a simmer over medium heat. Put the chocolate in a large heatproof bowl set over the pan and stir until the chocolate is melted.

5 Remove the bowl from the heat. Whisk in the olive oil, egg yolks, orange zest, vanilla, and hazelnut mixture. The batter will be thick.

6 In the bowl of a stand mixer fitted with the whisk attachment, beat the egg whites over medium-high speed until they begin to double in size and thicken. Slowly sprinkle in the remaining ½ cup (100 g) sugar, 1 tablespoon at a time, waiting a few seconds between additions. Continue beating until the egg whites are thick and glossy and hold their peaks. $\longrightarrow$

Ingredients

1⅓ cups (170 g) raw hazelnuts
1 cup (200 g) sugar, divided
2 tablespoons light buckwheat flour
½ teaspoon kosher salt
6 ounces (170 g) 70 percent chocolate, coarsely chopped
½ cup (110 g) extra-virgin olive oil, plus more for greasing
5 large eggs, separated
2 teaspoons finely grated orange zest
2 teaspoons vanilla extract
1 recipe Chocolate-Coffee American-Style Buttercream (page 45), optional

7   Fold one-third of the meringue into the chocolate mixture, mixing vigorously to lighten up the batter. Gently fold in the remaining two-thirds meringue until there are no visible white streaks.

8   Pour the batter into the prepared pan and bake for 30 to 35 minutes, until a toothpick inserted in the center comes out clean. Let the cake cool completely in the pan, then invert onto a platter and peel off the parchment. If you are frosting the cake with buttercream, you can pipe rose shapes on top or simply spread it all over and use a spatula to create a rippled effect. The cake will keep in the refrigerator for up to 3 days.

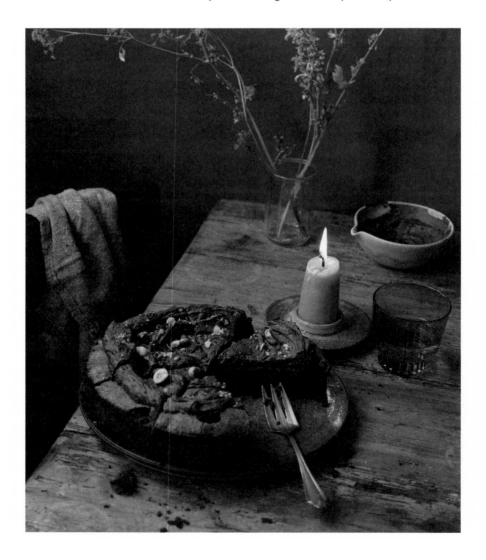

Chocolate Sourdough Cake with Chocolate Glaze

¾ cup (150 g) light brown sugar

½ cup (150 g) cold sourdough starter (page 25)

½ cup (110 g) extra-virgin olive oil, plus more for greasing

2 large eggs

2 tablespoons brewed espresso or very strong coffee, cooled to room temperature

¾ cup (75 g) almond flour

½ cup (70 g) superfine brown rice flour or light buckwheat flour

¼ cup (25 g) unsweetened cocoa powder

½ teaspoon baking soda

½ teaspoon kosher salt

4 ounces (110 g) 85 percent chocolate, chopped

1 recipe Chocolate Glaze (page 46)

Note: If you don't have any sourdough starter to discard, replace it with ½ cup (70 g) superfine brown rice flour plus 6 tablespoons water.

This easy-to-make, fairly healthy cake is in high rotation at my house. The sourdough starter doesn't need to be fed or fermented, so this recipe is perfect for when you need to discard some starter to revive it. It also adds tang to the cake, which works so well with chocolate. It is easily adaptable to make it vegan as well as free of refined sugar and grain. (See the variations below.) For something a bit more decadent, you can double the recipe, bake it as a sheet cake, and pipe pretty swirls of Chocolate Swiss Buttercream (page 42) on top, which makes a beautiful birthday or celebration cake.

MAKES ONE 8-INCH CAKE

1   Preheat the oven to 350 degrees F. Grease the inside of an 8-inch cake pan with olive oil and line the bottom with a circle of parchment paper.

2   In a large bowl, whisk together the light brown sugar, starter, olive oil, eggs, and espresso until smooth. Add both flours, cocoa powder, baking soda, and salt and whisk until the batter is smooth. Fold in the chopped chocolate.

3   Pour the batter into the prepared pan and bake for 30 to 35 minutes, or until a toothpick inserted in the center comes out clean. Let the cake cool in the pan for 15 minutes, then invert onto a wire rack and peel off the parchment. When the cake feels cool to the touch, spread the chocolate glaze all over it, letting it drip over the sides. The cake will keep tightly wrapped in the refrigerator for up to 3 days.

SUGAR-FREE

If you prefer to sweeten the cake with dates, use 5 ounces (150 g) pitted dates in place of the light brown sugar. Soak the dates in boiling water for 15 minutes, then puree them in a food processor with 3 tablespoons of the soaking liquid until it becomes a creamy, smooth paste.

EGG-FREE

To make this cake egg-free, stir together 2 tablespoons flaxseed meal and ¼ cup hot water. When gelled, add it to the batter in place of the eggs in step 2.

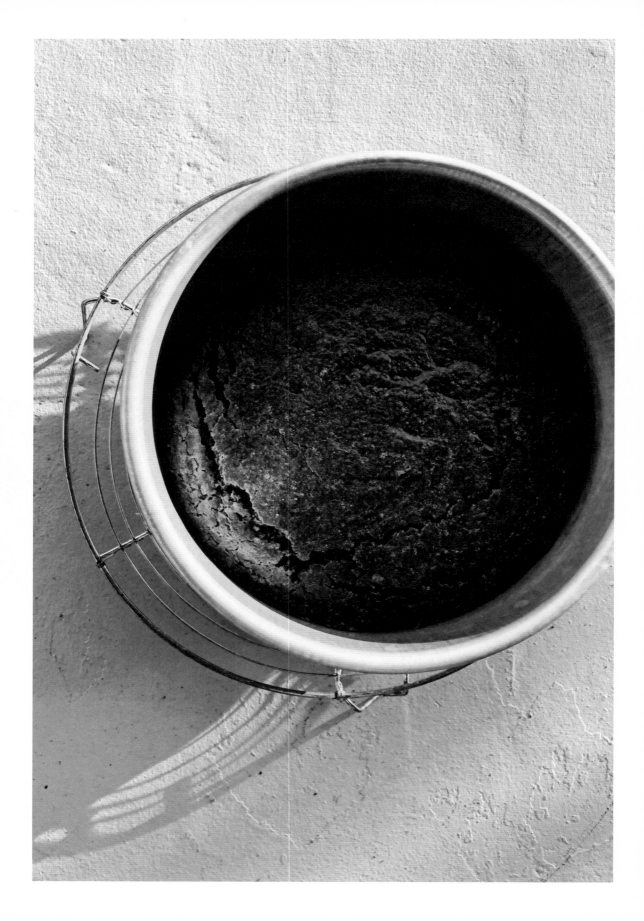

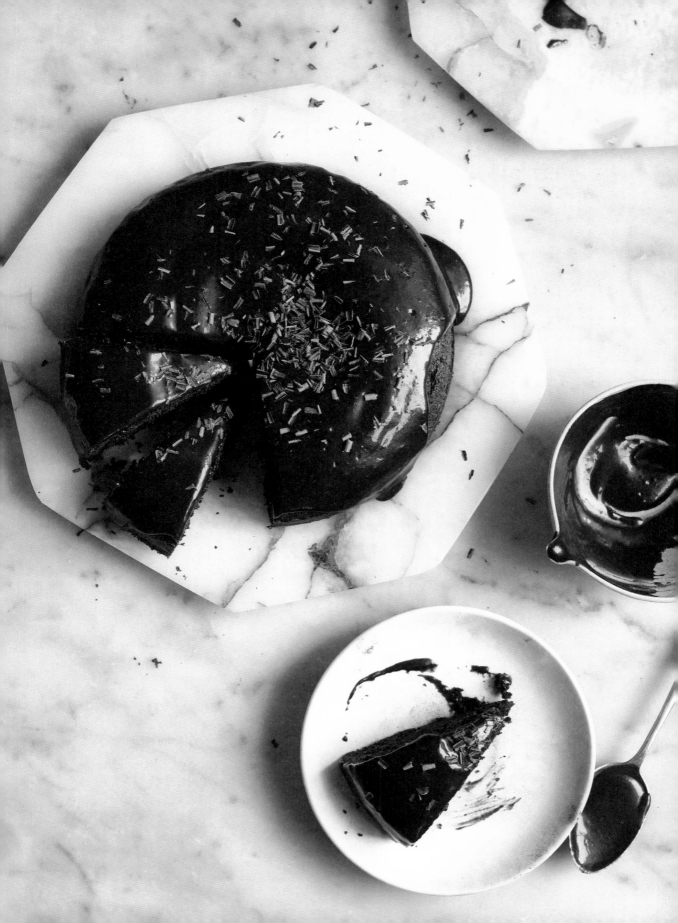

Lemon Curd and Honey Celebration Cake

1 recipe Lemon Curd (page 37)
2½ cups (250 g) almond flour
1½ cups (165 g) gluten-free
   oat flour
⅓ cup (45 g) tapioca starch
1 tablespoon baking powder
1 teaspoon kosher salt
½ teaspoon baking soda
¾ cup (150 g) sugar
2 teaspoons finely grated
   lemon zest
¾ cup (170 g) unsalted butter
   or dairy-free butter, at room
   temperature, plus more for
   greasing
4 large eggs, at room
   temperature
½ cup (170 g) honey
6 tablespoons freshly squeezed
   lemon juice
¼ cup (55 g) extra-virgin olive oil
3 cups Honey-Lemon Swiss
   Buttercream (page 42)

Everyone should have a favorite celebration cake recipe in their repertoire, and I hope this one will become yours. It is an unfussy yet flavorful cake with a lemon-curd filling and honey-lemon buttercream. It is light yet rich, just like a memorable party should be. I like to make the lemon curd and the cake the day before serving so they have time to settle and develop their flavors. When I'm ready to assemble, I whip the buttercream and put the cake together. You can be as intricate as you'd like with the decorations, but personally I love a naked cake with some edible flowers or small beeswax candles on top.

MAKES ONE 8-INCH FOUR-LAYER CAKE

1 Make the lemon curd at least 4 hours before you will use it as it needs time to chill completely. The recipe makes more than you'll need, so save the rest for another use.

2 Preheat the oven to 350 degrees F. Grease the insides of two 8-inch-wide by 2-inch-deep cake pans with butter and line the bottom with a circle of parchment paper.

3 To make the cake, in a large bowl, whisk together both flours, tapioca starch, baking powder, salt, and baking soda.

4 In the bowl of a stand mixer, rub the sugar and lemon zest between your fingers so the zest releases its natural oils and becomes fragrant. Attach the bowl to mixer and fit it with the paddle attachment. Add the butter and beat it over medium speed for 1 minute, until creamy. Add the eggs, one at a time, beating between additions. The mixture might look curdled, which is OK. Be sure to scrape the paddle, sides, and bottom of the bowl well.

5 In a medium bowl, whisk together the honey, lemon juice, and olive oil.

6 Add half of the dry ingredients to the mixer bowl. Beat on medium speed until the batter begins to come together and any curdled pieces of butter disappear. With the mixer running,

pour in the honey mixture and remaining half of the dry ingredients. Stop the mixer and scrape the bottom of the bowl well. Increase the mixer speed to medium-high and beat for another 30 seconds. The batter should be smooth. Divide it equally into the prepared pans and smooth out the tops.

7   Bake for 30 to 35 minutes, until golden brown and a toothpick inserted in the center comes out clean. Let the cakes cool completely in the pans. Run a knife around the edges, invert onto a wire rack, and peel off the parchments. You can make the cakes 1 day in advance and store them tightly wrapped in the refrigerator.

8   While the cakes are cooling, make the buttercream. Fit a large pastry bag with a medium-size plain tip (number 5 or 6). Fill with 1 cup of the buttercream.

9   Using a serrated knife, cut each cake in half crosswise. I press one hand on the top center of the cake and cut with the other hand as I turn the cake, which helps with cutting even layers. This cake is crumbly, which is what makes it so tender, so work carefully.

10   Place one cake layer, cut side up, on a cake stand. Using a spatula, spread a very thin layer of buttercream on top. Pipe a thin circle of buttercream all along the outer rim of the cake, creating a wall that is about ¼ inch tall for the lemon-curd filling. Spread ⅓ cup of the lemon curd over the center, staying inside the buttercream walls. Top with a second cake layer and gently press down. Repeat this process with the remaining cake layers, checking that they are centered as you build them up. Place the final cake layer cut side down.

11   Spread a thin layer of buttercream on the top and sides of the entire cake. Scrape off as much as possible. This will be your crumb coat. Refrigerate the cake for 15 minutes to firm up the buttercream. Coat the cake with another, thicker layer of buttercream. Decorate the top with flowers, candles, or any other decorations you like.

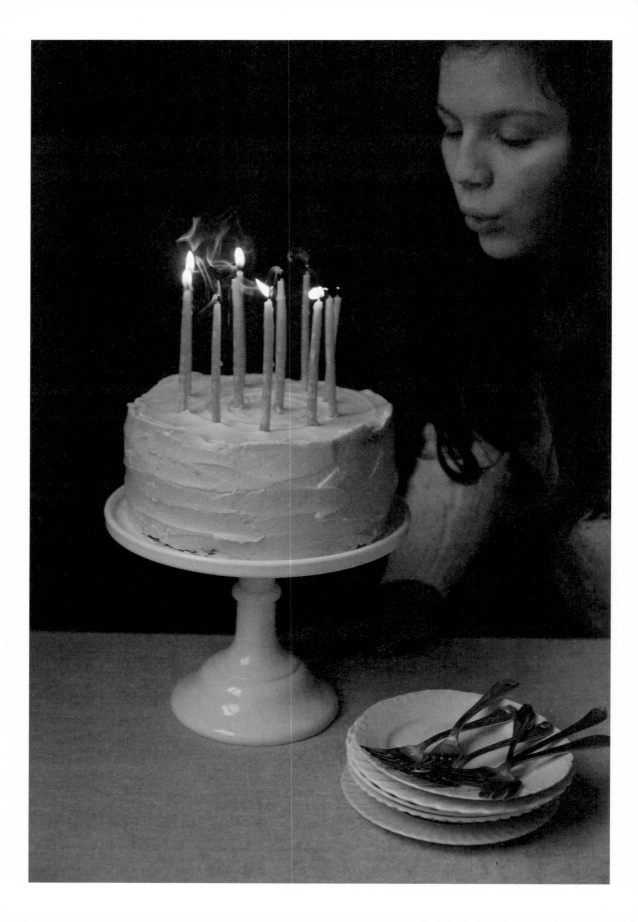

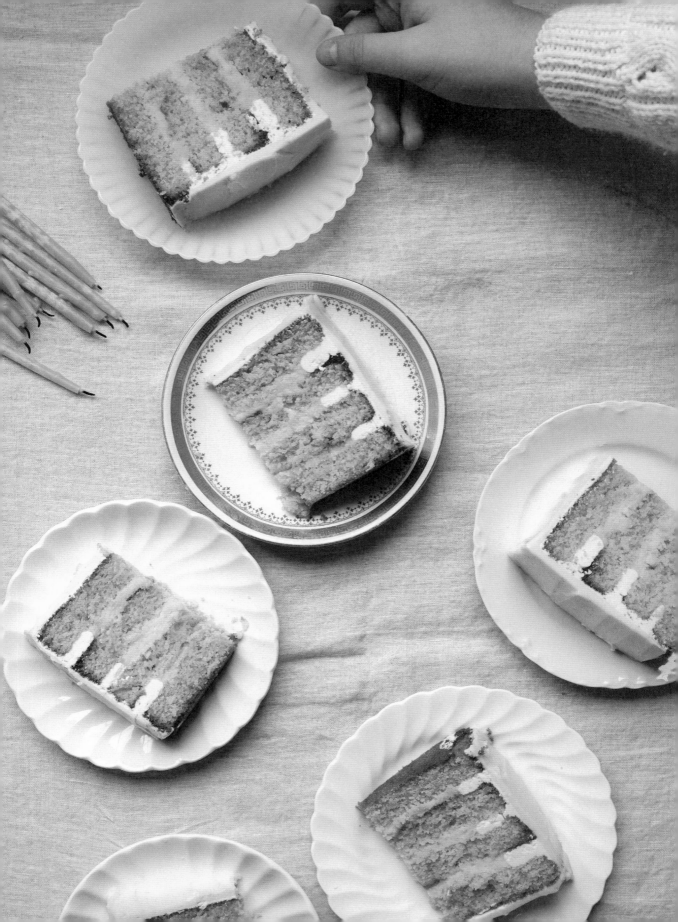

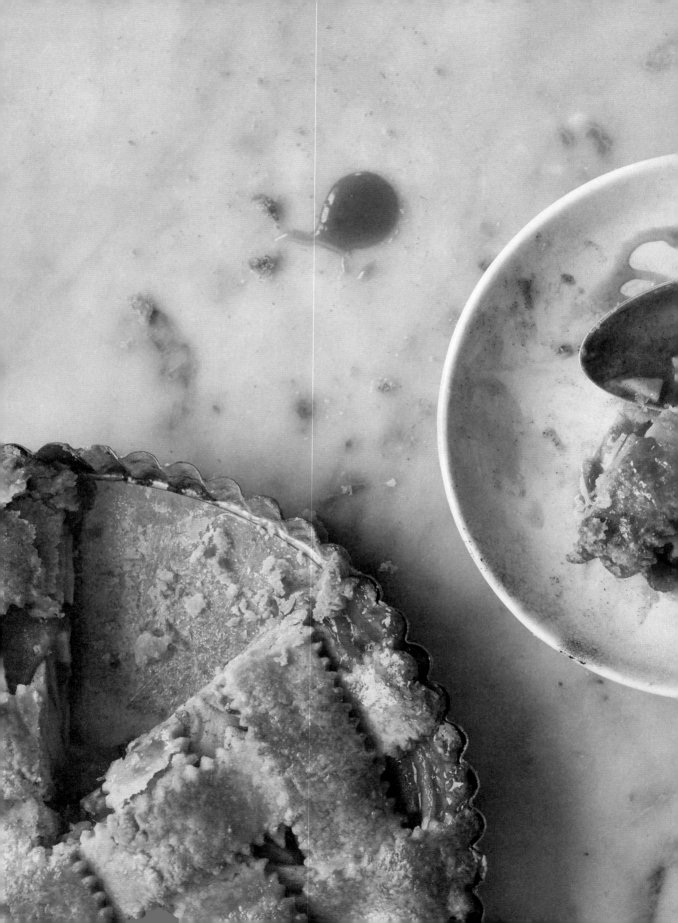

CHAPTER FOUR

The Flakiest Tarts, Pies, and Biscuits

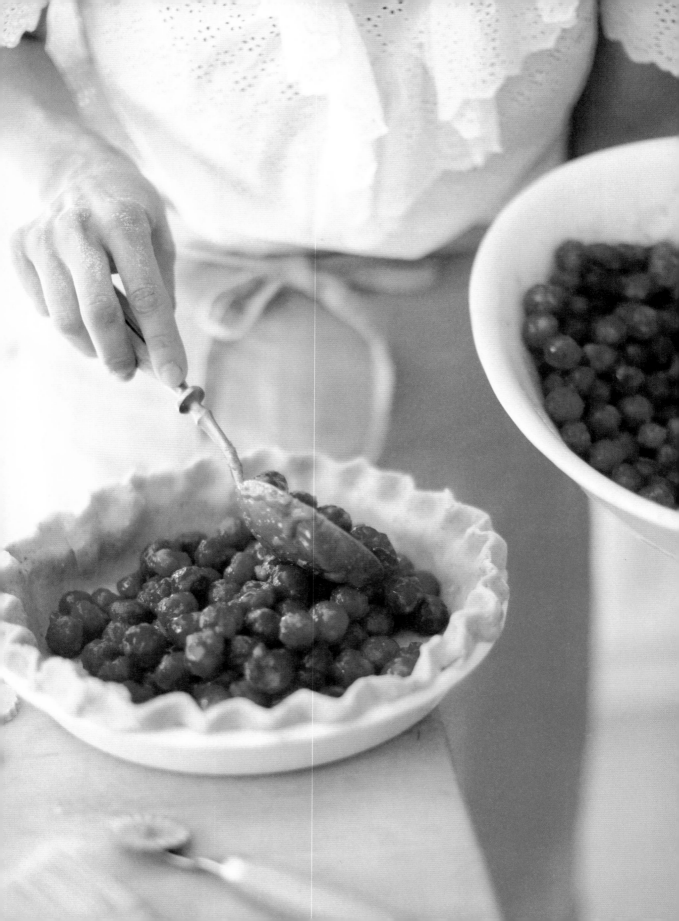

One of the most distinct scents from my youth is that of puff pastry caramelizing in the oven. A thousand laminated layers of butter, flour, and the right amount of salt pushing against each other, creating a flaky golden pastry. I believe a tart or a pie should have the irresistible balance between crunchy shell and creamy interior. They are still my favorite thing to make because the possibilities are endless through different combinations of crusts, fillings, fruits, and vegetables.

Unlike cakes and quick breads, where the absence of gluten isn't much of an issue, gluten-free pastry is a totally different game. Pastry relies on the fine balance between not overworking the dough in order to create flaky layers and having enough elasticity so it doesn't shatter. Gluten-free pastry is more fragile than its gluten-full counterpart, so you have to manipulate the dough a bit more gingerly. See page 158 for more tips on handling pastry.

You will find three pastry dough recipes in this chapter that are referenced throughout: Pie Dough (page 162), which is equivalent to your traditional *pâte brisée*; Buttery Rough Puff Pastry Dough (page 180), which is a simpler version of a standard puff pastry; and Chocolate-Buckwheat Pastry Dough (page 173), which is not very sweet, a little earthy, and perfect for creamy chocolate and custard fillings. Both the pie dough and the rough puff are equally great in sweet and savory preparations. If you are a beginning tart-maker, I recommend the forgiving rustic galettes, such as the Strawberry-Rhubarb-Almond Galette (page 161) or Plum-Chocolate Frangipane Galette (page 170). From there, move up to the recipes that require a bit more time and precision, like the Lemon Meringue Tartlets (page 175). Some of the recipes that follow are not quite tarts but in my mind belong in a similar category—the Jam-Filled Scones (page 194), Cheddar and Herb Scones (page 197), and Dutch Baby with Caramelized Apples and Lemon (page 186) are all examples.

Handling Gluten-Free Pastry Dough

It's been so long since I have rolled out a gluten dough that I cannot even remember what they feel like, beyond recalling how much more aggressive I could be with them. Gluten-free pastries are not as elastic, so you must take a bit more care. Here are some tips:

- Add ½ teaspoon xanthan gum to the Pie Dough (page 162) if you want to pull and stretch it a bit more or if you are going to use it to create more intricate decorations. This will help the dough hold its shape better.

- I have recently been making my pastry doughs with Cultured Cashew-Coconut Butter (page 33) and they work great. If you purchase dairy-free butter, I find that those specifically formulated for baking (they usually come in stick form) work better. The only issue I find is that these butters don't caramelize the same way due to lack of milk solids. So for pieces of dough that will be visible, such as galette edges or any lattice work you might apply to the top of a pie, make sure to brush the pastry with egg wash and a tiny sprinkle of sugar. This will help give a golden color to the pastry when baked.

- When the dough is too cold, it has a tendency to crack, so let it soften for about 10 minutes after you take it out of the refrigerator. To speed up the process, you can put the dough between two sheets of parchment paper or plastic wrap and pound it with a rolling pin to flatten and stretch it without rolling. If it continues cracking, gather it into a ball and give it a quick knead to help bring back some elasticity. I know this goes against a lot of the things we hear about pastry—not to overmanipulate it, that your hands will warm the dough too much. This is true, but I find that if dough cracks when it's still chilled, a quick knead will sometimes do the trick. This is a bit of intuition that you will develop as you become familiar working with gluten-free dough. It doesn't apply to puff pastry since it's important to keep the layers of dough and butter as intact as possible.

- If you are a beginner, I recommend that you try rolling the pastry between two sheets of parchment paper or plastic wrap. This will ensure you are not adding too much bench flour and that your dough doesn't stick to the surface.

- Move the dough around a lot. Every time I give it one pass with the rolling pin, I turn the dough 90 degrees and roll again. I make sure my surface and rolling pin are both dusted with flour.

- Doughs are very temperature sensitive and because they are crumbly, they can fall apart more easily when warm. If your dough is getting too soft, slide it onto parchment, place on a baking sheet, and refrigerate for a few minutes.

- Don't try to roll gluten-free pastry dough around a rolling pin to help transfer it to a tart pan. It doesn't have enough elasticity for that kind of stretch and will fall apart. Put the pan beside you, gently lift the dough with both hands, and quickly move it above and into the pan. Use your fingers to press it into the bottom and sides, then cut off excess dough by sliding a paring knife along the top of the pan.

- These dough recipes freeze really well. Wrap them tightly in parchment, put them inside a ziplock bag, and freeze them for up to 3 months. Thaw them in the refrigerator overnight before using.

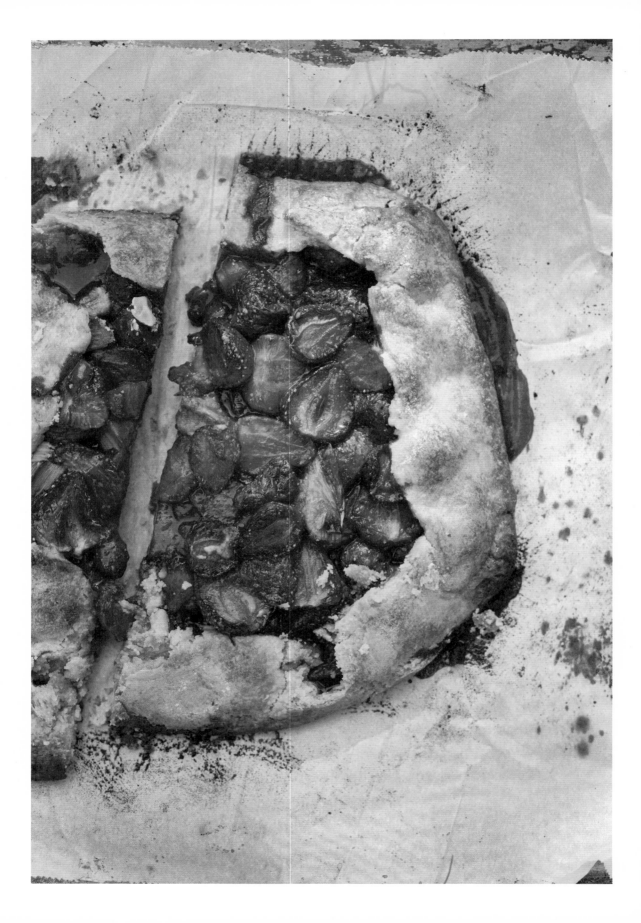

Strawberry-Rhubarb-Almond Galette

Strawberry and rhubarb is the quintessential early spring combination. I grow both in my garden. Choose strawberries that are very ripe and make sure the rhubarb is as red as possible so that it turns a beautiful rose color when baked. You can reduce the amount of sugar depending on how sweet your fruit is, and you might need to increase the amount of cornstarch if you are using very juicy fruit, especially previously frozen fruit.

MAKES ONE 7-INCH GALETTE

8 ounces (225 g) strawberries, hulled and halved

6 ounces (170 g) rhubarb (about 2 medium stalks), cut into 1-inch slices

¼ cup (50 g) sugar, plus more for sprinkling

1 tablespoon cornstarch

1 vanilla bean, split lengthwise and seeds scraped

Superfine brown rice flour, for dusting

½ recipe Pie Dough (page 162)

¼ cup (25 g) almond flour

1 large egg, lightly beaten

1 tablespoon raw sesame seeds (optional)

1   Preheat the oven to 400 degrees F. Line a baking sheet with parchment paper.

2   Toss the strawberries, rhubarb, sugar, cornstarch, and vanilla seeds together in a large bowl.

3   Dust a work surface with brown rice flour and roll the pie dough to approximately a ⅛-inch thickness and 11-inch diameter. Transfer the dough to the prepared pan. Sprinkle the almond flour in the center of the pastry and pile the fruit mixture on top, leaving a 2-inch border. Fold the pastry over the filling. It's OK if it cracks slightly—it's supposed to be rustic.

4   Brush the dough with the beaten egg and sprinkle sugar and sesame seeds over it. Bake the galette for 40 minutes, until the filling is bubbly and the crust is golden brown. Let the galette cool for 15 minutes before cutting. It's best eaten the same day, but it will keep in the refrigerator for up to 1 day.

Pie Dough

¾ cup (105 g) superfine
  brown rice flour
¾ cup (105 g) sorghum flour
⅔ cup (70 g) almond flour
½ cup (60 g) tapioca starch
2 tablespoons sugar
2 teaspoons (7 g) psyllium
  husk powder
½ teaspoon kosher salt
1 cup (225 g) cold unsalted
  butter, dairy-free butter, or
  Cultured Cashew-Coconut
  Butter (page 33), cut into
  ½-inch dice
1 large egg
2 to 3 tablespoons ice-cold
  water

You can make this pie dough by hand, if desired, by rubbing the flour and butter together, then folding in the rest of the ingredients with a spatula. For an egg-free version, add 1 tablespoon (7 g) flaxseed meal to the dry ingredients and increase the ice-water amount to 5 to 7 tablespoons.

MAKES TWO 9-INCH SINGLE-CRUST PIES
OR ONE 9-INCH DOUBLE-CRUST PIE

1   Combine the three flours, tapioca starch, sugar, psyllium powder, and salt in a food processor. Pulse a few times to aerate. Add the diced butter and pulse ten times, or until the butter is the size of peas.

2   In a small bowl, whisk the egg with 2 tablespoons of the ice water. Pour it into the food processor and pulse a few more times. The dough won't form a ball, so press it between your hands to feel the texture. It should be moist and hold together when pressed. Add more ice water, 1 teaspoon at a time, if the dough feels dry.

3   Turn the dough out onto a work surface, press all the pieces together with your hands, and give it a couple of kneads. The warmth of your hands can melt the butter, so work quickly.

4   Cut the dough into two equal pieces, shape each one into a disk, and wrap in parchment paper. Flatten them lightly and chill in the refrigerator for at least 30 minutes. The dough will keep in the refrigerator for 2 days or can be frozen for up to 3 months. If frozen, thaw in the refrigerator overnight.

SAVORY

For a savory dough, omit the sugar, increase the salt to 1 teaspoon, and add ¼ teaspoon freshly ground black pepper.

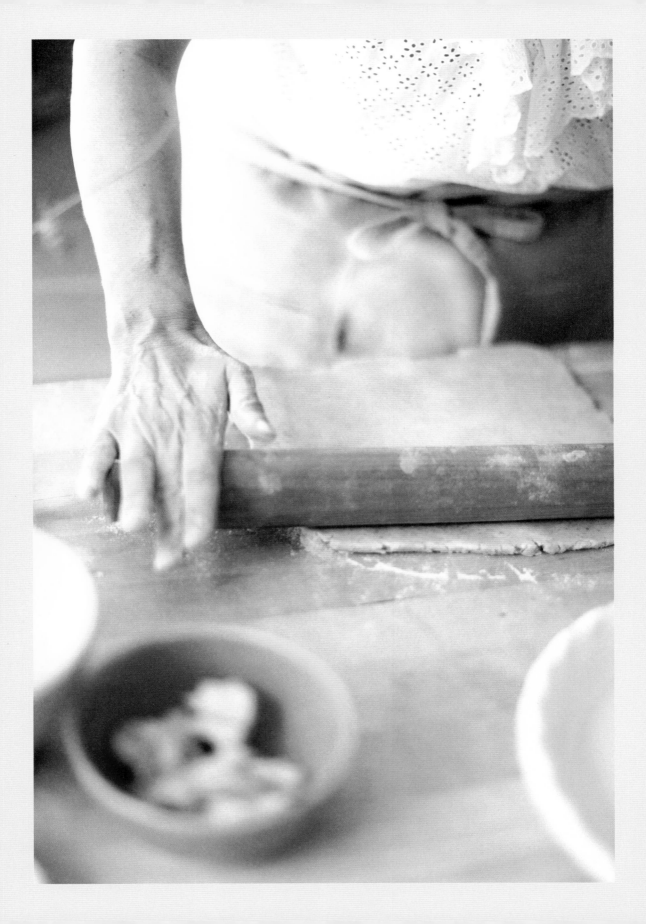

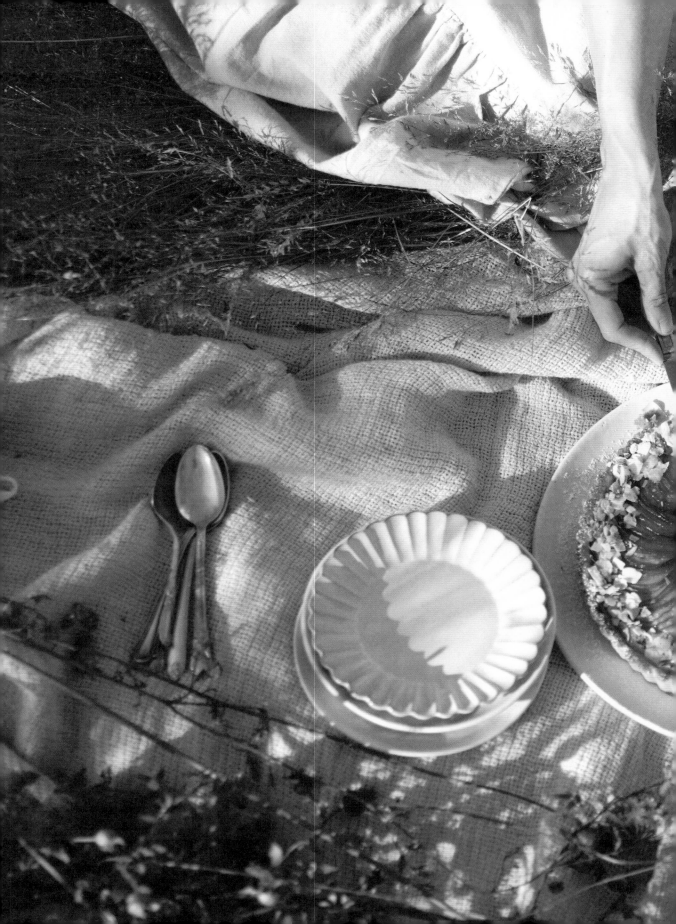

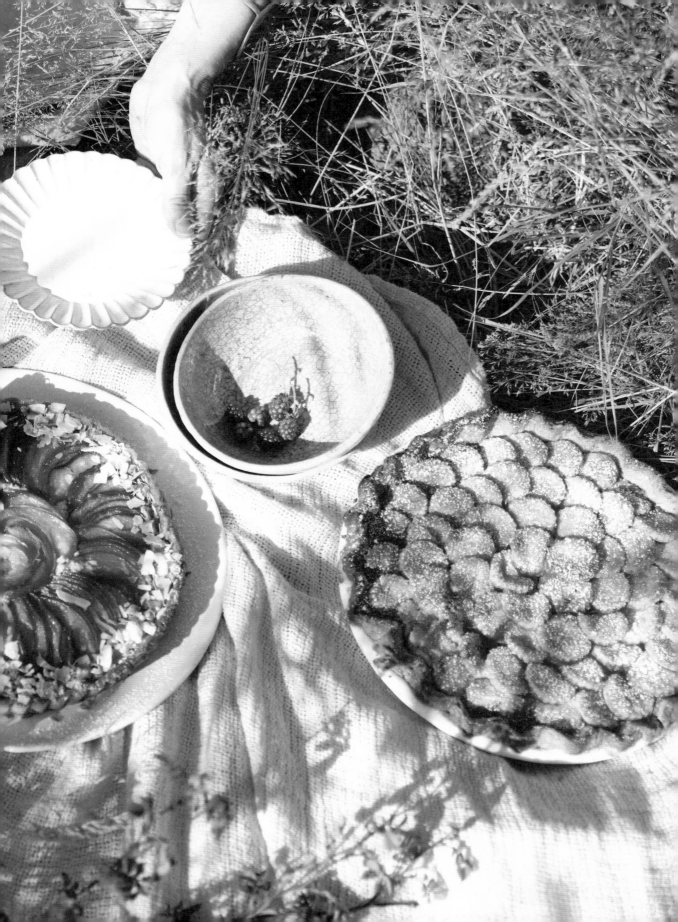

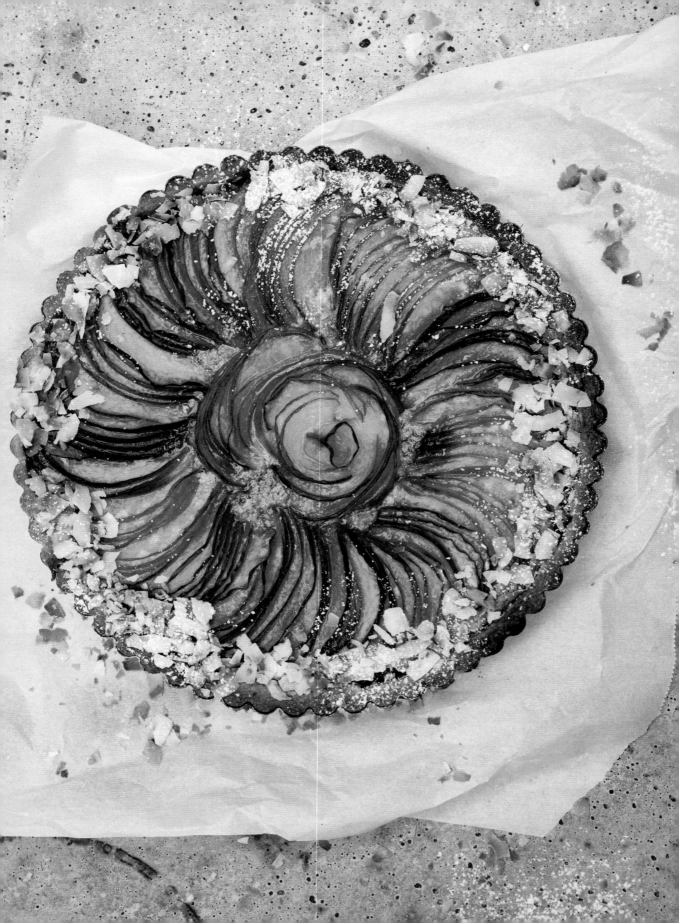

Peach and Sunflower-Coconut Frangipane Tart

Superfine brown rice flour,
  for dusting
½ recipe Pie Dough (page 162)
1 recipe Sunflower-Coconut
  Frangipane (page 38)
3 medium peaches
2 tablespoons toasted
  unsweetened coconut flakes
Powdered sugar, for dusting

The first time I recall eating a peach straight from the tree was on a hot August day. I must have been seven or eight. My uncle Jose vacationed in Sartaguda at that time, a small village in the arid plains of Navarre, and we would visit him there. It was midday. The hot, dry air felt heavy on my body. There was nothing but the sound of crickets in the middle of this orchard. The earth where rows and rows of peach trees stood was brown and cracked. My uncle lifted his arms and plucked a peach from a branch. Stem still attached, he asked me to smell it before biting into it. The aroma, sweetness, and juiciness of that one peach will remain burned in my memory. Stone fruits and frangipane are the perfect match, melting into one creamy filling.

MAKES ONE 9-INCH TART

1   Preheat the oven to 400 degrees F.

2   Dust a work surface with brown rice flour. Roll the pie dough to approximately a ⅛-inch thickness and 11-inch diameter. Carefully transfer the dough with both hands to a tart pan, pressing it into the bottom and sides. Trim any excess dough that hangs over the edge. Spread the frangipane evenly all over the dough.

3   Halve and pit the peaches, then thinly slice them. Arrange the slices in a slightly overlapping circular pattern on top of the frangipane.

4   Put the tart pan on a baking sheet and bake for 40 to 45 minutes, until the crust is golden brown. Let the tart cool in the pan for 15 minutes before unmolding. Top with the coconut flakes and dust with powdered sugar.

Cherry Marzipan Pie

1 recipe Pie Dough (page 162)
  with optional 1 teaspoon
  xanthan gum
2 pounds (900 g) cherries, pitted
½ to ¾ cup (100 to 150 g) sugar,
  depending on sweetness of
  fruit (see Note)
Zest and juice of 1 medium lemon
¼ teaspoon kosher salt
2 tablespoons cornstarch
2 tablespoons water
Tapioca starch, for dusting
½ cup (150 g) Marzipan (page 49),
  cut into ½-inch cubes
1 large egg, lightly beaten
Turbinado sugar or sprinkling
  sugar, for topping

Note: Sour cherries are best for
this recipe, but it can be made
with red or black cherries. Simply reduce the amount of sugar
from ¾ cup for sour cherries to
½ cup if using the sweeter red or
black varieties.

Cherries and almonds are a match made in heaven, and I
encourage you to make your own marzipan following the recipe
on page 49. It is so simple and will make this pie's filling extra
rich and delicious. You will notice that I call for xanthan gum to
be added to the dough. Doing so prevents the cutout dough
pieces on top from spreading too much while baking, but of
course, you can omit it.

MAKES ONE 9-INCH PIE

1 Make the pie dough according to the instructions, but add
1 teaspoon xanthan gum with the dry ingredients. Cut the
dough into equal halves and refrigerate them while preparing
the filling.

2 Combine the cherries, sugar, lemon zest and juice, and salt
in a medium pot and bring to a simmer over medium-high heat.
Stir frequently so the sugar doesn't burn, especially at the
beginning. Cook for 5 minutes, until the cherries are just beginning to soften. Using a slotted spoon, transfer the cherries to a
large bowl, leaving the liquid in the pot to continue simmering.

3 In a small bowl, whisk together the cornstarch and water
until dissolved. Add it to the simmering liquid while whisking.
Cook for 30 seconds to 1 minute, until thickened. Immediately
pour the thickened liquid over the cooked cherries. Stir well
and set aside to cool completely.

4 Dust a work surface with tapioca starch. Roll out one of the
pie dough halves ⅛ inch thick and carefully lift it with both
hands over a 9-inch pie plate. Press the dough into the bottom
and sides, allowing a bit of overhang, then crimp the edges.

5 Spoon the filling into the shell, dotting the marzipan
between. Refrigerate the pie while you work on the top.

6 Roll out the other piece of dough ⅛ inch thick and cut 1-inch
circles using a cookie cutter. You will need about 80 circles.
Reroll any scraps of dough, but if it gets too soft, chill again in
the refrigerator before proceeding.

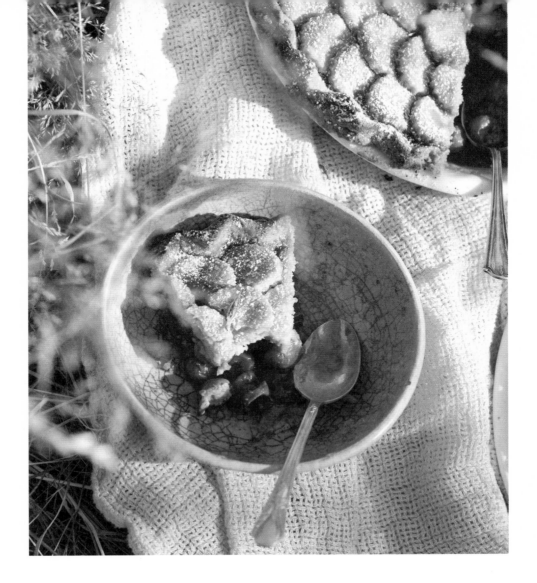

7   Preheat the oven to 425 degrees F. Remove the pie from fridge and top it with the dough disks, overlapping them slightly but leaving a bit of space between layers so some of the steam created while baking can escape. Once the topping is complete, freeze the pie for 10 minutes.

8   Put the pie plate on a baking sheet. Brush the dough with the beaten egg and sprinkle with turbinado sugar. Bake for 35 to 40 minutes, until the crust is golden brown and the filling is bubbling. Let the pie cool for 15 minutes before cutting. The pie will keep tightly wrapped in the refrigerator for 2 days.

Plum-Chocolate Frangipane Galette

The color of this galette reflects the mood I feel during those early fall days when plums signal the change in season. Choose dark-red or purple-fleshed plums for a dramatic effect and beautiful contrast against the chocolate. You can omit the sesame seeds and use some turbinado sugar to sprinkle on the crust instead, if desired.

MAKES ONE 7-INCH GALETTE

Light buckwheat flour, for dusting
½ recipe Chocolate-Buckwheat Pastry Dough (page 173)
1 recipe Chocolate, Brown Sugar, and Rum Frangipane (page 38)
1 pound (454 g) red plums, halved, pitted, and thinly sliced
1 large egg, lightly beaten
2 tablespoons raw sesame seeds

1 Preheat the oven to 400 degrees F. Position a rack in the bottom third of the oven. Line a baking sheet with parchment paper.

2 Dust a work surface and rolling pin with buckwheat flour. Roll the pastry dough to approximately a ⅛-inch thickness and 11-inch diameter. Carefully transfer the dough to the prepared pan.

3 Spread the frangipane all over the dough, leaving a 2-inch border. Top the frangipane with the sliced plums, then fold the edges of the dough over the fruit. If the dough feels soft, chill the galette for 15 minutes.

4 Brush the edges of the galette with the beaten egg and sprinkle with the sesame seeds. Bake for 35 minutes, until the filling is bubbling and the crust is flaky and baked throughout. Let the galette cool for 10 minutes, then serve warm. It is best eaten the same day but will keep in the refrigerator for 1 day.

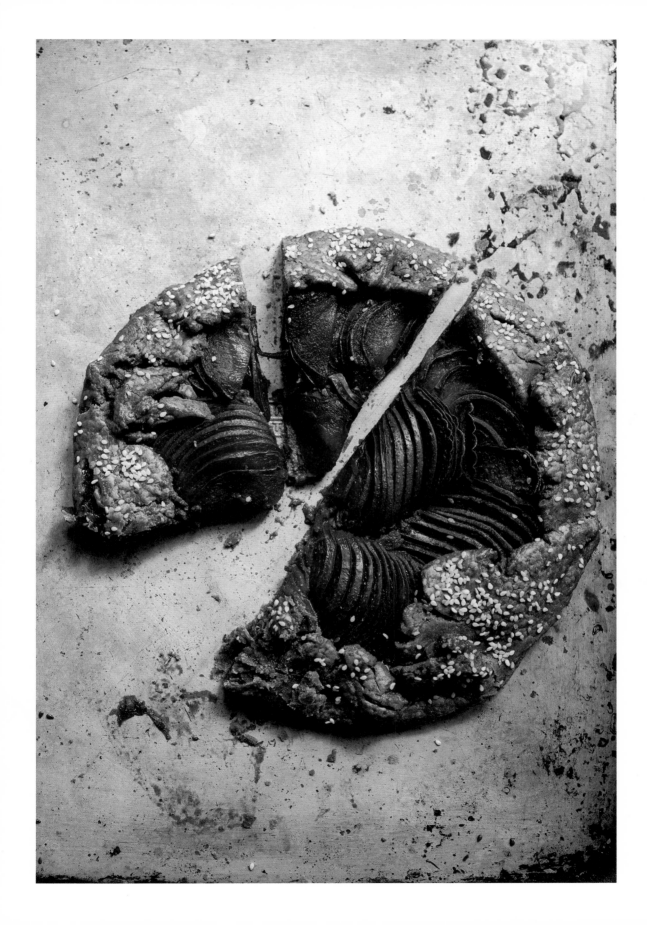

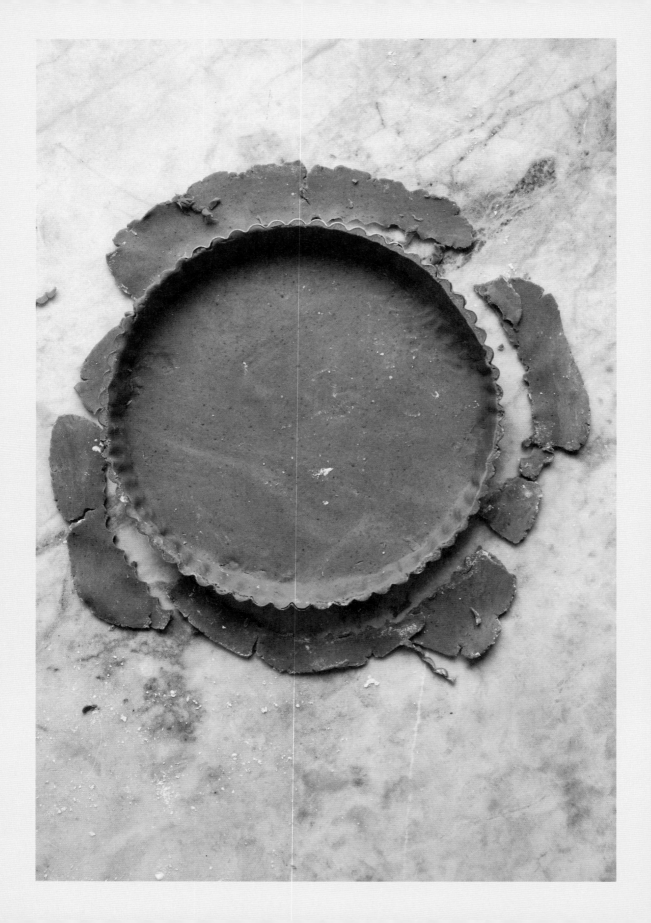

Chocolate-Buckwheat Pastry Dough

1 cup (140 g) superfine brown rice flour

1 cup (140 g) light buckwheat flour

½ cup (60 g) tapioca starch

3 tablespoons packed light brown sugar or coconut sugar

2 tablespoons unsweetened cocoa powder

2 teaspoons (7 g) psyllium husk powder

2 teaspoons (5 g) flaxseed meal

½ teaspoon kosher salt

1 cup (225 g) cold unsalted butter, dairy-free butter, or Cultured Cashew-Coconut Butter (page 33), cut into ½-inch dice

6 to 8 tablespoons ice-cold water

This dough is tender, holds its shape really well, and it has a deep, earthy flavor with the touch of buckwheat. I love it in the Plum-Chocolate Frangipane Galette (page 170) and also in the Chocolate-Cashew Mousse Tart (page 182). You can make this dough by hand, if desired: simply rub the butter and dry ingredients together between your fingers, then fold in the water.

MAKES TWO 9-INCH SINGLE-CRUST PIES OR ONE 9-INCH DOUBLE-CRUST PIE

1   Combine both flours, tapioca starch, brown sugar, cocoa powder, psyllium powder, flaxseed, and salt in a food processor. Pulse a few times to aerate. Add the diced butter and pulse ten times, or until the butter is the size of peas.

2   Start by adding 6 tablespoons of the ice water to the food processor and pulse a few times, until the dough starts coming together. The dough won't form a ball, so press it between your hands to feel the texture. It should be moist and hold together when pressed. Add more ice water, 1 teaspoon at a time, if the dough feels dry.

3   Turn the dough out onto a work surface, press all the pieces together with your hands, and give it a couple of kneads. The warmth of your hands can melt the butter, so work quickly.

4   Cut the dough into two equal pieces, shape each one into a disk, and wrap in parchment paper. Flatten them lightly and chill in the refrigerator for at least 30 minutes. The dough will keep in the refrigerator for 2 days or can be frozen for up to 3 months. If frozen, thaw in the refrigerator overnight.

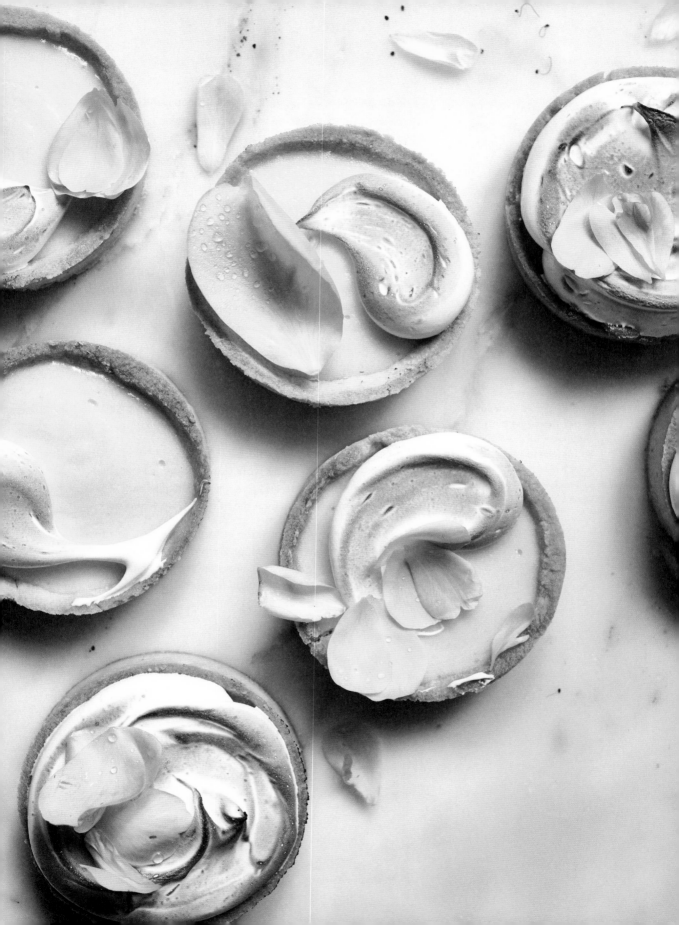

Lemon Meringue Tartlets

There is nothing more classic than a lemon meringue tart. The combination of sour lemon curd and sweet meringue cannot be messed with. You can make this in several small tartlet pans or in a large 9-inch tart pan. The ones I use are 3-inch plain rings (similar to those used to make English muffins), but you can also use small fluted tartlet pans with removable bottoms.

MAKES SEVEN 3-INCH TARTLETS OR ONE 9-INCH TART

Superfine brown rice flour,
  for dusting
½ recipe Pie Dough (page 162)
1 recipe Lemon Curd (page 37)
1 recipe Swiss Meringue
  (page 40)

1 Preheat the oven to 375 degrees F.

2 Lightly dust a work surface with brown rice flour. Roll the pie dough to approximately a ⅛-inch thickness. For tartlets, cut the pastry into disks that are about 4½ inches in diameter, then press the dough into tartlet pans. For a single tart, roll to 11-inch diameter and carefully transfer the dough with both hands to a tart pan, pressing it into the bottom and sides. Trim any excess dough that hangs over the edge.

3 Put the pans in the freezer for 15 minutes, then set them on a baking sheet. Bake for 25 minutes, until the crusts are lightly golden brown. Let them cool completely before unmolding.

4 Pour the lemon curd directly into the cooled crusts. Chill for at least 2 hours to set the curd.

5 Spoon the meringue over the curd, creating a large mound. Use a spatula to makes swirls in the meringue. Alternatively, you can pipe the meringue to create different patterns.

6 Caramelize the meringue using a blow torch. The tarts are best eaten the same day since the meringue and curd will begin to ooze and soften within 24 hours.

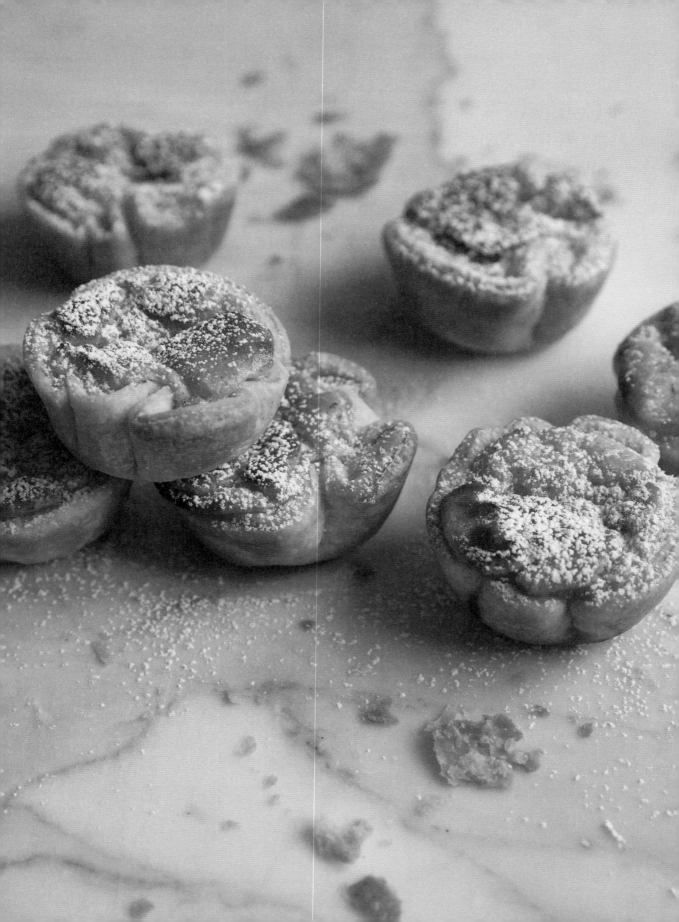

Rice Milk and Lemon Tartlets

Pasteles de Arroz y Limón

½ cup (100 g) white jasmine or other rice of choice

1½ cups cold water

1 to 2 large lemons

½ cup (100 g) sugar

1 vanilla bean, split lengthwise and seeds scraped

2 tablespoons sweet white rice flour or cornstarch

1 large whole egg plus 3 egg yolks

1 recipe Buttery Rough Puff Pastry Dough (page 180)

My family's pastry shop is known for their *pastel de arroz*, which translates in English to "rice tart." The funny thing, however, is that there is no rice in those tarts. They are simple cinnamon-flavored custard tarts encased in puff pastry and baked to golden perfection with some burnt spots on the surface. On rare occasions, my grandfather would make *pasteles de limón*, a lemon version of the traditional tarts, which my mother adored. I tried to re-create something similar, going back to the idea of using rice. With every batch I tested, I consulted with my mother through video-conferencing. This recipe connected me deeply with her and the memory of my grandfather.

Start the night before as you need to soak the rice before blending it. You can use 1¼ cups unsweetened rice, nut, oat, or even whole milk in place of the blended rice and water. You will need two muffin pans. If you only have one, keep the cut dough disks on a baking sheet in the fridge until ready to bake.

MAKES 18 TO 20 INDIVIDUAL TARTLETS

1   Soak the rice in 1 cup (225 g) of water at room temperature overnight or up to 24 hours. Drain the rice and blend with 1½ cups cold water in a high-speed blender, until you have a creamy milk. Strain this through a clean linen towel. You can also use a nut-milk bag, but I find the milk is a bit gritty this way. You should have approximately 1¼ cups of rice milk.

2   Finely zest 1 lemon into a medium bowl. Cut the lemon in half and juice it into a small bowl. You need ¼ cup of lemon juice, so you may need to juice the second lemon if you don't have enough. Set aside the juice.

3   Add the sugar and vanilla seeds to the bowl with the lemon zest and rub the mixture between your fingers until it feels sandy and smells fragrant. Whisk in the rice flour and lemon juice, followed by the egg, egg yolks, and rice milk. $\longrightarrow$

4 Pour the creamy mixture into a medium saucepan and cook over medium-high heat, whisking constantly, until it thickens, about 2 minutes. It should be the consistency of loose pastry cream. Be careful not to overheat it or the eggs could curdle. Transfer the cream to a clean bowl and whisk until most of the steam evaporates. Place some parchment paper directly on the surface of the cream and chill for at least 30 minutes.

5 Put a baking sheet inside the oven and preheat to 450 degrees F.

6 Cut the puff pastry in half. Work with each half separately so the dough doesn't get too soft. Roll the pastry to ⅛ inch thick and cut 4-inch disks using a cookie cutter. You can reroll the dough scraps. You should have enough for 18 to 20 disks.

7 I like to use a muffin pan for these, but you can use individual tartlet molds that are about 2 inches in diameter. Gently fill each muffin cavity with a disk of dough. It's OK if the edges fold. The tarts are supposed to be rustic, but be careful not to tear or puncture the dough or the filling will ooze out and stick to the pan when baking. Put the muffin pan in the freezer for 10 minutes.

8 Fill each tartlet two-thirds full, being careful not to overfill as it will spill in the oven. Put the muffin pan on the preheated baking sheet in the oven and bake for 15 minutes, then reduce the oven temperature to 375 degrees F and continue baking for another 10 to 15 minutes. The cream filling will puff up, then deflate, and turn golden brown in spots. Let the tartlets cool in the pan for at least 20 minutes. Once cooled, gently lift them out with the help of a knife tip. They can be eaten warm, at room temperature, or chilled. They are best eaten the same day.

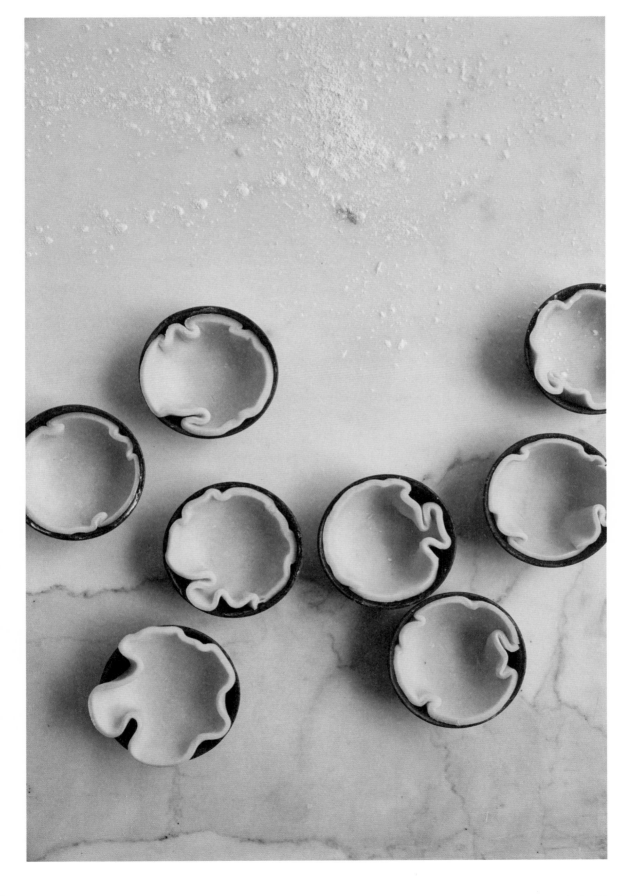

Buttery Rough Puff Pastry Dough

¾ cup (125 g) potato starch
½ cup (60 g) tapioca starch, plus more for dusting
½ cup (70 g) sorghum flour
⅓ cup (45 g) sweet white rice flour
1½ teaspoons xanthan gum
1 teaspoon kosher salt
1 cup (225 g) cold unsalted butter, dairy-free butter, or Cultured Cashew-Coconut Butter (page 33), cut into ½-inch dice
6 to 7 tablespoons ice-cold water

Rough puff pastry is a hybrid between pie dough and puff pastry. There is no butter packet like in a traditional puff. This recipe uses a variation of the *fraisage* method used in classic French pastry, where large pieces of butter are dragged across the work surface dusted with flour, creating a very flaky dough. This dough is then folded and laminated. You could also use this *fraisage* method to make the Pie Dough (page 162) or Chocolate-Buckwheat Pastry Dough (page 173) to work the butter into the flour without a food processor.

You can reroll any scraps of dough. Don't knead the dough back together, but instead simply layer the pieces of dough on top of each other and roll again to the desired thickness.

MAKES TWO 9-INCH SINGLE-CRUST PIES OR ONE 9-INCH DOUBLE-CRUST PIE

1 Whisk together both starches, both flours, xanthan gum, and salt in a large bowl. Toss in the diced butter to coat it in flour. Press the butter pieces and flour between your fingers, creating large, flat shards of butter.

2 Push the mixture into a mound, then make a well in the center and add 6 tablespoons of the ice water. Toss everything together until the dough starts to feel hydrated. It should be moist but not too wet—add the final tablespoon of water, if needed. Once the dough feels hydrated and lumpy, transfer it to a work surface and knead a few times to create a dough

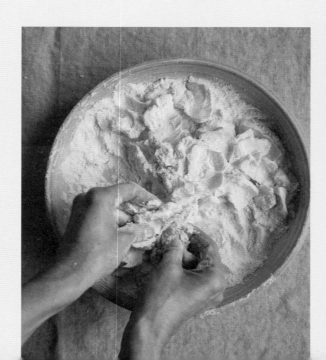
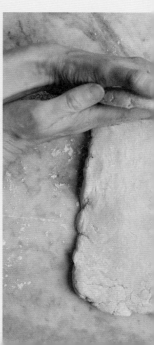

that sticks together. Use a bench scraper to help you bring it together, being careful not to work the butter into the flour too much. Wrap the dough in parchment or plastic wrap and refrigerate for 30 minutes.

3   Dust the work surface and a rolling pin with tapioca starch. Put the chilled dough on top and roll out a rectangle that is ½ inch thick. The exact size doesn't matter, but you want it to be about three times as long as it is wide. Avoid being too aggressive with rolling, which causes the butter to ooze out of the dough. Keep your surface and rolling pin dusted with starch, and turn the dough around as you are rolling it.

4   Create the first letter fold by folding a third of the dough over the middle third, then fold the other third over the top. The dough will likely crack around the fold edges, which is OK. Rotate the dough 90 degrees and roll it out ½ inch thick again. Give it another letter fold. Brush off any excess starch from the top of the dough, wrap again, and refrigerate for another 30 minutes.

5   Repeat this process two more times for a total of 6 letter folds. After the final fold, wrap the dough and refrigerate for at least 1 to 2 hours before using. This allows it to hydrate and lets the butter set. The dough will keep in the refrigerator for 2 days, or it can be frozen for up to 3 months. If frozen, thaw in the refrigerator overnight.

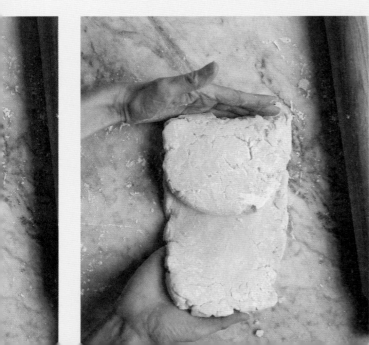
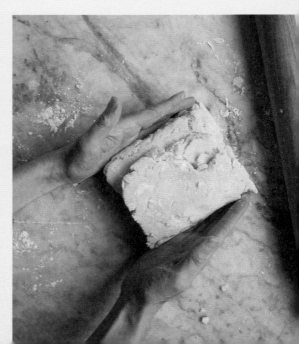

Chocolate-Cashew Mousse Tart

2 cups (250 g) raw cashews
1 (13½-ounce or 400-gram) can
   full-fat coconut milk
Light buckwheat flour, for
   dusting
½ recipe Chocolate-Buckwheat
   Pastry Dough (page 173)
¼ cup (80 g) maple syrup
1 tablespoon vanilla extract
1 tablespoon brewed espresso
   or very strong coffee
½ cup (50 g) unsweetened
   cocoa powder
½ teaspoon kosher salt
2 ounces (55 g) 70 percent
   chocolate, for garnish

Note: You can speed up the
cashew process in step 1 by
soaking them in boiling water for
2 hours (cover the bowl with a
plate to retain heat).

This tart is so silky, you'd never know there isn't heavy cream or eggs. It is important to blend the cashews in a high-speed blender. I am afraid a food processor won't do the job as it is likely to leave the cashews too coarse rather than as smooth as is needed. This tart comes together fairly quickly, but you will need time to soak the cashews and let the mousse set.

MAKES ONE 9-INCH TART OR A RECTANGULAR TART

1 Put the cashews in a medium bowl and cover them with 4 cups of water. Soak them in the refrigerator overnight. Refrigerate the can of coconut milk for at least 2 hours and see page 39 for how to collect the cream.

2 Preheat the oven to 400 degrees F. Dust a work surface with buckwheat flour. Roll the pastry dough to ⅛ inch thick and carefully transfer it to a tart pan with both hands. Press the dough into the bottom and sides of the pan, and trim any excess. Put the tart pan in the freezer for 15 minutes.

3 Set the tart pan on a baking sheet and bake for 20 minutes. Let the crust completely cool before adding the filling.

4 Drain the cashews and add them to a high-speed blender along with the maple syrup, vanilla, and coffee. Begin blending on low, then continue increasing the speed. Stop the blender to scrape the edges, then continue blending until you have a mixture that is as creamy as possible. It might take several tries to get all the cashews pureed, depending on the size of your blender container and its motor, but smoothness is key for this filling.

5 Open the can of coconut milk and scoop 1 cup (225 g) of the solidified cream on top. Reserve the coconut water in the can in case you need to loosen the cream a bit. Add the coconut cream, cocoa powder, and salt to the blender. Continue blending, again stopping the machine as needed to scrape and redistribute the ingredients. Add some of the reserved coconut water if the mousse seems too dry. Blend until completely smooth and creamy.

6 Spread the mousse evenly over the cooled dough and refrigerate for at least 2 hours, until set. Using a vegetable peeler, shave chocolate curls to garnish the tart before serving. The tart will keep loosely wrapped in the refrigerator for up to 3 days.

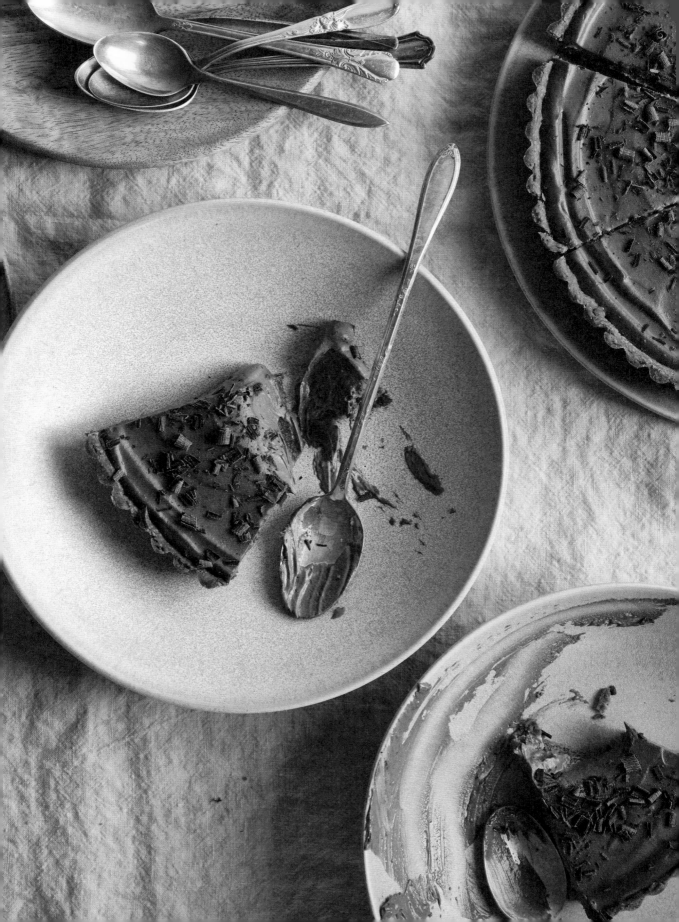

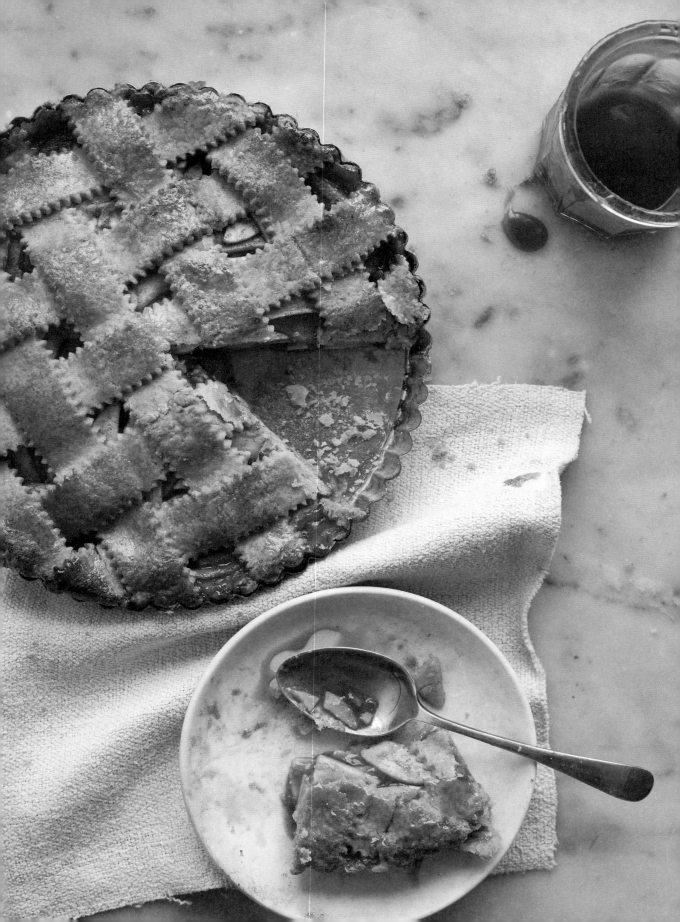

Apple and Pear Pie with Caramel

1½ pounds (680 g) Granny Smith apples, peeled, cored, and thinly sliced
1 pound (454 g) ripe Bosc pears, peeled, cored, and thinly sliced
½ cup (170 g) honey
3 tablespoons applesauce
2 tablespoons tapioca starch, plus more for dusting
1 tablespoon freshly squeezed lemon juice
1 vanilla bean, split lengthwise and seeds scraped
1 teaspoon ground cinnamon
¼ teaspoon kosher salt
1 recipe Pie Dough (page 162)
1 large egg
1 tablespoon sugar
1 recipe Coconut-Miso Caramel (page 46), for drizzling

It is hard to reinvent a classic apple pie, but this one, with the addition of pears, honey, and applesauce, results in a filling that becomes creamy while still retaining the bite of the apples. I top it with Coconut-Miso Caramel for added richness, but you could leave it off and simply serve the pie with a dusting of powdered sugar.

MAKES ONE 9-INCH DEEP-DISH PIE

1   In a large bowl, toss together the apples, pears, honey, apple-sauce, tapioca starch, lemon juice, vanilla seeds, cinnamon, and salt. Set aside.

2   Dust a work surface with tapioca starch. Cut the pie dough in two pieces, one slightly larger than the other. Roll the larger piece of dough to ⅛ inch thick. Gently lift it with both hands over a 9-inch deep-dish pie plate and press it into the bottom and sides, leaving some dough to hang over the edge.

3   Fill the shell with the apple and pear mixture, pressing down gently with your hands to compress the filling a bit.

4   Roll the remaining dough piece into a circle with a ⅛-inch thickness and 11-inch diameter. Using a pizza cutter or a sharp knife, cut 10 strips that are 1 inch thick. Lay 5 strips over the filling, leaving ½ inch between. Turn the pie plate 90 degrees, and lay the remaining 5 strips over the top in the same manner, creating a rustic lattice effect. Trim the excess dough with scissors and crimp the edges between your fingers, sealing the dough. Refrigerate the pie for 20 minutes.

5   While the pie is chilling, preheat the oven to 425 degrees F. In a small bowl, whisk together the egg with 1 tablespoon of water.

6   Put the pie plate on a baking sheet. Brush the egg all over the top of the dough, then sprinkle with sugar. Bake for 15 minutes, then reduce the oven temperature to 350 degrees F and bake for 45 to 50 more minutes, until the crust is golden brown and the filling is bubbling. Let the pie cool for 30 minutes before cutting. Drizzle the pie with the caramel when serving. The pie will keep tightly wrapped in the refrigerator for 2 days.

Dutch Baby with Caramelized Apples and Lemon

You might be wondering what a Dutch baby is doing in a tart and pie chapter. I initially wanted to include some sort of flan tart here, but I also wanted the recipe to be very simple—something that could be whisked in one bowl, then baked. And so I present this Dutch baby, which is somewhere between a pancake, a custard tart, and a flan. You can substitute pears or apricots for the apples.

MAKES 4 TO 6 SERVINGS

1 tablespoon sugar

Zest and juice of 1 large lemon

3 large eggs, at room temperature

½ cup (115 g) whole milk or oat milk

⅓ cup (45 g) light buckwheat flour or superfine brown rice flour

3 tablespoons potato starch

¼ teaspoon kosher salt

2 tablespoons unsalted butter or dairy-free butter, cut into ½-inch pieces

⅓ cup (105 g) maple syrup

2 medium Pink Lady apples, cored and cut into ½-inch slices

Powdered sugar, for dusting

1 Put a 10-inch cake pan or cast-iron pan into the cold oven, then preheat to 425 degrees F.

2 In a medium bowl, rub together the sugar and lemon zest until fragrant and sandy. Whisk in the eggs, milk, buckwheat flour, potato starch, and salt. Whisk vigorously until you have a very thin, crepe-like, lump-free batter.

3 Remove the pan from the oven and add the butter pieces, swirling them around until melted. Pour in the batter and bake for 20 to 22 minutes, until puffed up and golden brown.

4 Meanwhile, cook the apples. Heat a medium sauté pan over high heat. Pour in the maple syrup and cook for 2 minutes, until it is bubbly and begins to reduce. Add the apple slices and cook for 4 to 5 minutes, flipping them halfway through, until softened and caramelized. Add the lemon juice (about 2 tablespoons), cook for 20 seconds, and remove the pan from the heat.

5 As soon as the Dutch baby comes out of the oven, top with the caramelized apples and a generous dusting of powdered sugar. Serve immediately.

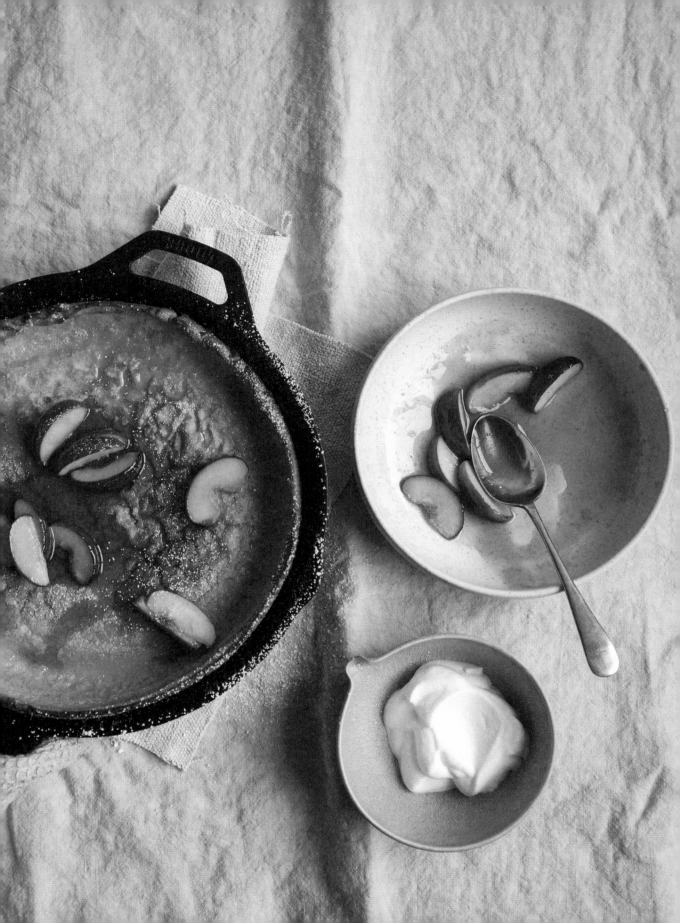

Peach and Blueberry Biscuit Cobbler

This cobbler is a summer favorite. Creamy, sweet fruit baked with flaky, slightly savory biscuits on top. It's a perfect dessert to bring to an outdoor gathering. You can make the filling and biscuits ahead of time and bake it right before serving so the filling is still bubbling when you bring it to the table. Serve the cobbler with a dollop of whipped cream or a scoop of vanilla ice cream.

MAKES 8 TO 10 SERVINGS

For the biscuits
¾ cup plus 2 tablespoons (120 g) sorghum flour

½ cup (60 g) tapioca starch, plus more for dusting

⅓ cup (60 g) potato starch

2¼ teaspoons baking powder

¼ teaspoon baking soda

¼ teaspoon kosher salt

½ cup (115 g) cold unsalted butter or dairy-free butter, cut into ½-inch pieces

½ cup plus 2 tablespoons (150 g) cold whole milk or oat milk

2 tablespoons freshly squeezed lemon juice

For the filling
1 pound (454 g) peaches, pitted and sliced

3 cups (400 g) blueberries

Zest and juice of ½ large lemon

⅓ cup (70 g) sugar, plus more for sprinkling

1 tablespoon vanilla extract

1 teaspoon ground cinnamon

¼ teaspoon kosher salt

¼ cup (30 g) cornstarch

2 tablespoons cold water

1 large egg yolk

1   To make the biscuits, stir together the sorghum flour, tapioca starch, potato starch, baking powder, baking soda, and salt in a medium bowl. Toss the butter in the flour and use your fingers to work the butter into the flour until the pieces are about the size of peas.

2   In a small bowl, stir together the milk and lemon juice. Gradually pour it into the flour mixture while stirring with a fork. It will be a lumpy mass. Turn the dough out onto a work surface lightly dusted with tapioca starch. Work it with your hands until it comes together, being sure not to knead it too much. Lightly dust the top with tapioca starch and roll it out ½ inch thick.

3   Cut the dough with a 1½-inch round cookie cutter and transfer the pieces to a tray or large platter. Dip the cookie cutter in tapioca starch often so it will easily release the dough. Reroll the dough scraps. You should have about 30 dough circles. Refrigerate them while you work on the filling. You can make these a day ahead and keep in the refrigerator.

4   Preheat the oven to 400 degrees F.

5   To make the filling, stir together the peaches, blueberries, lemon zest and juice, sugar, vanilla, cinnamon, and salt in a large saucepan. Cook over high heat until the sugar starts melting and the liquid starts to boil, 5 to 7 minutes.

6   In a small bowl, whisk the cornstarch and water. Once the fruit filling is boiling, add half of the slurry to the saucepan, stir, and continue cooking until thickened, about 2 minutes. Add a bit more of the slurry if the filling doesn't seem thick enough. Pour the filling into a 1½-quart gratin dish or a 9-inch deep-dish pie pan.

7   Top the filling with the chilled biscuits, making sure they touch but allowing small spaces between rows. In a small bowl, whisk together the egg yolk and 1 tablespoon of water. Brush the biscuits with the egg wash and sprinkle the tops with sugar.

8   Put the gratin dish on a baking sheet in the oven. Bake for 25 minutes, until the biscuits are golden brown and the filling is bubbling. Serve the cobbler warm or at room temperature. It is best eaten the same day.

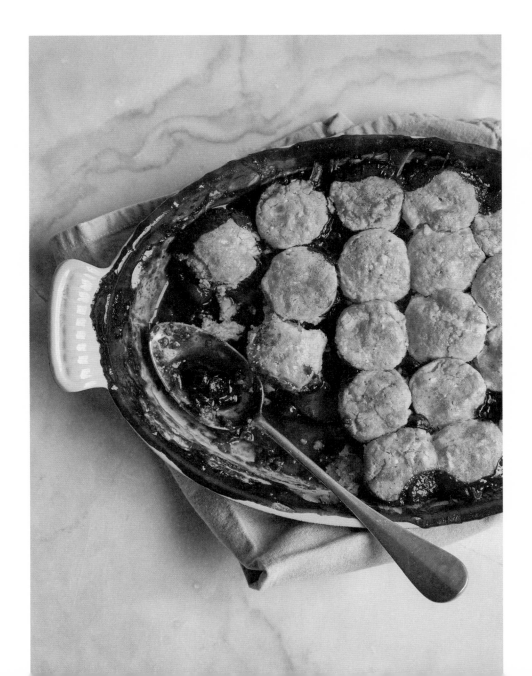

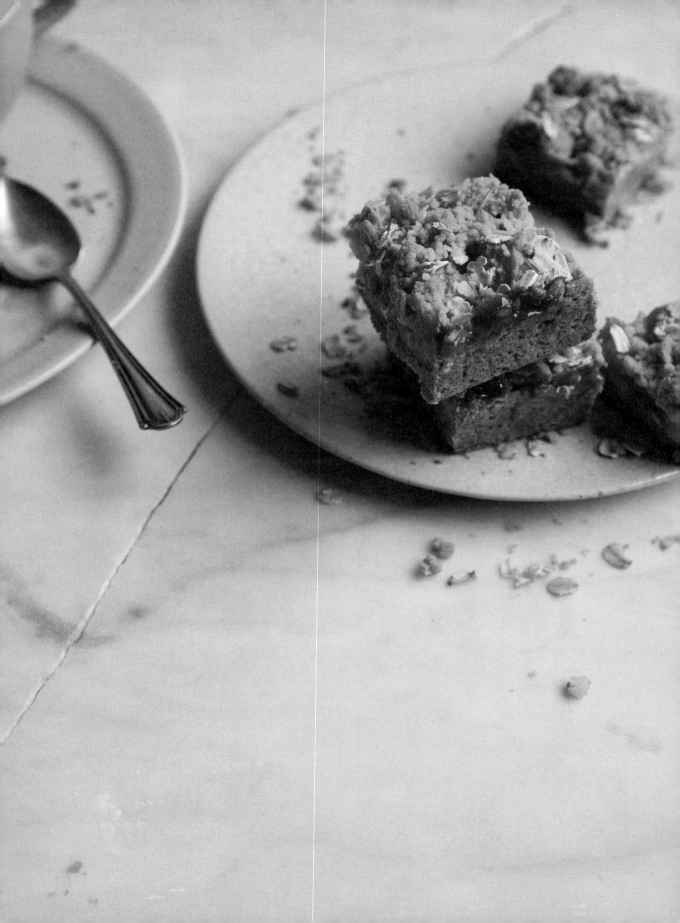

Quince-Chamomile Oat Bars

Quince is one of my favorite fruits. They are somewhat elusive as their season is very short and they are rarely available en masse. One must know a friend or neighbor with a quince tree or be lucky to find a farmer at the market who grows them. They resemble a wobbly pear, with hard skin, and are inedible raw. When ripe, their skin turns yellow and they smell of a mixture of apples, chamomile, and pineapple. Their scent is intoxicating. When cooked, they become one of the most luxurious fruits. For this tart, the quince are poached in chamomile, orange juice, and vanilla bean until fork-tender. Poached quince are delicious served on their own or with a sprinkle of Streusel (page 49) and some vanilla ice cream.

The crust is one of the most versatile in my repertoire. There is no rolling and you can essentially mix the dough in one large bowl and be done. I suggest making this recipe in an 8- or 9-inch square pan to cut perfect squares, but you can also use a 9-inch tart pan with removable bottom and simply cut into wedges.

MAKES 16 BARS

For the filling
Juice of 2 medium lemons
4 medium quince (about 2 pounds or 900 g)
1 quart (900 g) cold water
¾ cup (150 g) sugar
½ cup (115 g) freshly squeezed orange juice
2 chamomile tea bags
1 vanilla bean, split lengthwise and seeds scraped
1 tablespoon cornstarch or tapioca starch

For the dough
1 cup (140 g) light buckwheat flour or superfine brown rice flour
1 cup (110 g) gluten-free oat flour
½ cup (100 g) light brown sugar
¾ teaspoon kosher salt
½ cup (115 g) unsalted butter, dairy-free butter, or virgin coconut oil, cut into ½-inch pieces
2 to 3 tablespoons whole milk or oat milk
⅓ cup (45 g) gluten-free rolled oats

1   To make the filling, fill a medium bowl with cold water and add the lemon juice. Peel, quarter, and core the quince. Carve out any brown spots on the flesh. Drop the quince pieces into the lemon water as you cut to prevent oxidization.

2   Combine the water, sugar, orange juice, chamomile bags, and vanilla bean and seeds in a medium saucepan. Drain the quince pieces and transfer them to the pan. Bring the liquid to a simmer over medium-high heat, cover, then reduce the heat to low. Simmer the quince for 30 minutes, or until fork-tender. Let the quince cool completely in the poaching liquid. It will take on a rose color. You can cook the quince up to 3 days in advance and store in the poaching liquid in an airtight container in the refrigerator.

3   Discard the vanilla bean and tea bags from the poaching liquid. Place a strainer over a medium bowl and drain the quince. Measure ¾ cup (170 g) of the cooled poaching liquid. (You can save any extra to infuse cocktails.) $\longrightarrow$

4 In the saucepan where you cooked the quince, whisk together the poaching liquid and cornstarch. Bring the liquid to a rolling boil over medium-high heat and cook, whisking constantly, until thickened, 1 to 2 minutes. Remove the pan from the heat and fold in the quince. Set aside.

5 Preheat the oven to 375 degrees F. Line the inside of an 8-inch square pan with parchment paper, letting some hang over the sides. If you are using a tart pan with removable bottom, there is no need to line with parchment.

6 To make the dough, combine both flours, brown sugar, and salt in a medium bowl. Toss the butter with the flour mixture. Work the butter into the flour with your fingers until it is crumbly.

7 Pour 2 tablespoons of the milk over the mixture and stir with a spatula. Knead the dough with your hands a few times until it comes together. When pressed, it should feel like crumbly cookie dough. Add a bit more milk if it isn't sticking together.

8 Press three-quarters of the dough all over the bottom of the prepared pan and ¾ inch up the sides. Put the pan in the freezer for 5 minutes. Meanwhile, add the rolled oats to the remaining quarter of dough and toss together until you have crumbly pieces with oats mixed throughout.

9 Put the pan in the oven and bake for 15 minutes. Remove the pan and fill with the quince. Gently press down on the quince and top with the oat crumble. Bake for 30 to 35 minutes, until the top is golden brown and the filling is bubbling. Let the crumble cool in the pan completely, then use the parchment to lift it out. Cut the crumble into 16 equal pieces. Store them, tightly wrapped, in the refrigerator for up to 2 days.

VARIATIONS

To replace the quince filling, skip steps 1 through 4 and instead toss together the ingredients for each of the following variations in a medium bowl. Proceed with filling the crust in the final step as directed. Baking times may vary depending on the ripeness of the fruit, so bake until the crust is golden brown and the filling is bubbling.

APRICOT-BLUEBERRY-HONEY: 4 medium apricots (200 g), halved, pitted, and sliced + ½ cup (70 g) blueberries + 2 tablespoons honey + 1 tablespoon tapioca starch

SPICED APPLE-MAPLE: 3 juicy medium apples (300 g), peeled, cored, and thinly sliced + ¼ cup (80 g) maple syrup + 2 tablespoons freshly squeezed orange juice + 1 tablespoon finely grated fresh ginger + 1 tablespoon tapioca starch + 1 teaspoon ground cinnamon

SUMMER BERRY: 4 cups (600 g) mixed berries, such as sliced strawberries, blueberries, raspberries, blackberries, or currants + ¼ cup (50 g) sugar + 2 tablespoons tapioca starch + zest and juice of 1 lemon

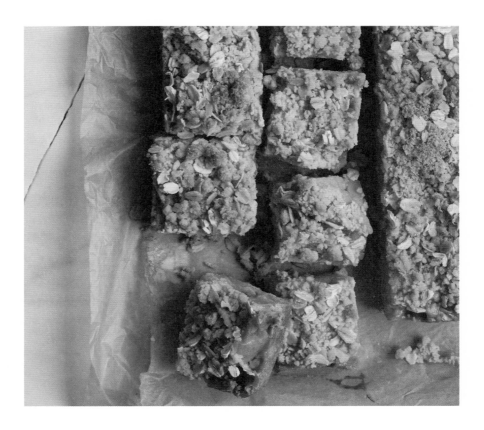

Jam-Filled Scones

½ cup (115 g) unsalted butter, dairy-free butter, or Cultured Cashew-Coconut Butter (page 33), frozen for at least 30 minutes

1 cup (140 g) superfine brown rice flour, plus more for dusting

½ cup (60 g) gluten-free oat flour

½ cup (60 g) tapioca starch

1 tablespoon sugar, plus more for sprinkling

2¼ teaspoons baking powder

¼ teaspoon baking soda

¼ teaspoon kosher salt

¼ teaspoon xanthan gum (optional)

½ cup plus 2 tablespoons (140 g) whole milk or oat milk

2 tablespoons freshly squeezed lemon juice

2 tablespoons Strawberry-Hibiscus Jam (page 52) or other jam of choice

These scones are a cross between a cakey scone and a layered biscuit. There is some jam spread between, which you can omit but it makes for a beautiful swirl effect. Traditional scone dough is shaped into a circle and cut into wedges, but the wedges are left in place and separated after baking. However, I prefer to cut the dough and separate the individual wedges so they have a chance to caramelize and develop a nice crust all around. I list xanthan gum as optional because these scones can be made without it, but adding it will allow you to layer the dough, which will hold a bit better while baking than without it.

MAKES 8 SCONES

1 Preheat the oven to 450 degrees F. Put the butter in the freezer.

2 Mix both flours, tapioca starch, sugar, baking powder, baking soda, salt, and xanthan gum in a large bowl. Grate the frozen butter into the flour mixture using a box grater. Toss the butter with the flour.

3 In a small bowl, whisk the milk and lemon juice and pour into the flour mixture. Stir with a fork until a loose, lumpy dough forms.

4 Dust a work surface with brown rice flour and turn the dough out onto it. Knead a few times until the dough comes together. Roll it into a ¼-inch-thick rectangle. Spread the jam all over, leaving a 1-inch border. Fold one-third of the dough over the center third, then fold the other third over the top. The jam will ooze out and become a bit of a mess—this is OK.

5 Transfer the dough to a piece of parchment and slide it onto a baking sheet. Pat the dough down to 1 inch thick, and shape into a circle about 7 inches wide. It doesn't have to be perfect.

6 Using a sharp chef's knife, cut the dough into 8 wedges. Space the scones evenly on the pan. Sprinkle the tops with a bit of sugar. Bake for 18 minutes, until golden brown. Let the scones cool on the pan for 15 minutes. They are best eaten the same day.

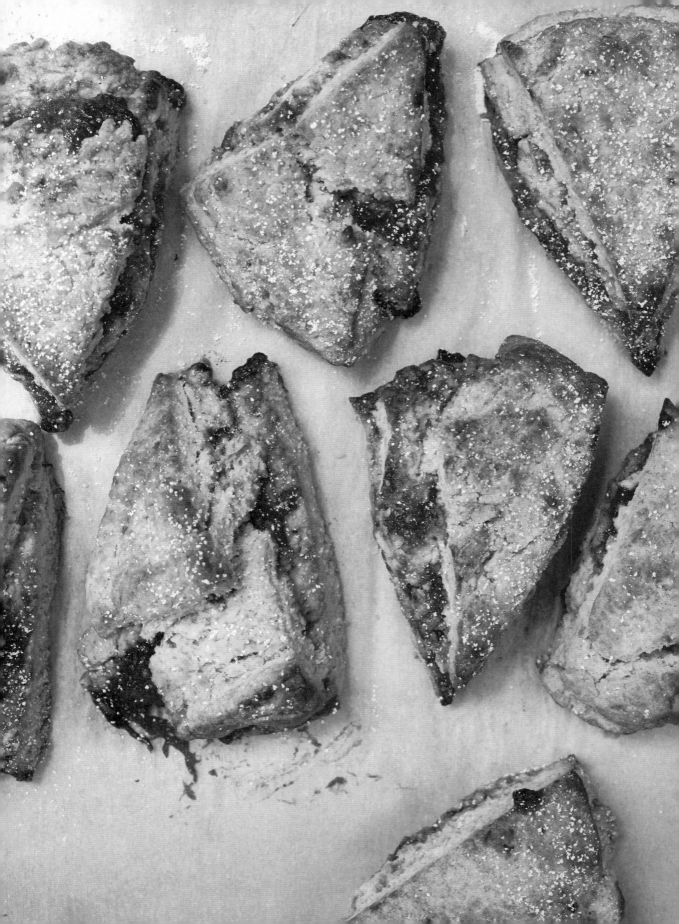

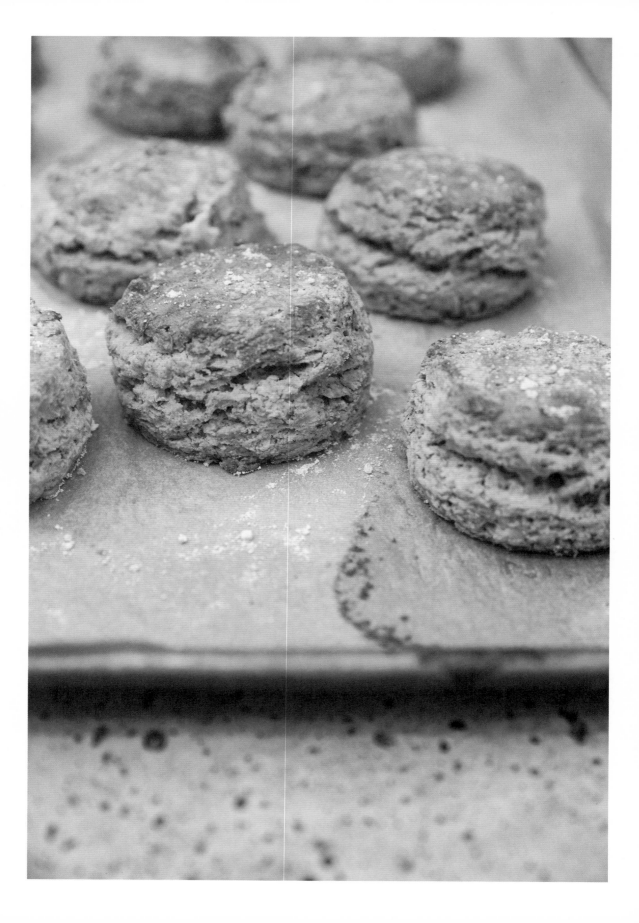

Cheddar and Herb Scones

This recipe is very similar to an Irish soda bread. The trick is to not overmix the dough so the gases created by the baking soda remain intact and the bread has an open crumb. You can add chopped kalamata olives in place of the cheese if you prefer. I have made these with dairy-free cheese alternatives, but nothing melts quite the same as real cheddar.

MAKES 12 SCONES

½ cup (115 g) unsalted butter, dairy-free butter, or Cultured Cashew-Coconut Butter (page 33), frozen for at least 30 minutes

1 cup (140 g) superfine brown rice flour

1 cup (110 g) gluten-free oat flour, plus more for dusting

½ cup (70 g) sorghum flour

½ cup (80 g) potato starch

½ cup (60 g) tapioca starch

3 tablespoons finely chopped fresh herbs (chives, parsley, oregano, rosemary)

2 tablespoons (20 g) psyllium husk powder

2½ teaspoons baking powder

1¼ teaspoons kosher salt

½ teaspoon baking soda

2 ounces (60 g) cheddar cheese, coarsely grated

1¼ cups (300 g) whole milk or oat milk, plus more for brushing

2 large eggs

2 tablespoons apple cider vinegar

1 Preheat the oven to 450 degrees F. Line a baking sheet with parchment paper. Put the butter in the freezer.

2 In a large bowl, whisk together the three flours, both starches, herbs, psyllium powder, baking powder, salt, and baking soda. Stir in the grated cheese. Grate the frozen butter into the flour mixture using a box grater. Toss the butter with the flour.

3 In a small bowl, whisk together the milk, eggs, and vinegar and pour into the flour mixture. Stir with a fork until a loose, lumpy dough forms.

4 Dust a work surface with oat flour and turn the dough out onto it. Knead a few times until the dough comes together. Press the dough into a disk about 9 inches wide and ¾ inch thick.

5 Using a 2¾-inch cookie cutter, cut out the scones and transfer them to the prepared pan. You can gently knead together any dough scraps and cut again, but don't work the dough too much. You should have 12 scones.

6 Brush the tops of the scones with milk and dust with a bit of oat flour. Bake for 20 to 22 minutes, until golden brown. Serve warm. They are best eaten the same day.

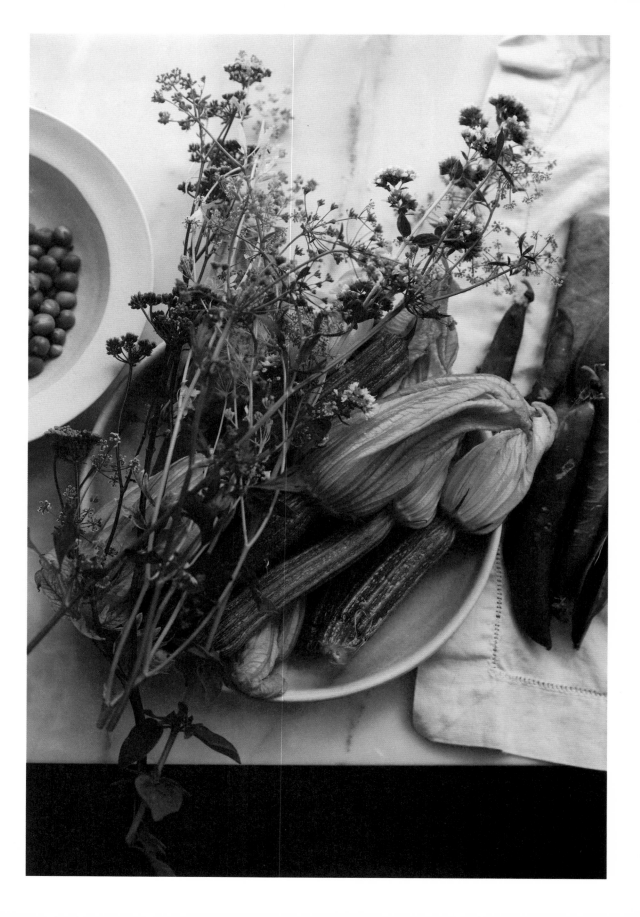

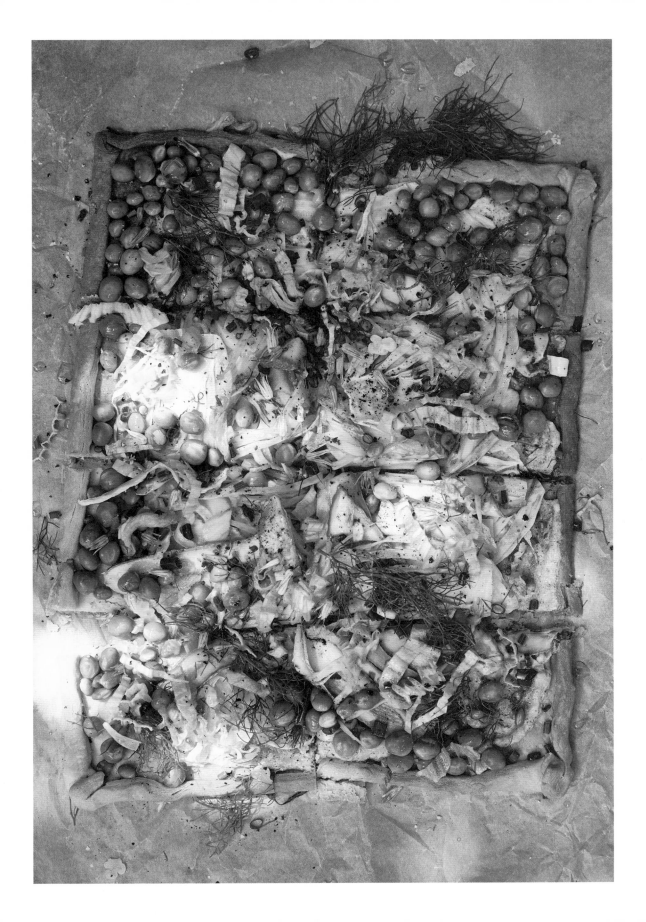

Zucchini, Fennel, and Pea Tart with Eggless Aioli

This recipe falls somewhere between a tartine and a galette. One thin, flaky layer of buttery puff pastry is topped with thinly shaved spring vegetables and a creamy almond aioli. I serve it for brunch or a light lunch and make double the aioli to serve on the side. I recommend using a mandoline to cut the vegetables so they are paper thin. If you don't have one and your vegetables are a bit thicker, blanch them in boiling water for a minute before topping the tart with them. Prepare the puff pastry first as it needs to chill for at least 1 hour before rolling.

MAKES 4 TO 6 SERVINGS

For the aioli
1 cup (100 g) raw sliced almonds
6 to 7 tablespoons water, at room temperature
6 tablespoons extra-virgin olive oil
2 tablespoons Dijon mustard
1 large clove garlic
¾ teaspoon kosher salt

For the tart
Tapioca starch, for dusting
½ recipe Buttery Rough Puff Pastry Dough (page 180) or Savory Pie Dough (page 162)
1 small zucchini, thinly sliced
½ medium fennel bulb, thinly sliced
¾ cup (100 g) shelled peas
2 tablespoons extra-virgin olive oil
½ teaspoon kosher salt
¼ cup tender fresh herbs (chives, fennel fronds, parsley, basil, mint)
Zucchini blossoms (optional)

1   To make the aioli, puree the almonds, 6 tablespoons of the water, olive oil, Dijon, garlic, and salt in a high-speed blender until creamy, thick, and as smooth as possible, about 2 minutes. Add another tablespoon of water if needed. Stop the blender, scrape the sides, and puree again until light in color. You should have about 1 cup. The aioli will keep for 3 days in an airtight container in the refrigerator.

2   Preheat the oven to 425 degrees F. Line a baking sheet with parchment paper.

3   To make the tart, lightly dust a work surface with tapioca starch and roll the pastry dough into a rectangle that is approximately 11 by 13 inches and ⅛ inch thick. Cut the edges with a sharp knife to get a nice rectangle. Fold up the edges about ½ inch to create a border all around. Place the dough on the prepared pan and refrigerate for 15 minutes.

4   Using a fork, prick the center of the dough, then bake for 25 minutes, until golden brown. Remove from the oven and dollop the aioli all over the crust, spreading it gently (the tender dough might tear if you are too aggressive). Top with the zucchini, fennel, and peas. Drizzle with the olive oil, sprinkle with the salt, and bake for another 10 minutes. Top with the herbs and zucchini blossoms and serve immediately.

Roasted Mushroom, Spinach, and Olive Slab Pie

---

1 recipe Buttery Rough Puff Pastry Dough (page 180)

1¾ pounds (800 g) assorted mushrooms (maitake, oyster, chanterelle), cut or torn into large pieces

2 small red onions, cut into ½-inch slices

6 tablespoons extra-virgin olive oil

6 sprigs thyme, plus more for topping

3 cloves garlic, peeled and smashed

1½ teaspoons kosher salt

1 teaspoon freshly ground black pepper, plus more for topping

1 teaspoon dried oregano

2 cups (100 g) fresh spinach, coarsely chopped

1 cup (125 g) pitted kalamata olives, coarsely chopped

2 tablespoons finely chopped chives

1 heaping tablespoon Dijon mustard

1 tablespoon good-quality balsamic vinegar

Tapioca starch, for dusting

5 ounces (145 g) Gruyère or dairy-free cheese, coarsely grated (optional)

1 large egg, lightly beaten

Roasted mushrooms encased in buttery puff pastry is probably my favorite thing to have for lunch on a cold winter's day. This very rustic tart is shaped into a slab, then cut into squares or triangles. It reminds me of the empanadas I grew up eating. Prepare the puff pastry first as it needs to chill for at least 1 hour before rolling.

MAKES 8 SERVINGS

1 Preheat the oven to 425 degrees F. Toss together the mushrooms, onions, olive oil, thyme, garlic, salt, pepper, and oregano on a baking sheet until the mushrooms are well coated. Bake for 30 minutes, stirring halfway through, until the mushrooms are golden brown with crispy edges. Stir in the spinach, olives, chives, Dijon, and balsamic and toss to coat all ingredients evenly. Set aside to cool.

2 Line a rimmed baking sheet with parchment paper. Cut the pastry dough roughly in half—one piece should be slightly larger than the other. Lightly dust a work surface with tapioca starch and roll the larger dough piece into a rectangle that is 9 by 13 inches and ⅛ inch thick. Fill the prepared pan with the dough, pinching any cracks together and pushing the dough up the sides of the pan. Don't worry about imperfection—it's supposed to be rustic. Spread the cooled mushroom mixture evenly over the dough, and scatter the cheese over the top.

3 Roll out the second dough piece to 9 by 13 inches and ⅛ inch thick. Drape the dough over the mushrooms. Crimp the edges of the dough together. Refrigerate the baking sheet for 15 minutes.

4 Brush the pie with the beaten egg. Cut ½-inch slits in the top of the dough to let steam escape during baking. Sprinkle with some pepper and thyme leaves. Bake for 30 to 35 minutes, until golden brown. Let the pie cool for 10 minutes, then cut into squares. Serve warm with a simple salad.

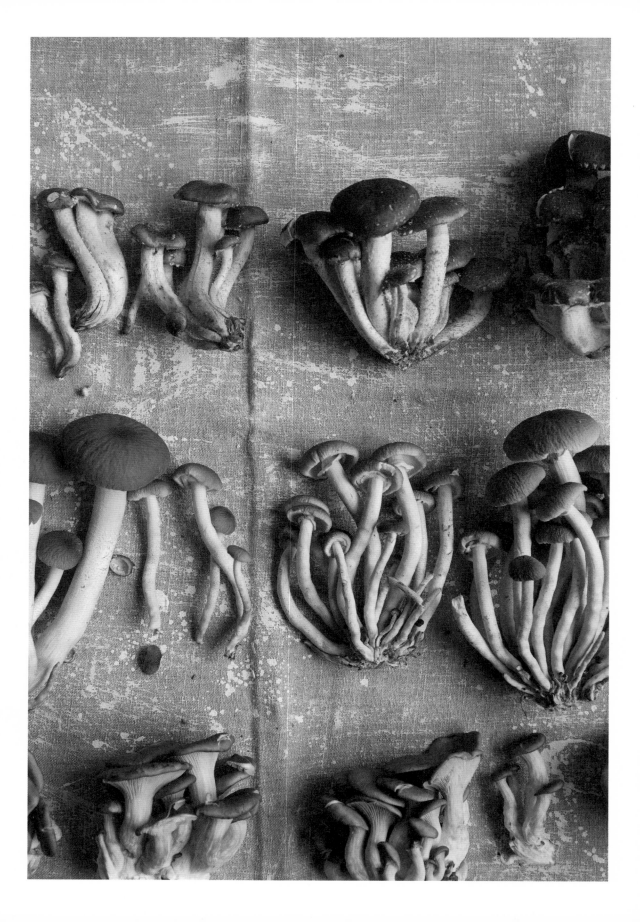

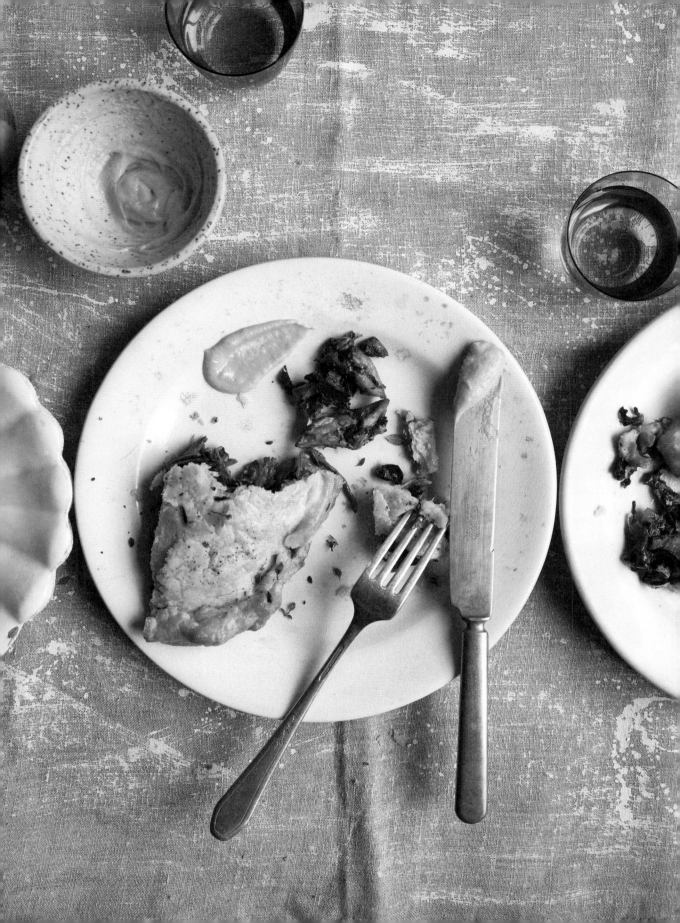

Crispy Potato, Leek, and Kale Focaccia Pie

1 recipe Spiced Sourdough
   Flatbreads (page 106)
Superfine brown rice flour,
   for dusting
2 medium (10 ounces or 300 g)
   Yukon Gold potatoes, well
   scrubbed
6 tablespoons extra-virgin
   olive oil, divided
2 medium leeks (white and light-
   green parts only), thinly sliced
   (about 2 cups)
2 cloves garlic, thinly sliced
¾ teaspoon kosher salt, divided
3 cups loosely packed finely
   chopped Lacinato kale leaves
   (about 4 large), tough ribs
   removed
1 to 2 tablespoons finely
   chopped preserved lemon
   (optional)
2 teaspoons fresh thyme leaves
Freshly ground black pepper
1 ounce (30 g) finely grated
   Parmesan (optional)

This recipe could live in the bread chapter or right here with the rest of the savory tarts. It uses the Spiced Sourdough Flatbread as a base and is something in between a pizza, a focaccia, and a pie. Regardless of what we call it, it is a delicious crowd-pleaser. I like to make the flatbread recipe a day in advance and keep it tightly wrapped in the refrigerator to develop flavor. Use thin-skinned potatoes so there is no need to peel them.

MAKES 8 SERVINGS

1 Make the flatbread dough, but don't cut it in half. You can use it right away or wrap it tightly in plastic wrap and refrigerate for up to 24 hours.

2 Set a pizza stone at the bottom of the oven and position an oven rack just above it. Preheat the oven to 425 degrees F. Dust a baking sheet with brown rice flour.

3 Using a mandoline, cut the potatoes into very thin slices—they should be so thin that they bend when you hold them—as if for potato chips. Put the potato slices in a large bowl and cover completely with cold water for 15 minutes. Drain the potatoes really well and lay them out on a large kitchen towel. Pat dry with another towel. The slices should have crisped up and not bend after soaking and drying.

4 Heat a large sauté pan over medium heat. Add 3 tablespoons of the olive oil, leeks, garlic, and ¼ teaspoon of the salt. Cook, stirring occasionally, until the leeks are soft and slightly caramel-ized, about 5 minutes. Add the kale and continue cooking until it wilts, about 3 minutes. Remove the pan from the heat and stir in the preserved lemon. Let the mixture cool for 10 minutes.

5 Dust a work surface with brown rice flour. Roll the flatbread dough into a rectangle that is approximately 11 by 14 inches and ¼ inch thick. Be gentle when rolling because the dough is fragile and can tear. Transfer the dough to the prepared pan.

6 Spread the vegetable mixture over the dough. Arrange the potato slices in rows on top, overlapping them slightly. Drizzle with the remaining 3 tablespoons olive oil, making sure to coat all the potatoes, then sprinkle with the thyme, remaining ½ tea-spoon salt, and pepper.

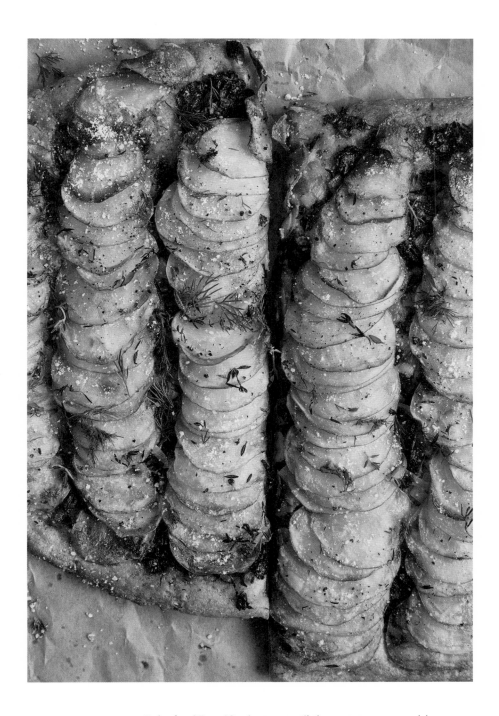

7   Bake for 35 to 40 minutes, until the potatoes are golden brown and crispy and the bottom of the dough is also golden brown. Remove the pan from the oven and immediately sprinkle with the Parmesan. Cut into 8 slices and serve hot.

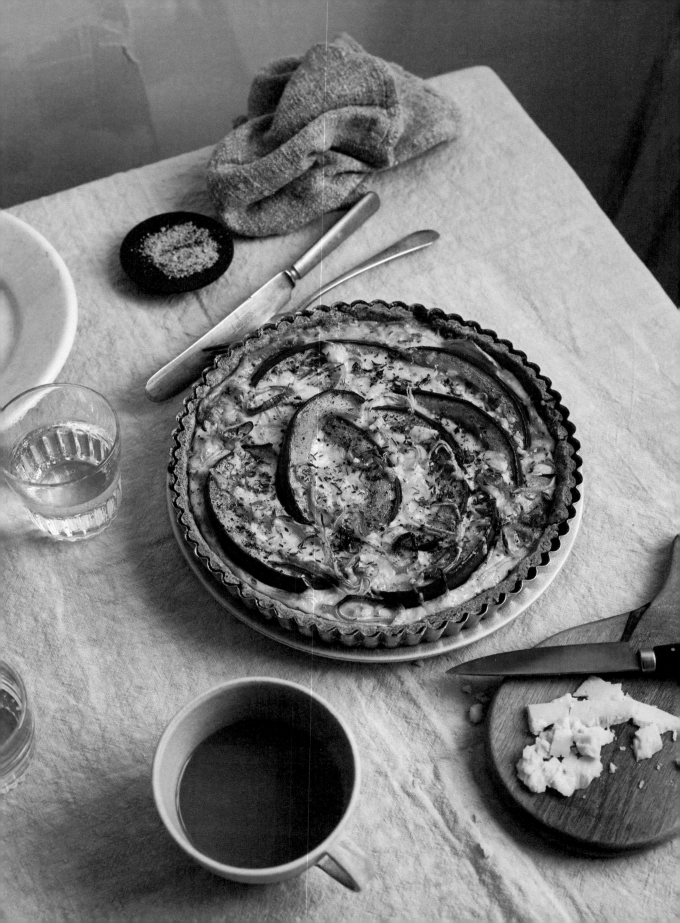

Squash, Onion, and Cheddar Quiche

Tapioca starch, for dusting
½ recipe Savory Pie Dough
   (page 162)
½ medium winter squash, such
   as kabocha or red kuri, peeled,
   seeded, and cut into ½-inch
   wedges
4 tablespoons extra-virgin
   olive oil, divided, plus more
   for brushing
1 teaspoon kosher salt, divided
½ teaspoon freshly ground
   black pepper
2 medium shallots, thinly sliced
¼ teaspoon fennel seeds
2 teaspoons Dijon mustard
3 large whole eggs plus
   2 egg yolks
¾ cup (170 g) half-and-half or
   canned full-fat coconut milk
2 tablespoons finely chopped
   fresh Italian parsley
Small pinch of freshly grated
   nutmeg
3 ounces (90 g) English-style
   cheddar cheese, coarsely
   grated, divided
½ teaspoon dried thyme
½ teaspoon dried oregano

As I like to think of it, a quiche is the perfect vessel for eating your vegetables. Savory custard encased in a flaky exterior makes for an ideal snack or light meal all day long. You can use this basic recipe and change up the vegetables. I love cooked beets, steamed broccoli, roasted cauliflower, corn, or any roasted leftovers from the fridge. I love using white English-style cheddar cheese, but grated Gruyère or sliced Taleggio are also great. For a dairy-free version that doesn't rely on vegan cheese, whisk a tablespoon of miso into the custard for a similar depth of flavor.

MAKES ONE 9-INCH QUICHE

1   Preheat the oven to 400 degrees F.

2   Dust a work surface and rolling pin with tapioca starch. Roll the pie dough ⅛ inch thick and carefully transfer it with both hands to a 9-inch tart pan with removable bottom. Press the dough into the bottom and sides and trim any excess. Chill the dough for at least 30 minutes.

3   On a baking sheet, toss together the squash, 2 tablespoons of the olive oil, ½ teaspoon of the salt, and pepper. Bake for 25 minutes, until the squash is tender and golden brown. Set aside.

4   Reduce the oven temperature to 375 degrees F. Put the tart pan on a baking sheet and bake for 15 to 20 minutes, until lightly golden brown. Set aside to cool.

5   Heat a medium sauté pan over medium heat and add the remaining 2 tablespoons olive oil, shallots, and ¼ teaspoon of the salt. Cook, stirring occasionally, until the shallots are tender and begin to caramelize, about 5 minutes. Add the fennel seeds and cook for another minute. Remove from the heat and stir in the Dijon. Set aside.

6   In a small bowl, whisk together the eggs, egg yolks, half-and-half, parsley, and nutmeg. Pour the custard into the pie crust. Sprinkle half of the cheese over the top, then arrange the squash slices in a circle (cut them if they are too long). Top with the shallots and remaining cheese. Sprinkle the thyme and oregano over everything.

7   Bake the quiche for 30 to 35 minutes, until golden brown and puffed up. Serve warm with a side of greens.

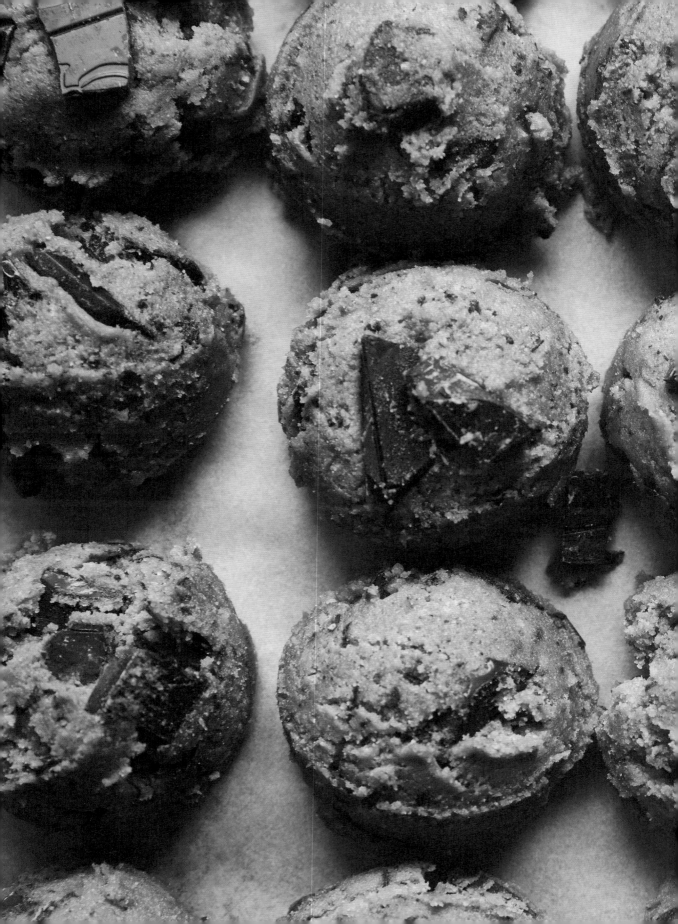

CHAPTER FIVE

Crispy, Chewy, and Crunchy: The Cookies

An oozing chocolate chunk cookie shared on social media will ignite many oohs and aahs. A cookie can lift people out of the depths of sadness, boredom, or anxiety. I have seen it with my own eyes. Cookies spark a strong reaction in people, and everyone has opinions on what makes a perfect cookie, especially chocolate ones. But I have to confess something to you, dear reader—I am hardly overtaken by a cookie craving. It has never been a thing for me, except the occasional sandy shortbread that leans extra salty. So when writing this chapter exclusively on cookies, I relied heavily on others to help me decipher if the cookie at hand, as written and developed, sparked the perfect reaction of "Oh, yes, this is what I needed all along."

When I began deciding what to include, I tried to imagine what a perfect spread of cookies would look like, one that reflected the wide array—crispy exterior and chewy interior like the Salted Chocolate Chunk Cookies (page 223), crumbly such as the Pistachio and Rose Water Sandies (page 214), crunchy like the Biscotti (page 227), light and delicate such as the Candied-Sesame and Cacao Nib Meringues (page 234), or the thin and crispy Almond–Cacao Nib Lace Cookies (page 238).

Another thing I had in mind while crafting these recipes was creating a balance between indulgence and nourishment. The Peanut Butter–Banana Cookies (page 217), the Date-Caramel and Chocolate Shortbread Squares (page 213), and the Chocolate-Tahini Truffles (page 231) are arguably even good for you.

There's a little something for everyone.

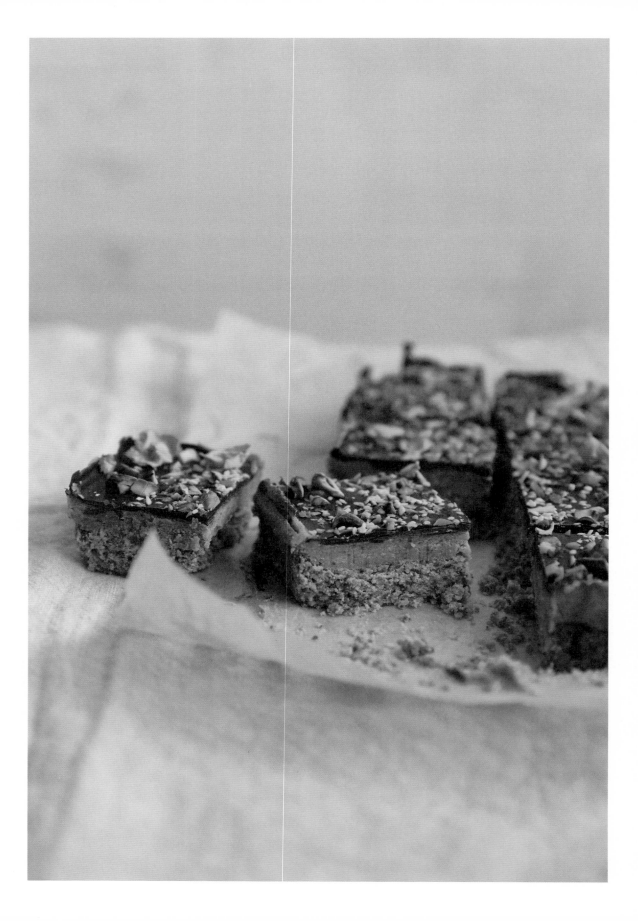

Date-Caramel and Chocolate Shortbread Squares

This is my take on a millionaire's shortbread, inspired by food writer Anna Jones. Here, pecan shortbread is topped with date caramel and a thin layer of chocolate, nuts, and seeds. Date caramel is my latest obsession: I use it as a dip as well as a filling for tarts that I dollop with whipped coconut cream. It is more of a paste than a traditional caramel, but it smells and tastes just like the classic, with the benefit of being naturally sweet.

MAKES 16 SQUARES

1 recipe Date-Nut Crust
    (page 267), made with pecans
⅓ cup (90 g) canned full-fat
    coconut milk
⅓ cup (90 g) plus 1 teaspoon
    melted virgin coconut oil,
    divided, plus more for greasing
1 teaspoon vanilla extract
½ teaspoon flaky sea salt, plus
    more for topping
8½ ounces (240 g) plump pitted
    Medjool dates (about 13)
6 ounces (170 g) 70 percent
    chocolate, finely chopped
½ cup (50 g) toasted nuts
    (pistachios, hazelnuts, pecans,
    walnuts), coarsely chopped
1 tablespoon raw sesame seeds
1 teaspoon dried rose petals
    (optional)

1   Preheat the oven to 350 degrees F. Grease the inside of an 8-inch square pan with coconut oil and line with parchment paper, letting some hang over the sides.

2   Firmly press the crust into the bottom of the prepared pan, reaching all corners and making sure it is evenly spread. Bake for 22 to 25 minutes, until golden brown. Remove from the oven and let it cool while you prepare the rest of the layers.

3   To make the date caramel, in a medium saucepan, combine the coconut milk, ⅓ cup (90 g) of the coconut oil, vanilla, and sea salt. Bring to a simmer over medium heat. Add the dates, simmer for 1 minute, then remove from the heat. Let the dates steep in the coconut milk for 10 minutes, then puree in a food processor. Be patient—it will take 3 to 5 minutes for the dates to puree to a fine and creamy texture. Scrape the date caramel onto the cooled crust and spread it evenly.

4   To make the chocolate glaze, in a medium heatproof bowl, combine the chopped chocolate and remaining 1 teaspoon coconut oil. Fill a small saucepan one-quarter full with water and bring to a simmer over medium heat. Place the bowl on top and stir until the chocolate is melted and shiny. Pour it over the date caramel and spread it evenly.

5   Sprinkle the nuts, sesame seeds, rose petals, and a pinch of flaky sea salt over the top of the chocolate. Transfer the pan to the refrigerator for 2 hours, or until the chocolate and caramel harden. Lift the cookie bar from the pan using the parchment, and cut it lengthwise into 4 equal pieces, then cut each piece into quarters. You should have 16 (2-inch) squares. The caramel is quite gooey, so the bars are a bit messy when soft. Once cut, store them in the refrigerator, tightly wrapped, for up to 5 days.

Pistachio and Rose Water Sandies

½ cup (70 g) raw unsalted shelled pistachios
½ cup (70 g) superfine brown rice flour
½ cup (50 g) oat flour
⅓ cup (40 g) tapioca starch
¼ cup plus 2 tablespoons (45 g) powdered sugar, plus more for rolling
2 teaspoons dried rose petals (optional)
½ teaspoon kosher salt
½ cup (115 g) unsalted butter or dairy-free butter, cut into ½-inch dice, at room temperature
1 tablespoon rose water

Harinados were, and still are, my favorite cookie sold in my family's pastry shop. They are a buttery and rather crumbly cookie, similar to shortbread but dusted in powdered sugar. They are traditionally flavored with almond, vanilla, and a touch of cinnamon, but in this adaptation, I use pistachios and rose water for a more fragrant version. If you don't have pistachios, you could easily make them with lightly toasted and skinned hazelnuts, or even almonds. You can also use vanilla extract in place of rose water and omit the rose petals.

MAKES 16 SANDIES

1   Preheat the oven to 350 degrees F. Line a baking sheet with parchment paper.

2   In a food processor, combine the pistachios, brown rice flour, oat flour, tapioca starch, powdered sugar, rose petals, and salt and pulverize into a fine powder.

3   Add the butter and rose water and continue processing until the dough sticks together when pressed between your hands.

4   Using an ice cream scoop or your hands, remove 1-tablespoon portions and shape them into balls. Place on the prepared pan, leaving at least 1 inch between.

5   Bake the sandies for 10 to 12 minutes, being careful not to overbake them. They might appear a bit underdone, but they firm up fairly fast once cooled. Let the cookies cool on the pan for 5 minutes, or until they are set enough to handle, then roll them in powdered sugar. The sandies will keep for up to 5 days in an airtight container.

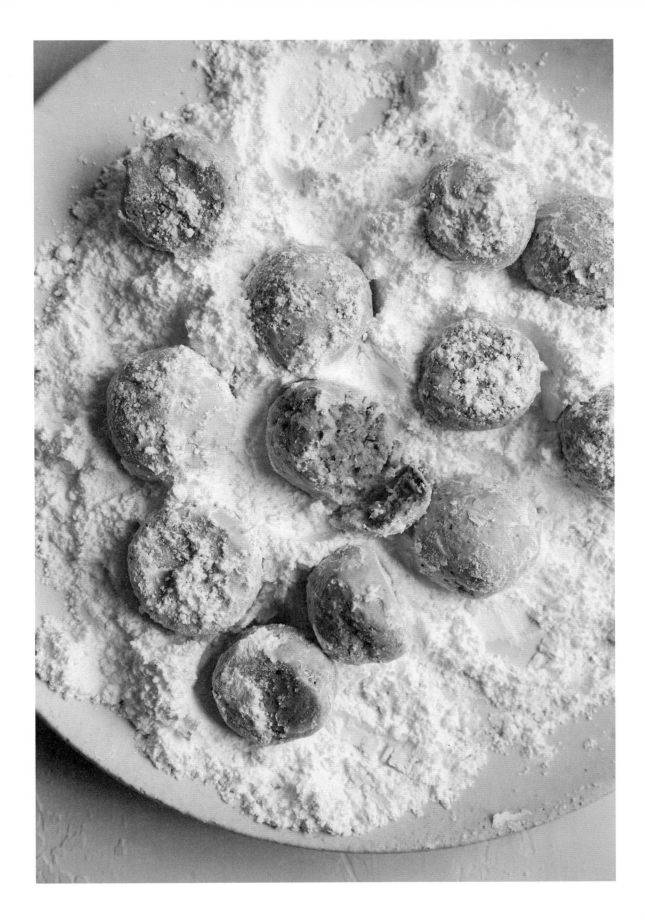

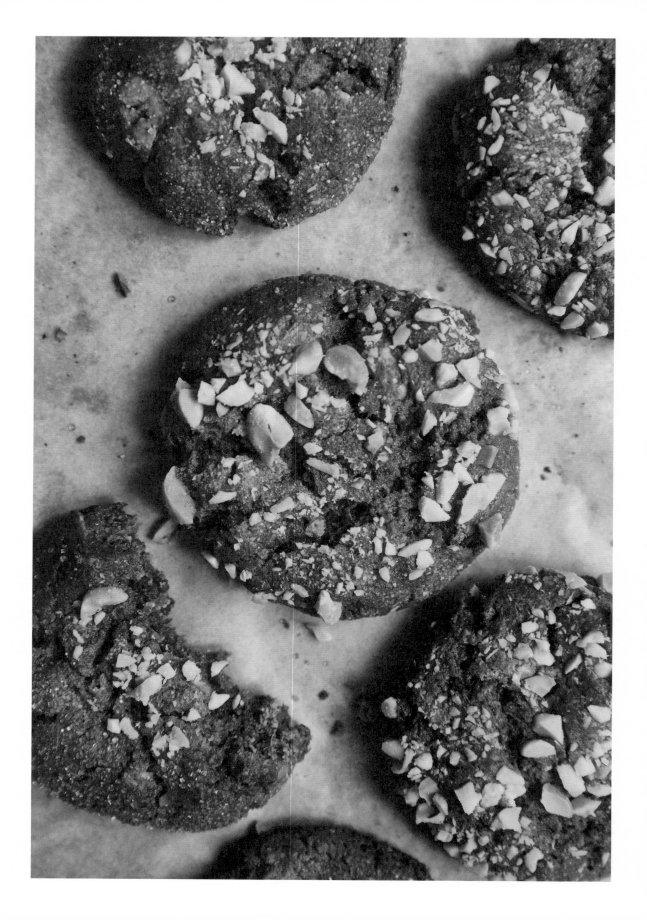

Peanut Butter– Banana Cookies

½ cup (75 g) salted roasted peanuts
2 tablespoons sugar (optional)
1 cup (240 g) unsweetened chunky peanut butter
⅔ cup (120 g) coconut sugar
¼ cup finely mashed banana (about 1 medium)
2 tablespoons maple syrup
2 teaspoons vanilla extract
½ teaspoon baking soda
½ teaspoon kosher salt

You would never know how decadent these cookies are by looking at the ingredient list. Because they are vegan and free of gluten and refined sugar, I feel good making these often for a nourishing snack. The coconut sugar perfectly complements the peanut and banana here. I have made several versions of these cookies with only maple syrup, but the crisp factor is not there when the coconut sugar is left out.

MAKES 14 COOKIES

1   Preheat the oven to 375 degrees F. Line two baking sheets with parchment paper.

2   Coarsely chop the peanuts. Reserve half of them and continue chopping the remaining half into very small pieces. Put the finely chopped peanuts in a small bowl, add the sugar, and set aside. The sugar adds a bit of crunch to the exterior of the cookie, but it's not essential.

3   Stir together the reserved coarsely chopped peanuts, peanut butter, coconut sugar, banana, maple syrup, vanilla, baking soda, and salt in a medium bowl. The dough will be thick and sticky. Let it sit for 15 minutes. As the baking soda reacts, the dough will thicken a bit.

4   Scoop 1 heaping tablespoon of dough into the bowl of finely chopped peanuts. Roll the dough around to coat, then roll it into a ball in your hands. Place on a baking sheet and repeat with the remaining dough. Leave 2 inches between cookies as they will spread while baking. Flatten them slightly with your fingers.

5   Bake for 8 to 10 minutes, until the cookies crack and their edges begin to look crispy. Do not overbake as they will continue to dry out while cooling. Cool on the pan for 10 minutes, then transfer to a wire rack. The cookies will be crispy on the outside and chewy on the inside. They will keep for 5 days in an airtight container.

Gooey Almond Butter, Nut, and Seed Blondies

1 cup (125 g) nuts and seeds, coarsely chopped, plus more for topping
¾ cup (105 g) sorghum flour
¼ cup (30 g) tapioca starch
¾ teaspoon kosher salt
½ teaspoon baking powder
½ teaspoon baking soda
1 cup (200 g) light brown sugar
½ cup (115 g) unsalted butter or dairy-free butter, melted and cooled to room temperature
¼ cup (65 g) almond butter
1 large egg
2 teaspoons vanilla extract
Flaky sea salt, for topping (optional)

I tested so many variations of this recipe, trying to achieve what in my opinion is a perfect blondie—slightly cakier than a cookie, but definitely more of a cookie than a cake. These blondies are crispy around the edges and gooey inside. I like texture and chewiness, so my version is about 75 percent nuts and 25 percent seeds. For nuts, I recommend almonds, hazelnuts, walnuts, pecans, or pine nuts. For seeds, I frequently use sesame, sunflower, pumpkin, and sometimes even a bit of fennel or coriander. There is no chocolate called for here, but you could replace a portion of the nuts with coarsely chopped bittersweet chocolate if desired.

MAKES 16 BLONDIES

1   Preheat the oven to 350 degrees F. Line an 8-inch square pan with parchment paper, letting some hang over the sides.

2   In a large bowl, whisk together the nuts and seeds, sorghum flour, tapioca starch, salt, and baking powder and soda.

3   In a medium bowl, whisk together the brown sugar, both butters, egg, and vanilla. Add to the dry ingredients and stir to combine. The mixture will have the consistency of thick cake batter or loose cookie dough. Pour it into the prepared cake pan and spread it to reach all corners. Sprinkle with more nuts and seeds and a pinch of flaky salt.

4   Bake for 30 to 35 minutes, until the blondies are golden brown with crispy edges, and a toothpick inserted in the center comes out clean. Let the blondies cool completely in the pan, then lift out onto a cutting board and cut into 16 squares. Store the blondies in an airtight container for up to 3 days.

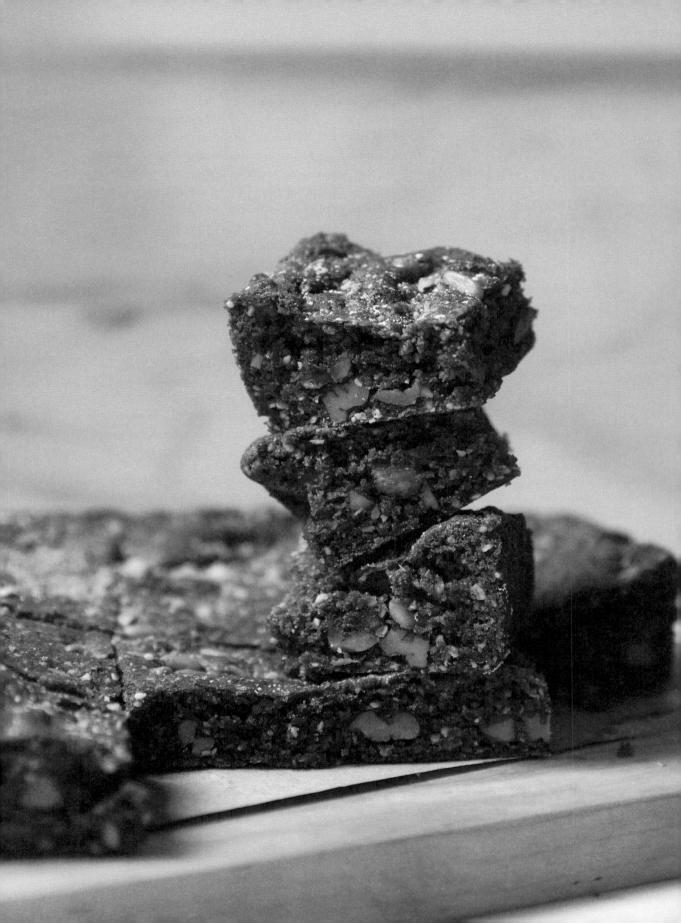

Orange-Flower Water and Almond Crinkles

Macarrones de Azahar y Almendra

———

1½ cups (150 g) almond flour

1 cup (120 g) powdered sugar, plus more for dusting

2 teaspoons freshly squeezed lemon juice

1 teaspoon orange-flower water

1 teaspoon finely grated orange zest

1 large egg, lightly beaten

These cookies are an amalgamation of various recipes I have made throughout my life: my family's *macarrones de almendra*, which are still made at the pastry shop; the macarons at Maison Adam in Saint-Jean-de-Luz; and Moroccan *ghriba* or *ghoriba*. They are very simple to put together—a mixture of almonds, sugar, and egg—and as the name indicates, they are cracked on the outside and chewy on the inside. If you prefer not to use orange-flower water, substitute with 2 additional teaspoons of finely grated orange zest. You can flavor the crinkles with vanilla, cinnamon, rose water, lemon zest, or anything you prefer.

MAKES 15 COOKIES

1 Preheat the broiler on high. Line a baking sheet with parchment paper.

2 Mix the almond flour, powdered sugar, lemon juice, orange-flower water, orange zest, and half of the beaten egg in a medium bowl. Add a bit more egg until the dough is moist and sticky, almost like thick cake batter. Let the dough sit at room temperature for 10 minutes.

3 Spread some powdered sugar on a plate. Wet your hands and scoop 1 tablespoon of dough into them. Roll it into a 1-inch ball with your palms, then roll it in the powdered sugar. Place the dough on the baking sheet and repeat with the remaining dough.

4 Put the baking sheet in the hot oven, turn it off, and bake the cookies undisturbed for 12 to 15 minutes, until they are cracked and golden brown. Remove from the oven and let the cookies cool on the pan for 10 minutes. They will keep for 1 week in an airtight container.

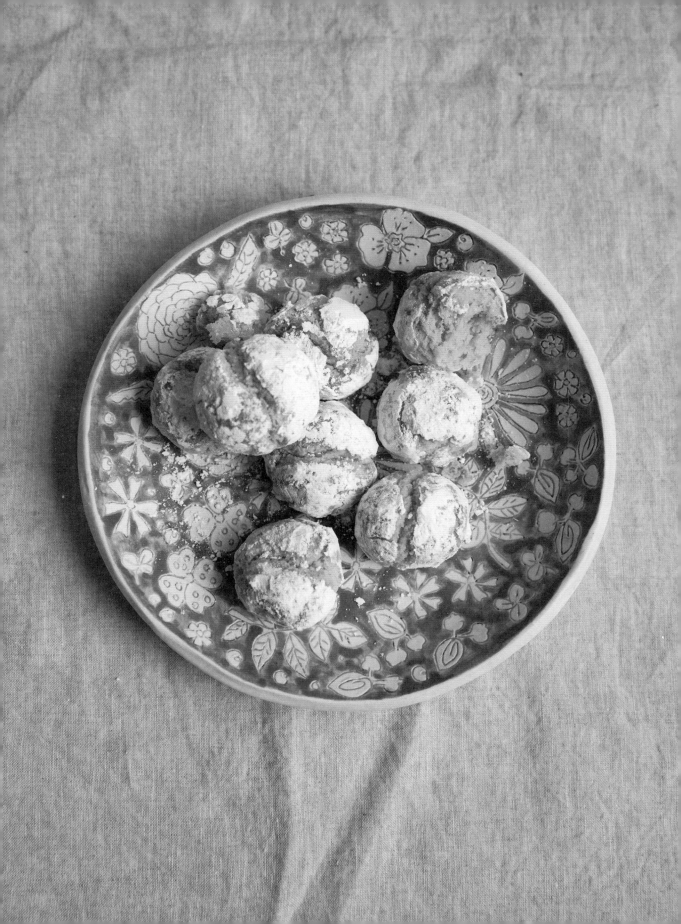

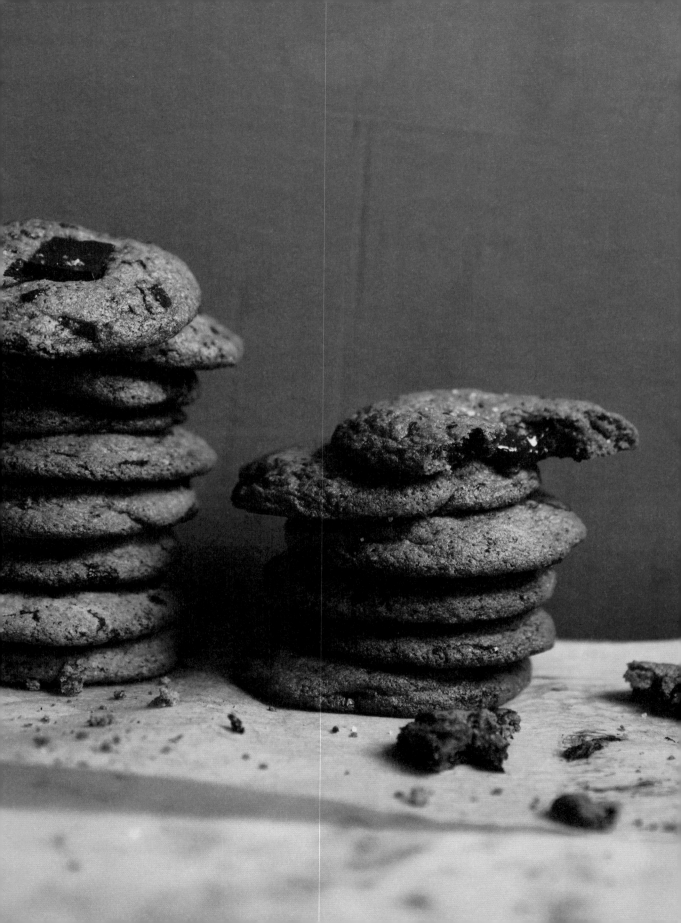

Salted Chocolate Chunk Cookies

Do we really need another salted chocolate chunk cookie, I asked myself when I set out to develop this chapter. After all, there are thousands of recipes out there. I tested at least a dozen variations of this one, each time altering small amounts of the ingredients to achieve the texture that I felt was perfect—a combination of a crispy edge and a gooey and chewy interior. The result, at least in my opinion, is exceptional.

MAKES 15 COOKIES

½ cup (115 g) very soft unsalted butter or dairy-free butter
½ cup (140 g) tightly packed dark brown sugar
¼ cup (50 g) sugar
2 teaspoons vanilla extract
1 large whole egg plus 1 egg yolk
1 cup (140 g) superfine brown rice flour
½ cup (50 g) almond flour
⅓ cup (40 g) tapioca starch
½ teaspoon kosher salt
¼ teaspoon baking soda
7 ounces (200 g) 70 percent chocolate, coarsely chopped
Flaky sea salt, for topping

1   In a large bowl, using a spatula or wooden spoon, stir together the butter, both sugars, and vanilla until smooth. Stir in the egg and egg yolk until well incorporated.

2   In a small bowl, whisk together both flours, tapioca starch, salt, and baking soda. Fold the dry ingredients into the butter mixture until all the flour has been incorporated.

3   Fold in the chocolate chunks until they are evenly distributed throughout the dough. Refrigerate the dough, covered, for at least 2 hours or preferably overnight, to enhance the flavor and hydrate the dough.

4   Preheat the oven to 375 degrees F. Line two baking sheets with parchment paper.

5   Using a 1½-ounce ice cream scoop, place 6 dough mounds on each baking sheet, leaving at least 3 inches of space between. Sprinkle the tops with a small pinch of flaky sea salt.

6   Bake for 11 to 13 minutes, until the edges of the cookies are golden brown but the centers are still soft. The cookies will continue firming up when cooling, so to have a soft chewy center, it is important to not overbake them. Cool on the pan for at least 5 minutes. You should be able to lift the cookies without them falling apart. Scoop and bake the remaining dough. Store the cookies in an airtight container for up to 3 days—if they make it that long.

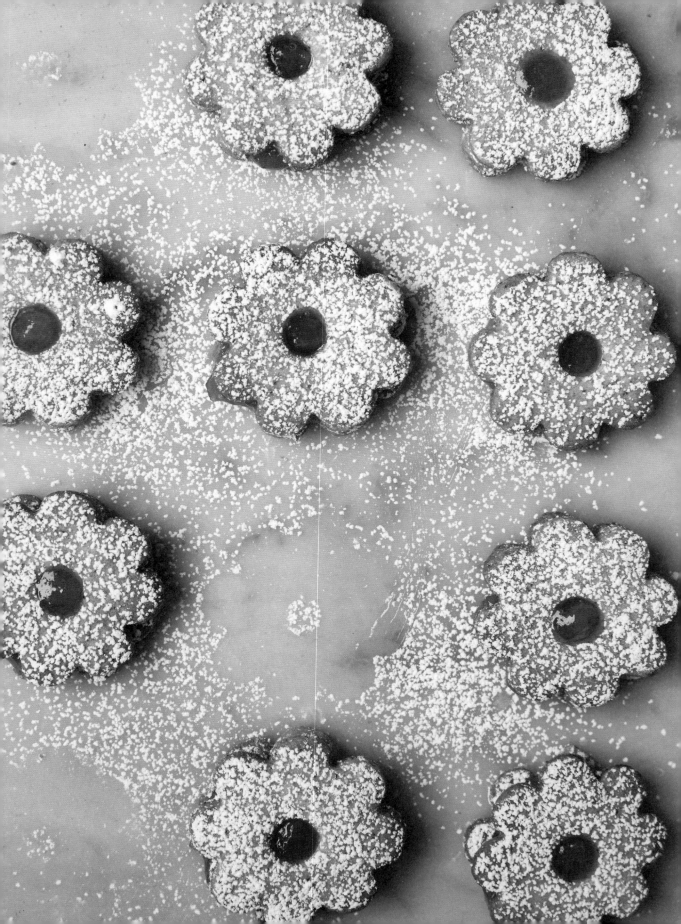

Sugar Cookies with Jam

1 cup (225 g) unsalted butter or dairy-free butter, at room temperature
1 cup (120 g) powdered sugar
2 teaspoons vanilla extract
1 large whole egg plus 1 egg yolk
2 cups (200 g) almond flour
1 cup (140 g) sorghum flour
½ cup (80 g) potato starch
½ cup (60 g) tapioca starch, plus more for dusting
½ teaspoon xanthan gum (optional but helps with rolling)
½ teaspoon baking powder
½ teaspoon kosher salt
¾ cup Honey-Apricot Jam (page 55), Strawberry-Hibiscus Jam (page 52), or other jam of choice, for filling
Powdered sugar, for dusting

This is the dough that I rely on most for cutout cookies. It is buttery, crispy, and sandy. It is also not overtly sweet, and the salt and almonds add a savory touch. I grew up with this kind of cookie, always filled with homemade jam or buttercream. Use any fruit preserves or jam you like, but make sure it's on the thicker side so it doesn't ooze out or make the cookies soggy. You can use a ½-inch round cookie cutter to cut a hole in the center of half of the cookies so when they are sandwiched together, the jam shows through.

MAKES ABOUT 32 SANDWICH COOKIES
(64 INDIVIDUAL COOKIES)

1   In the bowl of a stand mixer fitted with the paddle attachment, beat the butter, powdered sugar, and vanilla on medium speed until smooth and creamy. Scrape the paddle and sides of the bowl, then add the egg and egg yolk and continue mixing until smooth.

2   In a small bowl, stir together both flours, both starches, xanthan gum, baking powder, and salt. Add to the mixer bowl and beat together until you have a very creamy, smooth, and soft yet quite sticky dough.

3   Scrape the dough onto a large piece of parchment and wrap it up, then flatten it and shape it into a rectangle. Refrigerate the dough for at least 2 hours to firm and hydrate it.

4   Preheat the oven to 350 degrees F. Line two baking sheets with parchment paper.

5   Remove the dough from the refrigerator and cut it in half. Rewrap one half of the dough and refrigerate it while you roll out and cut the other.

6   Dust the top of the dough and a rolling pin with some tapioca starch, and have more nearby. On a work surface, roll the dough to slightly thicker than ⅛ inch. Keep the dough moving and dusted with tapioca at all times. The dough is pliable and can soften easily in a warm kitchen, so work quickly. ⟶

7 Using a 2-inch round or fluted cookie cutter, cut out disks of dough. Cut a ¼-inch hole from the center of half of the cookies, if desired. Transfer the cookies to the prepared baking sheets, leaving 1 inch of space between—the cookies will expand a bit while baking but not much. If the dough softens while you work, put it in the freezer for 5 minutes to firm up again. If you have any leftover dough, wrap and refrigerate it. The dough can be rerolled multiple times as long as it is chilled.

8 Bake for 12 to 14 minutes, until lightly golden brown. Rotate the baking sheets halfway through to ensure even baking. Let the cookies cool on the pan for 5 minutes, then transfer them to a wire rack. Repeat the rolling out, cutting, and baking with the second half of the dough.

9 When the cookies are cooled, spoon 1 teaspoon of jam on top of one and press another cookie on top, creating a sandwich. Fill only the cookies that will be eaten the same day. The rest can be kept in an airtight container for up to 5 days; fill them as they will be eaten. Dust the tops with powdered sugar before serving.

Biscotti

1 cup (140 g) superfine brown
  rice flour
¾ cup (105 g) sorghum flour
¼ cup (30 g) tapioca starch
1 teaspoon baking powder
¾ teaspoon kosher salt
2 large eggs
⅓ cup (130 g) honey
¼ cup (55 g) extra-virgin olive oil
  or melted unsalted butter
Finely grated zest of 1 medium
  lemon
2 teaspoons vanilla extract
7 ounces (200 g) nuts, seeds,
  and/or dried fruit of choice
  (see page 228)

Biscotti remind me of my mother as they are her most-requested cookie from me. When she comes to visit, I always make a large batch for her. I store them in glass jars and serve them with coffee in the afternoon. This recipe is very lightly sweetened with honey. I like how subtle and delicate it is. If you prefer a sweeter version, increase the amount of honey to ½ cup (170 g). Play around with flavors and nut-and-dried-fruit combinations—I offer some suggestions on page 228.

MAKES 30 BISCOTTI

1   Preheat the oven to 350 degrees F. Line a baking sheet with parchment paper.

2   In a large bowl, mix the brown rice flour, sorghum flour, tapioca starch, baking powder, and salt.

3   In a small bowl, whisk together the eggs, honey, olive oil, lemon zest, and vanilla. Add to the dry ingredients and mix until you have a sticky, cookie-like dough. Fold in the nuts, seeds, and dried fruit.

4   Scrape the dough onto the baking sheet and, using wet hands, shape it into a flat log about 13 inches long and 2½ inches wide.

5   Bake for 30 to 35 minutes, until golden brown. The dough will crack a bit on the surface. Remove from the oven to cool for at least 30 minutes. It's easiest to cut the dough when it's completely cooled. You can stop at this point and store the tightly wrapped dough at room temperature for up to 1 day.

6   Reduce the oven temperature to 300 degrees F. Using a very sharp or serrated knife, cut the dough into ½-inch slices and lay them down on the same baking sheet. The dough is fragile, so cut carefully.

7   Bake until the biscotti are dry, 20 to 25 minutes. Transfer them to a wire rack to cool completely. Store the biscotti in an airtight container for up to 1 week. ⟶

APRICOT-PISTACHIO

3½ ounces (100 g) coarsely chopped dried apricots + 3½ ounces (100 g) raw shelled pistachios

CHOCOLATE-ANISE

Decrease the amount of brown rice flour by 1 tablespoon and add 6 ounces (170 g) chopped 70 percent chocolate + 1 tablespoon toasted aniseed + 1 tablespoon unsweetened cocoa powder + 1 teaspoon finely grated orange zest

ALMOND-CHERRY

3½ ounces (100 g) dried cherries + 3½ ounces (100 g) chopped toasted almonds + 2 teaspoons kirsch (optional)

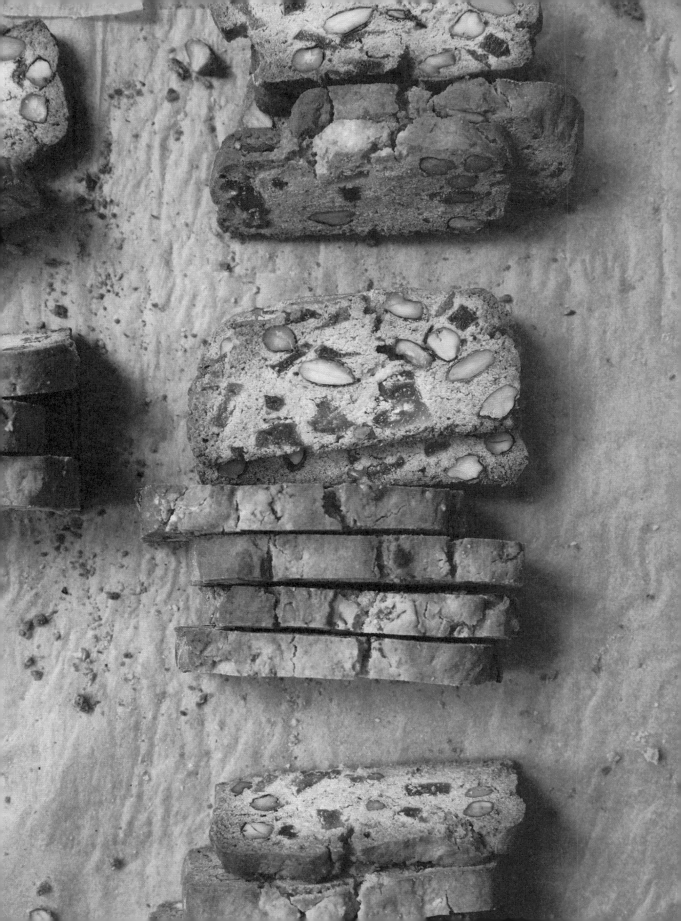

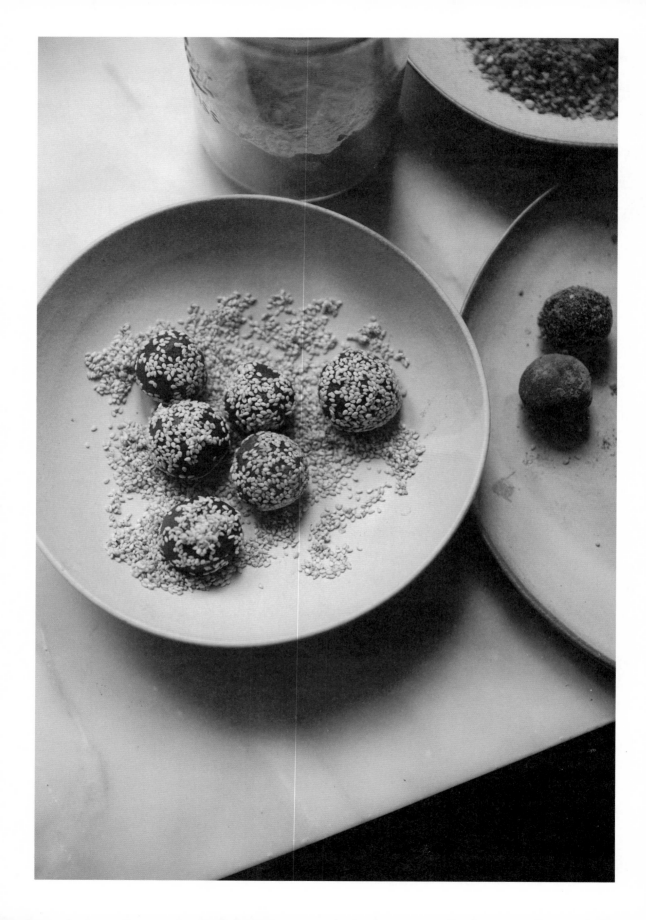

Chocolate-Tahini Truffles

8 ounces (225 g) 70 percent
  chocolate, coarsely chopped
2 tablespoons unsalted butter or
  dairy-free butter
1 cup (240 g) well-stirred tahini
¼ cup (80 g) maple syrup
1 vanilla bean, split lengthwise
  and seeds scraped, or
  2 teaspoons vanilla extract
1 teaspoon finely grated
  orange zest
1 teaspoon flaky sea salt
Toasted sesame seeds,
  for rolling
Unsweetened cocoa powder,
  for rolling
Finely chopped raw pistachios,
  for rolling

I realize these are not cookies, but I like to serve and gift them just as I do cookies. This recipe is a slightly savory take on a traditional truffle with nutritious ingredients that can serve as a treat as well as a little afternoon energizing pick-me-up.

MAKES 30 TRUFFLES

1 Put the chocolate and butter in a large heatproof bowl. Fill a medium saucepan with about 2 inches of water and bring to a simmer over medium-high heat. Place the bowl over the saucepan and stir the chocolate and butter until melted.

2 Remove the bowl from the saucepan. Stir in the tahini, maple syrup, vanilla seeds, orange zest, and salt until well incorporated. Cover the bowl and chill for at least 2 hours, until the mixture has firmed up and is scoopable.

3 Put the sesame seeds, cocoa powder, and pistachios each on their own small plates. Scoop out 1-inch balls of the chocolate and roll in different toppings until coated. Store them in an airtight container in the refrigerator for up to 1 week.

Double Chocolate Fennel-Buckwheat Crinkle Cookies

My grandmother loved a sliver of chocolate with a cup of aniseed tea, similar in flavor to fennel, after lunch. If you are intrigued by the combination of flavors, I encourage you to make this recipe. These cookies are crispy and gooey at the same time—a cross between a brownie and a cookie.

MAKES 16 COOKIES

1 Preheat the oven to 375 degrees F. Line two baking sheets with parchment paper. Crush the fennel seeds to a powder in a mortar and pestle or clean coffee grinder.

2 Fill a medium saucepan one-quarter full with water and bring to a simmer over medium-high heat. In a large heatproof bowl, combine the fennel, 7 ounces (200 g) of the chocolate, butter, and almond butter, and place over the simmering water. Stir until the chocolate is nearly all melted, then remove from the heat. The residual heat will continue melting the chocolate.

3 In the bowl of a stand mixer fitted with the whisk attachment, combine the eggs, brown sugar, and vanilla and beat on high speed until the eggs are pale and very thick, about 5 minutes. Pour in the melted chocolate and beat on medium speed until thick, about 1 minute.

4 In a small bowl, stir together the buckwheat flour, cocoa powder, baking soda, and salt. Fold this into the batter using a spatula. Scoop 1½-tablespoon mounds of dough onto each baking sheet, leaving 2 inches of space between. Lightly press small pieces of the remaining 1 ounce (25 g) chocolate into the top of each cookie.

5 Bake for 8 to 9 minutes, until the edges of the cookies are crispy but the centers are soft. Be careful not to overbake. They might look a little underdone, but they will set while cooling. Cool on the pan for 10 minutes, or until you are able to pick the cookies up without them falling apart. They will keep for 3 days in an airtight container.

1 to 1½ teaspoons fennel seeds

8 ounces (225 g) 70 percent chocolate, coarsely chopped, divided

¼ cup (55 g) unsalted butter or dairy-free butter

3 tablespoons almond butter

2 large eggs

1 cup (200 g) light brown sugar

2 teaspoons vanilla extract

¾ cup (105 g) light buckwheat flour

3 tablespoons unsweetened cocoa powder

½ teaspoon baking soda

½ teaspoon kosher salt

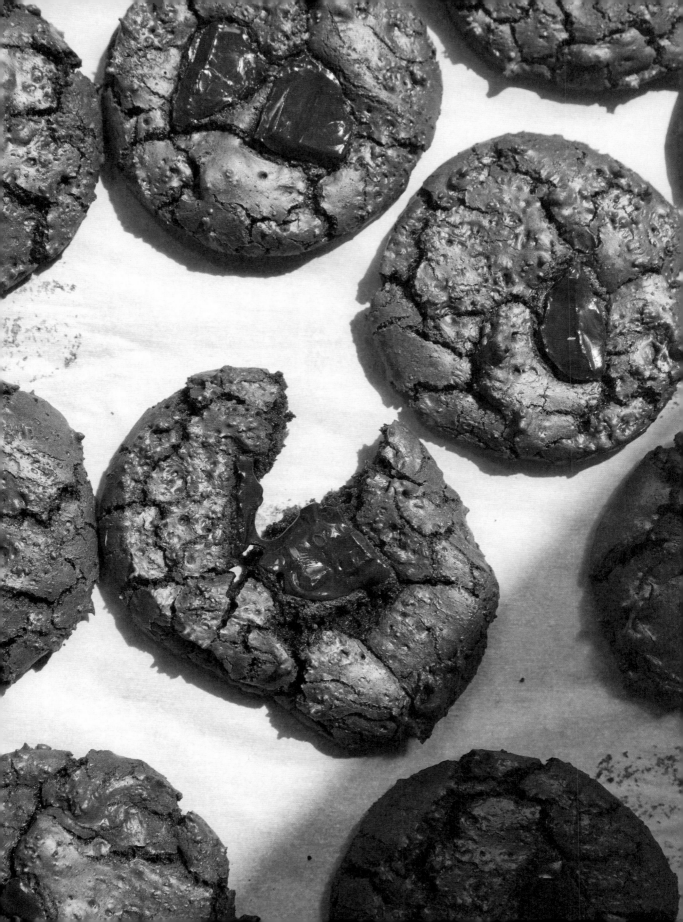

Candied-Sesame and Cacao Nib Meringues

Taking a bite out of one of these baked meringues—with their crispy exterior and marshmallow-like interior—makes me feel like I'm five years old again. I remember silver trays piled high with them sitting on the wood-and-glass counter at the pastry shop. I was mesmerized by their intricate swirls and pointy tops. This is an homage to those simple baked meringues, though I've added candied sesame seeds and cocoa nibs to mine.

MAKES 8 TO 10 MERINGUES

2 tablespoons sugar
2 tablespoons water
¼ cup (30 g) raw sesame seeds
3 large egg whites
1½ cups (180 g) powdered sugar
½ teaspoon kosher salt
¼ cup (35 g) cacao nibs
2 teaspoons vanilla extract

1   Preheat the oven to 350 degrees F. Line two baking sheets with parchment paper.

2   In a small sauté pan, combine the sugar and water. Bring to a boil over medium-high heat. When the sugar dissolves and the syrup simmers, add the sesame seeds, stirring constantly. The water will evaporate and the seeds will begin to caramelize. Cook for 3 to 5 minutes to a nice golden amber, then immediately remove the pan from the heat and spread the sesame seeds evenly on one of the baking sheets to cool completely. Once cooled, break the candied sesame into small pieces.

3   Combine the egg whites, powdered sugar, and salt in the bowl of a stand mixer. Fill a medium saucepan one-quarter full with water and bring to a simmer over medium heat. Place the mixer bowl over the simmering water and whisk by hand until the sugar is dissolved and the egg whites feels warm to the touch.

4   Attach the bowl to the mixer fitted with the whisk attachment and beat the egg whites on medium-high speed until stiff and glossy, about 4 minutes. The meringue will be shiny and should really hold peaks firmly. Using a spatula, gently fold in the cacao nibs, vanilla, and candied sesame, reserving 1 tablespoon of the sesame seeds for topping.

5   Spoon 8 to 10 mounds of meringue onto the second baking sheet and sprinkle the tops with the reserved candied sesame. Put the baking sheet in the oven and keep the door ajar with the help of a wooden spoon. Bake for 20 to 25 minutes, until the meringues have cracked, the exterior is crispy, and the interior is moist. Cool on the pan for at least 20 minutes. They will continue drying as they cool. The meringues will keep for up to 1 week stored in an airtight container.

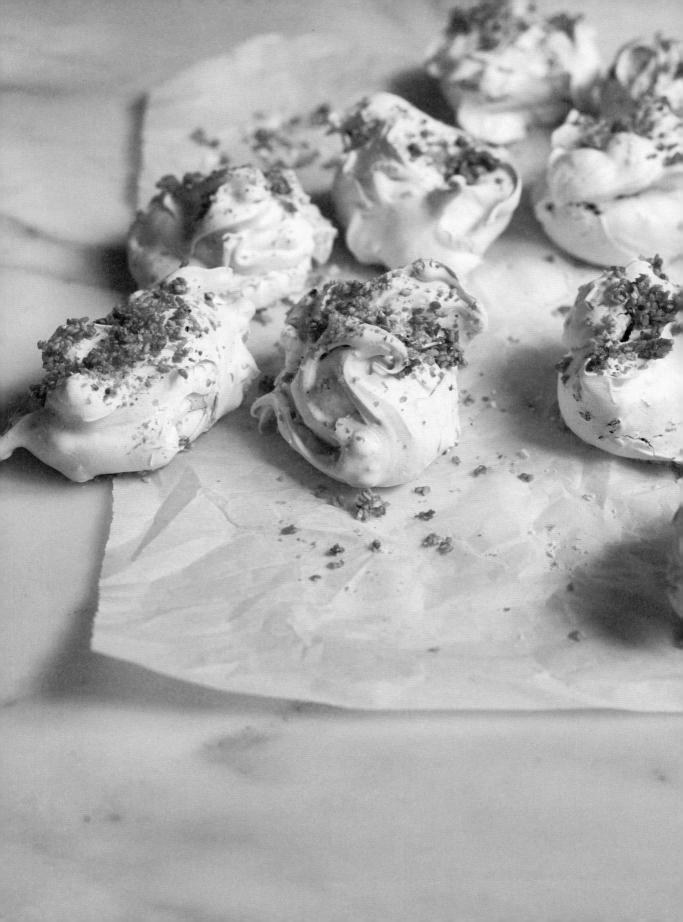

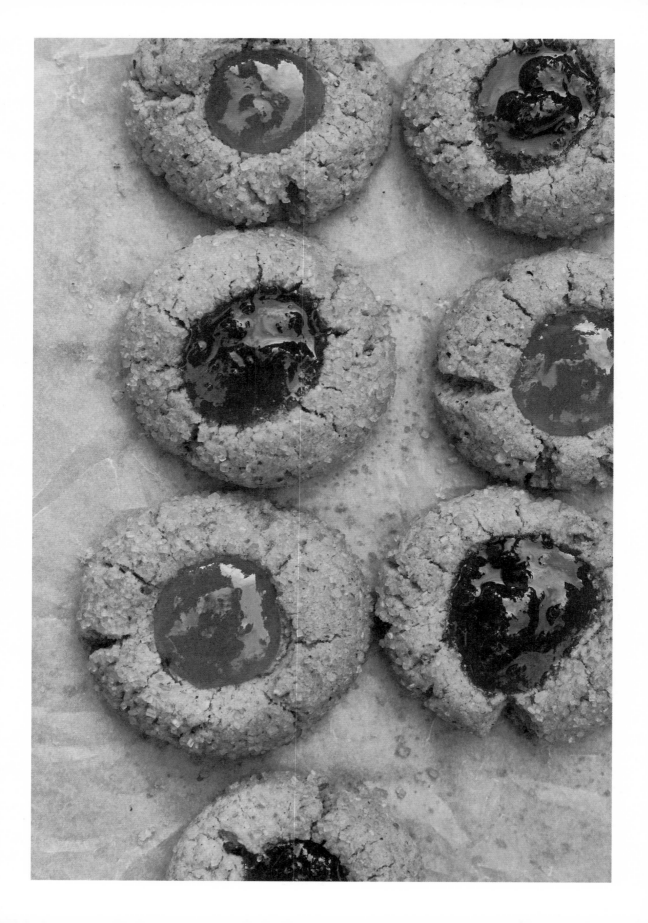

Toasted Hazelnut Thumbprint Cookies

These thumbprint cookies have a soft center with a very crispy exterior, similar to a sandy cookie but with added crunch from the coarse sugar. The kitchen smells deliciously warm while toasting the hazelnut flour and as the cookies bake. I fill them with a variety of fruit jams and chocolate.

MAKES 16 COOKIES

¾ cup (75 g) hazelnut flour
½ cup (115 g) unsalted butter or dairy-free butter, at room temperature
½ cup (100 g) light brown sugar
1 teaspoon vanilla extract
1 large egg yolk
1 cup (140 g) light buckwheat flour
2 tablespoons tapioca starch
½ teaspoon ground cinnamon
½ teaspoon kosher salt
⅓ cup (80 g) turbinado or raw sugar, for rolling
½ cup Honey-Apricot Jam (page 55), Strawberry-Hibiscus Jam (page 52), or Chocolate Glaze (page 46)

1   Preheat the oven to 375 degrees F. Line a baking sheet with parchment paper.

2   Heat a medium sauté pan over medium heat. Evenly spread the hazelnut flour in the pan and cook, stirring constantly, until it is toasted and fragrant, 2 to 3 minutes. Be careful not to burn it. Spread the hazelnut flour on a plate to cool completely.

3   In the bowl of a stand mixer fitted with the paddle attachment, beat the butter, brown sugar, and vanilla extract on medium speed until creamy, about 2 minutes. Add the egg yolk and continue mixing until incorporated.

4   In a small bowl, stir together the toasted hazelnut flour, buckwheat flour, tapioca starch, cinnamon, and salt. Add to the mixer bowl and beat on medium speed until the dough comes together and is smooth, about 1 minute.

5   Spread the turbinado sugar on a small plate. Scoop 1½-tablespoon mounds of dough, shape them into 1-inch balls, and roll them in the sugar. Place the cookies on the prepared baking sheet, leaving 1½ inches between. Using your thumb, press down in the center of the cookies to create an indentation. This is where the filling will go after baking.

6   Bake the cookies for 8 minutes. Remove from the oven and press down on the centers again with the end of a wooden spoon. Return the cookies to the oven and bake for another 4 to 5 minutes, until the edges feel firm but the centers are still soft. Be sure not to overbake or the cookies will dry out. Let them cool on the pan for 5 minutes, or until you can lift them without them falling apart. Fill the center with jam or chocolate glaze. Only fill the cookies that will be eaten immediately; unfilled cookies will keep in an airtight container for up to 3 days.

Almond–Cacao Nib Lace Cookies

These are one of my favorite cookies in this book. This is my take on traditional Florentine, or lace, cookies—perfectly thin, crispy, and elegant—without the loads of butter and sugar. They literally take fifteen minutes to make from start to finish and keep for days in an airtight container. They are great on their own or crumbled over vanilla ice cream.

MAKES 20 COOKIES

½ cup plus 1 tablespoon (55 g) almond flour

⅓ cup (70 g) sugar

⅓ cup (45 g) raw sliced almonds, coarsely chopped

⅓ cup (45 g) cacao nibs

1 tablespoon tapioca starch

1 teaspoon finely grated orange zest

¼ teaspoon baking soda

¼ teaspoon kosher salt

¼ cup (55 g) melted virgin coconut oil

2 tablespoons canned full-fat coconut milk

1 Preheat the oven to 350 degrees F. Line two baking sheets with parchment paper.

2 In a medium bowl, stir together the almond flour, sugar, almonds, cacao nibs, tapioca starch, orange zest, baking soda, and salt. Add the coconut oil and milk and stir together until all ingredients are fully incorporated.

3 Scoop 1½ teaspoons of dough and quickly shape it into a ball in your hands. Place 5 or 6 cookies on each baking sheet, leaving at least 3 inches of space between because they spread widely.

4 Bake for 8 to 10 minutes, or until golden brown. The cookies tend to spread unevenly; if that bothers you, use a 4-inch cookie cutter to help round them. As soon as the cookies come out of the oven, while they are still soft, place the cookie cutter over them (making sure the cookie is completely inside) and gently apply a circular motion. The edges should round up. Let the cookies cool on the pan for 5 minutes to firm up, then carefully lift with a spatula and transfer to a wire rack to cool completely. The cookies will keep for up to 1 week in an airtight container at room temperature.

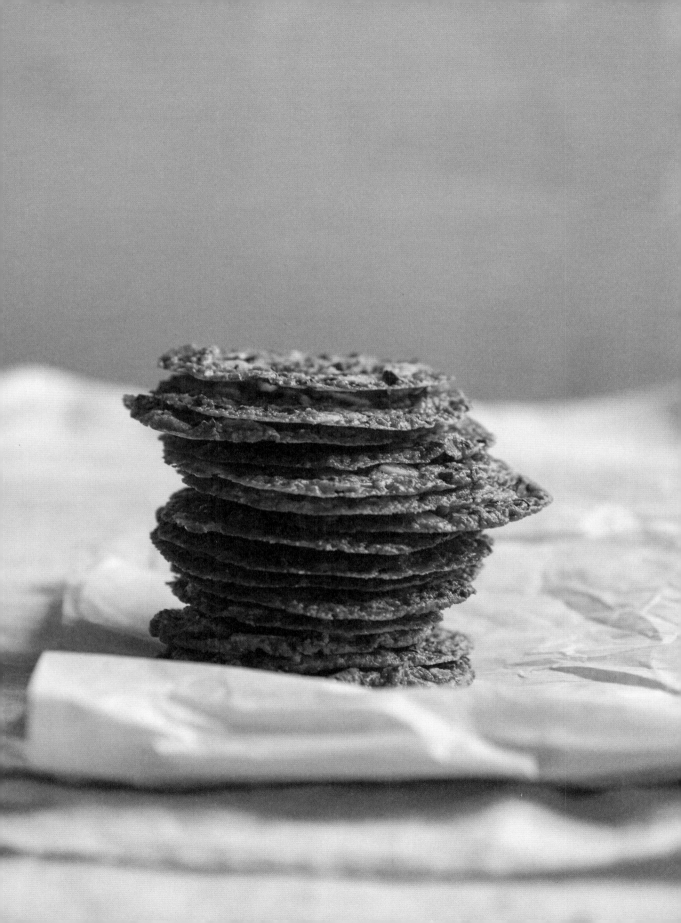

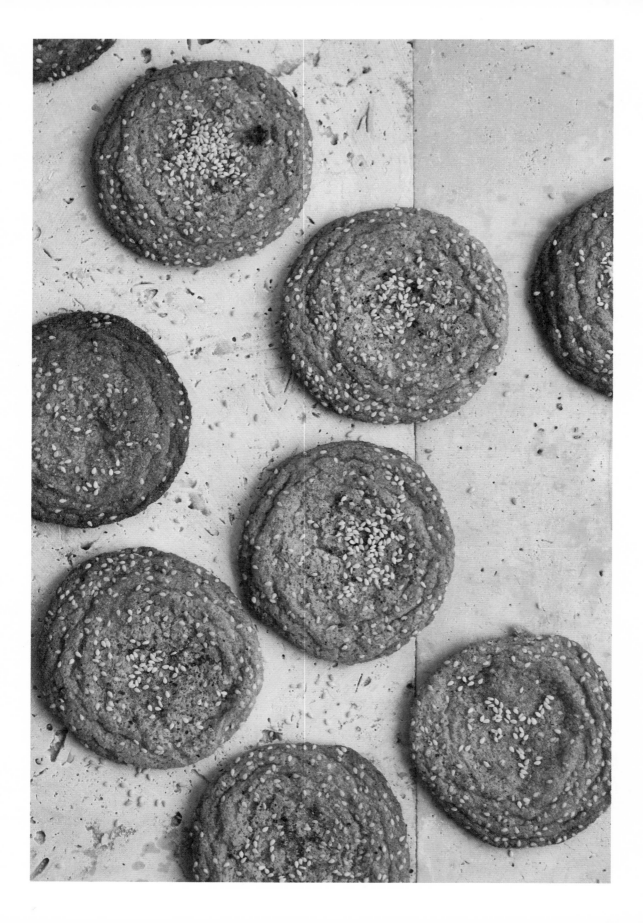

Sesame Snickerdoodles

---

6 tablespoons (85 g) unsalted
   butter or dairy-free butter, at
   room temperature
¼ cup (65 g) well-stirred tahini
½ cup (100 g) plus 2 tablespoons
   sugar, divided
¼ cup (50 g) light brown sugar
1 teaspoon vanilla extract
1 large egg
¾ cup (105 g) sorghum flour
¼ cup (40 g) potato starch
¼ cup (25 g) almond flour
1 teaspoon cream of tartar
½ teaspoon baking soda
½ teaspoon kosher salt
¾ teaspoon ground cinnamon,
   divided
2 tablespoons raw white
   sesame seeds

The perfect snickerdoodle is wrinkly, with very crispy edges but a soft and chewy center. This version, made with tahini and sesame seeds, borders on the savory-sweet territory that I love so much. Personally, I like to up the salt to ¾ teaspoon and even add a touch of freshly ground black pepper, but I kept a conservative amount of salt in the ingredient list and left the black pepper out here. I encourage you to try it for a cookie that has a slight floral spice to it. As always with cookies of this kind, be sure not to overbake or you will miss out on the chewy center.

MAKES 16 COOKIES

1   In the bowl of a stand mixer fitted with the paddle attachment, beat the butter, tahini, ½ cup (100 g) of the sugar, brown sugar, and vanilla for 3 minutes on medium speed, or until very light and airy. Add the egg and beat for another 2 minutes.

2   In a small bowl, whisk together the sorghum flour, potato starch, almond flour, cream of tartar, baking soda, salt, and ¼ teaspoon of the cinnamon. Add to the mixer bowl and beat on medium speed until the dough is very smooth and airy, about 30 seconds. Put the mixer bowl in the refrigerator for 15 minutes.

3   Preheat the oven to 400 degrees F. Line two baking sheets with parchment paper.

4   In a small sauté pan, toast the sesame seeds over medium heat until light golden brown, 1 to 2 minutes. Be careful not to burn them—they go from light golden brown to dark fairly quickly, so keep an eye on them. Transfer to a small bowl to cool, then stir in the remaining 2 tablespoons sugar and ½ teaspoon cinnamon.

5   Scoop 1½-tablespoon mounds of dough and roll in the sesame seed mixture. Place on the baking sheets, leaving 3 inches of space between. I am able to fit 6 cookies on each sheet.

6   Bake for 8 to 9 minutes, until the cookies are light golden brown, the tops have cracked, and the edges are crispy. The centers should stay soft as they firm up while cooling. Cool on the baking sheet for 10 minutes, or until you can lift the cookies without them falling apart. Finish baking the remaining dough. The cookies will keep for 3 days in an airtight container.

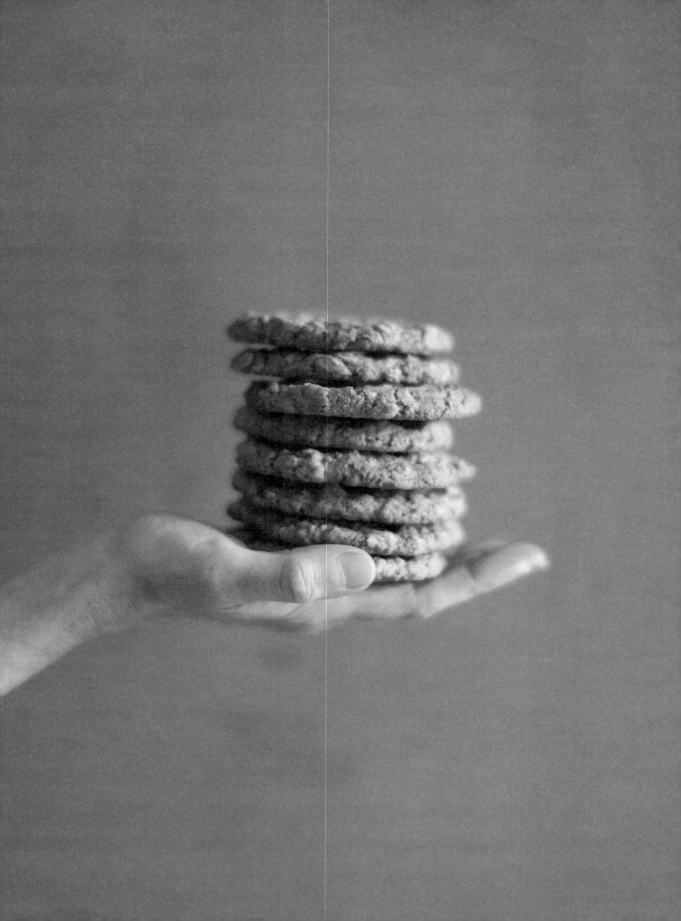

Gingery Oat, Sunflower, and Coconut Cookies

This is a hearty version of an oatmeal cookie loaded with rolled oats, sunflower seeds, and coconut, and spiced with a generous amount of fresh ginger. I kept it simple, but feel free to add other warming spices, such as cinnamon or nutmeg. If I had to pick one cookie for ice cream sandwiches, this one would be it because it is chewy, very textural, and holds its own alongside ice cream.

MAKES 15 COOKIES

½ cup (115 g) unsalted butter or dairy-free butter, at room temperature
½ cup (100 g) sugar
½ cup (120 g) tightly packed light brown sugar
1 tablespoon finely grated fresh ginger
1 teaspoon vanilla extract
1 large egg
1 cup (90 g) gluten-free rolled oats
¾ cup (105 g) sorghum or superfine brown rice flour
½ cup (70 g) raw sunflower seeds
½ cup (50 g) unsweetened finely grated coconut
¼ cup (30 g) tapioca starch
½ teaspoon baking soda
¼ teaspoon baking powder
¼ teaspoon kosher salt

1 Preheat the oven to 350 degrees F. Line two baking sheets with parchment paper.

2 In the bowl of a stand mixer fitted with the paddle attachment, beat the butter, both sugars, ginger, and vanilla on medium speed until smooth, about 1 minute. Scrape the paddle and sides of the bowl, then add the egg and continue mixing until creamy.

3 In a medium bowl, stir together all the remaining ingredients and add to the mixer bowl. Mix on medium speed until all the flour is incorporated into the butter.

4 Using a 3-tablespoon ice cream scoop, drop 4 balls of the dough onto each baking sheet, leaving plenty of space between as the cookies will spread significantly while baking.

5 Bake for 13 to 14 minutes, until golden brown. Let the cookies cool on the pan for 5 minutes, otherwise they will fall apart, then transfer them to a wire rack. Bake the remaining dough. The cookies will keep for up to 3 days in an airtight container at room temperature.

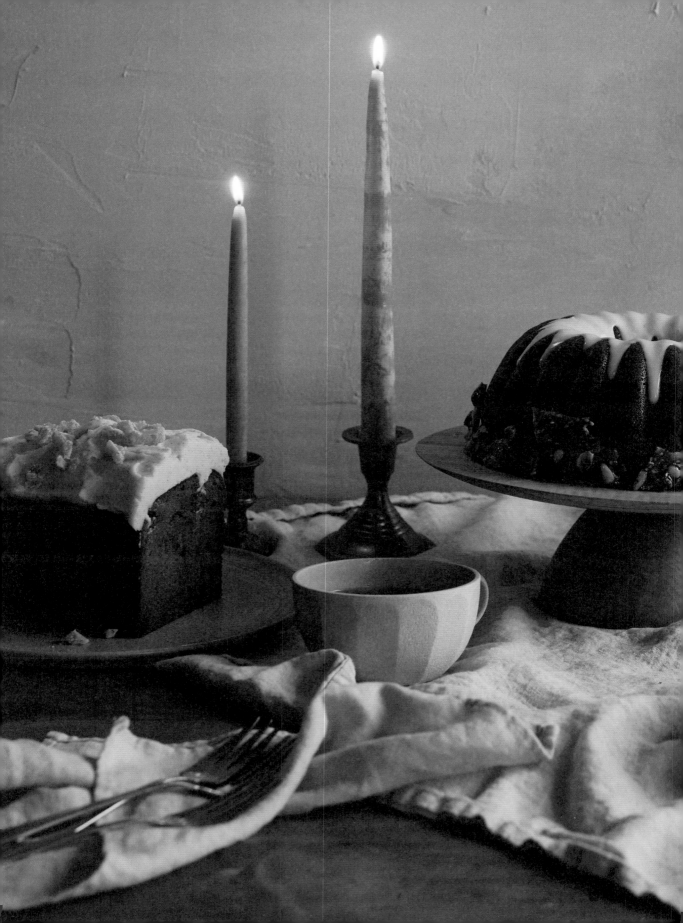

CHAPTER SIX

Holiday Baking

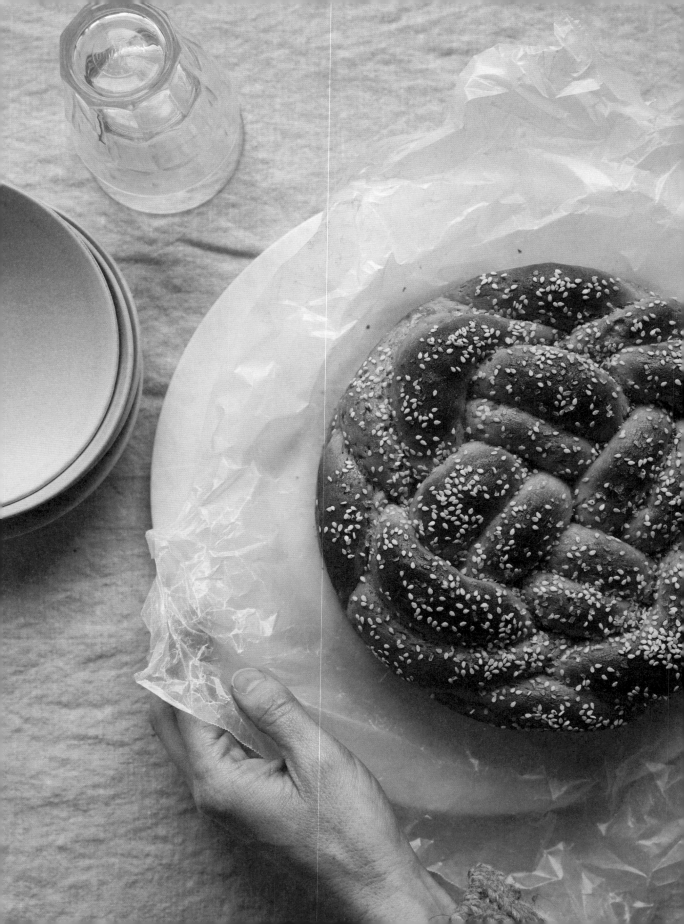

As far as I remember, holidays in my family meant work. The nature of the pastry business was (and still is) to work when everyone else took time off to celebrate. I enjoyed the hustle and bustle of holiday time, particularly leading up to Christmas. Fifty-pound burlap sacks of raw almonds were delivered to the shop. It was my grandmother's job to blanch and peel every single almond that was to be used for marzipan, cookies, and cakes. She recruited the grandchildren to help with the task. My mom and all of her siblings worked around the clock the last week before Christmas. On Christmas Eve, even as a wee girl, I went to the shop bright and early to help deliver pastries or simply talk to the customers waiting in line. I was somewhat of an usher and enjoyed the responsibility assigned to me. At 6 p.m. sharp, when the shop closed, everyone collapsed into their chairs.

Our holiday baking tradition was clearly very European. A vast array of *turrón*, marzipan figurines, *tarta de ponche* (syrup-and-liqueur-soaked sponge cake with egg yolk custard, covered in marzipan), and apple custard tarts encased in rich puff pastry. I have to confess that none of these confections are a big part of my personal holiday baking, but I do feel nostalgic for them.

The recipes in this chapter are influenced by the many people I have met and worked for throughout the years, all filtered through my family's heritage. Some were passed down, some I have learned along the way. You will notice the recipes are heavy in nuts and honey because those are, historically, the ingredients ancient baking traditions have used to celebrate nature and seasons.

Many of these recipes make thoughtful gifts because they keep well for days, such as Chocolate-Hazelnut Toffee (page 252), Buttery Shortbread (page 255), and Apricot and Pecan Rugelach (page 248). Others are beautiful centerpieces, such as the Chocolate Bûche de Noël (page 276), Braided Challah (page 261), and Cranberry Linzertorte (page 271).

It is my hope that some of these recipes will become part of your family traditions as well.

Apricot and Pecan Rugelach

½ cup (70 g) sorghum flour

¼ cup (40 g) potato starch

¼ cup (30 g) tapioca starch, plus more for dusting

½ teaspoon xanthan gum

¼ teaspoon kosher salt

½ cup (115 g) cold unsalted butter or dairy-free butter, cut into ½-inch pieces

½ cup (115 g) cold cream cheese or dairy-free cream cheese spread, cut into ½-inch pieces

½ cup Honey-Apricot Jam (page 55) or other jam of choice

3 tablespoons sugar

¾ teaspoon ground cinnamon

½ cup (75 g) pecans, very finely chopped

1 large egg, lightly beaten with 2 teaspoons water

Rugelach dough is somewhere in between cookie and pastry dough. The cream cheese makes it flaky and tender. These rugelach are filled with apricot and pecan, but you can use any other fruit jam and nut you like. You can shape the rugelach into crescents, but because the dough is delicate and warms quickly, I find it easier to roll it into a log and then cut. Another tip: the dough by itself is perfect to use for a tart or galette.

MAKES 16 RUGELACH

1   To make the dough, in a medium bowl, whisk together the sorghum flour, potato starch, tapioca starch, xanthan gum, and salt. Toss the butter and cream cheese in the flour to coat it, then use your fingers to work them into the flour until you have large lumps of dough. Turn out onto a work surface and lightly knead the dough a couple of times until it comes together. Cut the dough in half, shape into disks, and wrap each piece in parchment paper. Chill the dough for at least 2 hours.

2   While the dough chills, prepare the filling. If the apricot jam is chunky, puree it in a food processor until somewhat smooth. Transfer it to a small bowl and set aside. In another small bowl, whisk together the sugar and cinnamon. Set aside.

3   Lightly dust a work surface and rolling pin with tapioca starch, and have more nearby. Remove one dough half from the refrigerator. If it's too cold to roll, let it sit at room temperature for 5 minutes. Roll the dough into an 8-inch square, approximately ⅛ inch thick. The dough will be sticky, so move it often and dust the surfaces with tapioca starch again as needed. Don't let the dough become too soft or it will be hard to roll. Trim the edges to create a nice square.

4   Brush the dough with half of the apricot jam, then sprinkle with half of the pecans, and one-third of the cinnamon-sugar. Place a piece of parchment paper over the top and gently press down so the pecans stick to the jam. Roll the dough into a tight log and press down gently on the seam to seal. Put the log in the freezer. Repeat the rolling out, filling, and rolling up with the second piece of dough and remaining filling. Freeze the logs for 15 minutes.

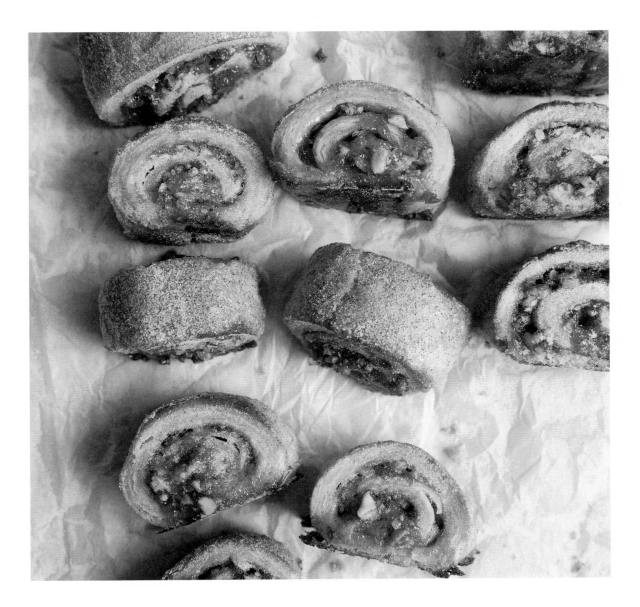

5   Preheat the oven to 350 degrees F. Line a baking sheet with parchment paper.

6   Brush the dough logs with the egg wash, then sprinkle all sides with the remaining one-third cinnamon-sugar. Cut each log into 1-inch-thick rounds and place them standing upright, seam side down, on the baking sheet.

7   Bake for 20 to 25 minutes, until golden brown. Let the rugelach cool for 10 minutes before removing them from the baking sheet. They will keep for up to 5 days in an airtight container.

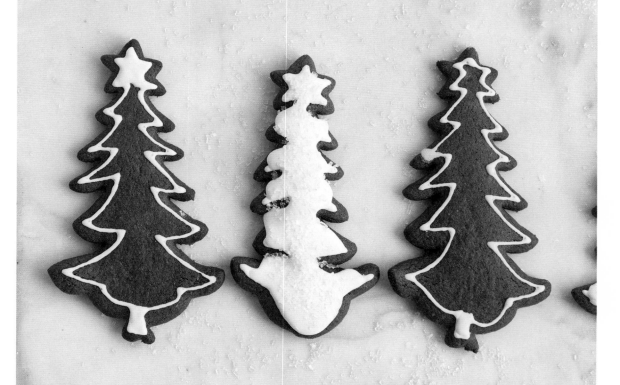

Gingerbread Cutout Cookies

The scent of the warm spices in these gingerbread cookies is intoxicating. Gingerbread cookies are sometimes too hard for my liking, but almond flour makes these tender. Use this recipe to create gingerbread houses, but be sure to roll out the dough on the thicker side (¼ to ⅓ inch thick) and bake a little bit longer so it dries out. My trick is to turn off the oven after baking and leave the gingerbread in for another 10 to 15 minutes to dry.

MAKES 26 TO 32 COOKIES

1¼ cups (175 g) light buckwheat flour
1 cup (100 g) almond flour
¾ cup (120 g) potato starch
½ cup (60 g) tapioca starch
1½ teaspoons ground cinnamon
1½ teaspoons ground ginger
½ teaspoon ground nutmeg
½ teaspoon xanthan gum
½ teaspoon kosher salt
¼ teaspoon ground cloves
¼ teaspoon baking soda
6 tablespoons (85 g) unsalted butter or dairy-free butter, at room temperature
¾ cup (150 g) light brown sugar
½ cup (160 g) molasses
1 large egg
1 cup Royal Icing (page 256)

1 In a medium bowl, whisk together both flours, both starches, cinnamon, ginger, nutmeg, xanthan gum, salt, cloves, and baking soda.

2 In the bowl of a stand mixer fitted with the paddle attachment, beat the butter and brown sugar on medium speed until creamy and smooth, about 2 minutes.

3 Add the molasses and beat again until smooth. Add the egg and beat until just incorporated. Aerating the dough can cause it to puff up too much. Add the dry ingredients and mix until you have a soft, sticky dough.

4 Divide the dough in half and wrap each piece in parchment paper or plastic wrap. Chill the dough for at least 2 hours, or preferably overnight, so it is well hydrated. (The dough can be tightly wrapped and frozen at this point. Thaw in the refrigerator before baking.)

5 Preheat the oven to 350 degrees F. Line two baking sheets with parchment paper.

6 Roll out the dough ⅛ inch to ¼ inch thick and use cookie cutters in the desired shapes. Arrange the cookies on the baking sheets, leaving 1 inch between. Put the baking sheets in the refrigerator for 15 minutes to firm the dough so the cookies retain their shapes when baked. The dough can be rerolled several times.

7 Bake for 9 to 11 minutes, until the edges turn golden brown and the centers are slightly soft. Let the cookies cool on the baking sheets for 10 minutes, then transfer to a wire rack. Once completely cooled, decorate with royal icing. Store the cookies in an airtight container for up to 5 days.

Chocolate-Hazelnut Toffee

¾ cup (100 g) raw hazelnuts
1 cup (225 g) unsalted butter
    or dairy-free butter, cut into
    1-inch cubes
¾ cup (150 g) sugar
½ cup (100 g) light brown sugar
¼ cup (55 g) water, at room
    temperature
½ teaspoon kosher salt
2 teaspoons vanilla extract
¼ teaspoon baking soda
4 ounces (115 g) 70 percent
    chocolate, very finely
    chopped

This chocolate and hazelnut toffee is one of my favorite treats to gift during the holidays. Crack the toffee into shards and package it in small paper boxes. As with most candymaking, be sure to use a calibrated candy thermometer to cook the sugar to the right temperature—not too soft and not too hard.

MAKES ONE 9-BY-13-INCH SHEET

1   Preheat the oven to 325 degrees F. Line a 9-by-13-inch rimmed baking sheet with parchment paper and set aside.

2   On a second, unlined baking sheet, spread the hazelnuts and roast for 15 to 20 minutes, until fragrant and golden brown. When they are cool enough to handle, transfer them to a large kitchen towel and rub together to loosen their skins. Once they are mostly peeled (it's OK if they still have some skin), transfer them to a food processor and pulse several times to roughly chop. I like to have some small and medium pieces mixed throughout. Set aside.

3   In a medium saucepan, stir together the butter, both sugars, water, and salt. Cook over medium-high heat, undisturbed, until a candy thermometer reads 300 degrees F, about 15 minutes. The mixture will be dark brown and begin to smell like it might burn. Remove the pan from the heat and add the vanilla carefully—it will splatter. Stir in the baking soda until it is distributed throughout, but don't overmix. You want to preserve the bit of gas that the baking soda produces.

4   Pour the toffee onto the prepared baking sheet and spread it evenly with a spatula. Sprinkle the top with the chopped chocolate. The heat of the toffee will melt it. Spread it evenly with the spatula. Distribute the chopped hazelnuts evenly across the top and lightly press down so they stick to the chocolate.

5   Let the toffee cool completely at room temperature for at least 4 to 5 hours. I like to find a cold corner of my house and tuck it away. You can speed up the process by chilling in the refrigerator for 10 to 15 minutes. Break the toffee into bite-size pieces. Store it in an airtight container for up to 1 month.

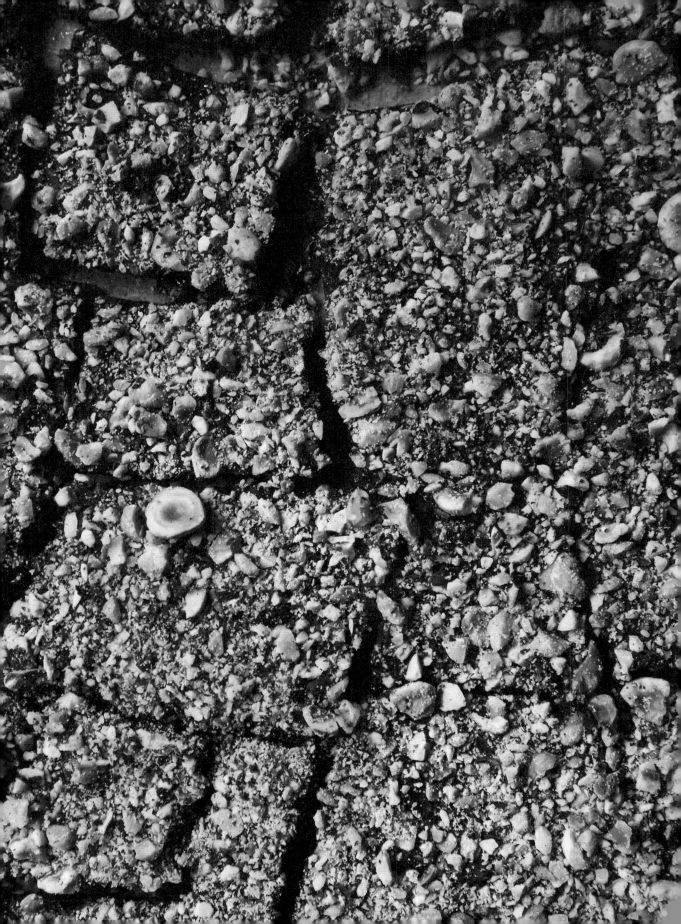

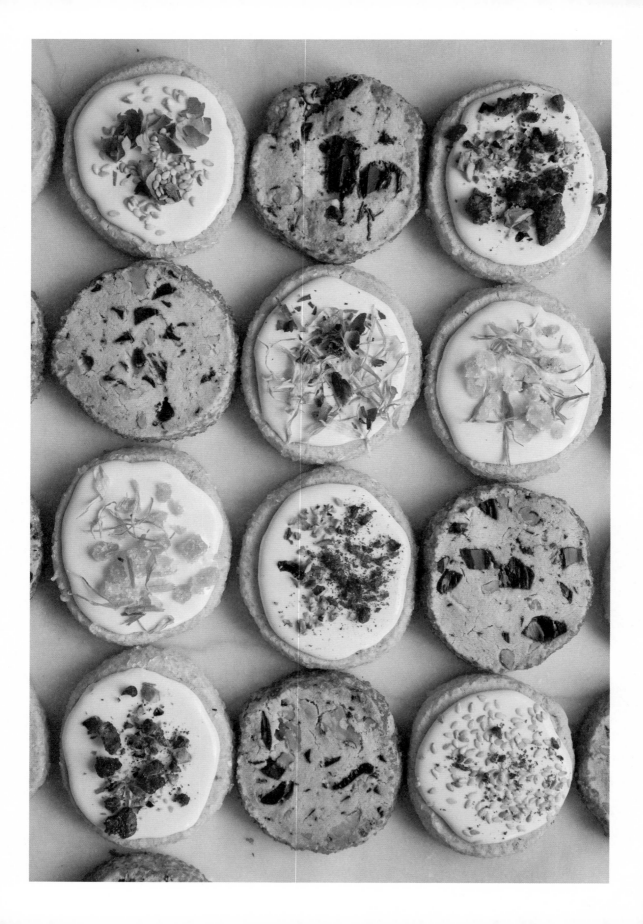

Buttery Shortbread

1 cup (225 g) unsalted butter or dairy-free butter, at room temperature
¾ cup (90 g) powdered sugar
2 teaspoons vanilla extract
2 large egg yolks
1 cup (105 g) gluten-free oat flour
¾ cup (105 g) sorghum flour
½ cup (80 g) sweet white rice flour
½ cup (60 g) tapioca starch
1 teaspoon kosher salt
Coarse sugar, for rolling

Harinados or *mantecadas* are some of my favorite Christmas-time cookies in Spain. Traditional ones are made with lard, and even though they are sweets, they also taste a touch savory. I love them. The texture of this shortbread reminds me of those *mantecadas*—a little sandy, crumbly, but with a bit of snap. You can make them simply, just with vanilla, or follow some of the suggested variations on page 256.

MAKES 30 COOKIES

1 In the bowl of a stand mixer fitted with the paddle attachment, combine the butter, powdered sugar, and vanilla. Beat the butter and sugar on medium speed until creamy and smooth, about 2 minutes. Scrape the sides, bottom, and paddle, then add the egg yolks and mix again until smooth.

2 In a small bowl, whisk together all the flours, tapioca starch, and salt. Add to the mixer and beat on medium speed until the dough comes together.

3 Scrape the dough onto a piece of parchment paper set on a work surface and use it to shape the dough into a rounded log 1½ inches in diameter. Wrap the log tightly and refrigerate for 30 minutes or so, until the dough has hardened slightly but is still pliable, then give the log another roll. This will ensure that the dough doesn't develop a flat bottom, and results in perfect cookie circles. Return the dough to the refrigerator to chill for another 1½ hours.

4 Preheat the oven to 350 degrees F. Line two baking sheets with parchment paper. Spread some coarse sugar on a clean surface and roll the chilled dough over it, pressing so the sugar sticks. Cut the log into ¼- to ⅓-inch-thick disks and arrange on the prepared baking sheets, leaving about 2 inches between cookies, as they will spread a little.

5 Bake for 12 to 14 minutes, rotating the pans halfway through, until the edges begin to set and turn golden brown. Do not overbake or the cookies will dry out. They might appear a bit too soft, but they crisp up as they cool. Let the cookies cool on the baking sheet for 10 minutes, or until they can be lifted without crumbling. Store them in an airtight container for up to 5 days. $\longrightarrow$

PECAN-CHOCOLATE

Finely chop ½ cup (75 g) pecans and coarsely chop 3 ounces (85 g) 70 percent chocolate. Fold both into the shortbread dough at the end of step 2. Roll the log of dough in turbinado sugar before slicing.

GLAZED

Spread a thin layer of Royal Icing (recipe below) on the cookies, then sprinkle with ½ teaspoon finely chopped toasted nuts or candied flowers. Let the glaze set for 30 minutes before handling the cookies.

Royal Icing

2⅔ cup (320 g) powdered
    sugar, sifted
2 large egg whites
¼ teaspoon cream of tartar

Substitute pasteurized eggs if you are concerned about using raw egg whites.

MAKES 1 CUP

1 Use a spatula to stir all the ingredients in a medium bowl until you have a thick, smooth paste. Let the icing rest for 10 minutes, then check that it is the desired consistency—add more powdered sugar for a drier icing or a touch of water for a thinner one. Make sure the cookies are cooled before glazing. The icing will keep tightly wrapped in the refrigerator for up to 5 days. Bring the icing to room temperature before using.

Hot Cross Buns

1¼ cups (300 g) whole milk or oat milk, heated to 105 degrees F, plus more if needed

2 teaspoons (8 g) active dry yeast

2½ tablespoons (25 g) psyllium husk powder

1 cup plus 1 tablespoon (110 g) gluten-free oat flour

1 cup (120 g) tapioca starch, plus more for dusting

¾ cup (120 g) potato starch

½ cup (100 g) sugar, divided

2 teaspoons finely grated lemon zest

2 teaspoons finely grated orange zest

1 teaspoon kosher salt

1 teaspoon ground cinnamon

½ teaspoon ground cardamom

3 large eggs, divided

¾ cup (90 g) dried currants

4 tablespoons very soft unsalted butter or dairy-free butter, plus more for greasing

2 tablespoons plus 1 teaspoon water, divided

1 cup (120 g) powdered sugar

4 teaspoons cold whole milk or oat milk

I didn't grow up with hot cross buns, but we did enjoy something similar called *mokots*. It is the Basque version of an enriched sweet dough that is served on Easter Sunday. The Basque *mokots* is shaped into a crown and has a cooked egg nestled in the center, which represents rebirth and renewal. These traditional hot cross buns are scented with citrus, cardamom, cinnamon, and currants. They are perfectly tender and slightly sweet.

MAKES 12 BUNS

1   In a medium bowl, whisk together the heated milk and yeast. Proof until the yeast bubbles and a thin layer of foam forms on top, about 10 minutes. Whisk in the psyllium powder and let it gel for 5 minutes.

2   In the bowl of a stand mixer fitted with a dough hook, whisk together the oat flour, tapioca starch, potato starch, ¼ cup (50 g) of the sugar, lemon and orange zests, salt, cinnamon, and cardamom. Add the psyllium gel. Begin mixing on medium speed.

3   In a small bowl, lightly beat 2 of the eggs and add them to the mixer. Mix for 1 minute, until the eggs are incorporated, then add the currants. At this point the dough might look a bit dry. Continue mixing for another 2 minutes, then add the butter, 1 tablespoon at a time, waiting for each one to be incorporated before adding the next. Mix the dough for another minute until it's sticky and all ingredients are well combined. The dough shouldn't feel dry, but if it does, add 1 additional teaspoon of lukewarm milk until you have a sticky, pliable dough.

4   Grease a large bowl with butter. Scrape the dough into the bowl and turn it to coat so the surface is no longer sticky. Cover the bowl with a clean kitchen towel and proof for 45 minutes to 1 hour, until doubled. $\longrightarrow$

5   Line a 9-by-13-inch rimmed baking sheet with parchment paper. Lightly dust a work surface with tapioca starch. Turn the dough out onto it and cut into 12 equal pieces (each about 80 grams). Roll each piece into a ball and arrange on the baking sheet, making sure the dough is nearly touching. This way the rolls will attach to each other while baking and rise up. Cover the dough with a clean kitchen towel and proof for 30 minutes, or until doubled and the dough pieces nearly touch.

6   Meanwhile, preheat the oven to 375 degrees F. In a small bowl, lightly beat the remaining egg with 1 teaspoon of water. When the dough is ready, brush all over with the egg wash. Bake the buns for 25 to 30 minutes, until golden brown.

7   While the buns are baking, make the glaze. Combine the remaining ¼ cup (50 g) sugar and 2 tablespoons water in a small saucepan. Heat over medium-high heat until the sugar has melted and the syrup boils. As soon as the buns come out of the oven, brush the tops with this glaze. Let the buns cool completely on the baking sheet.

8   Make the icing by whisking the powdered sugar and cold milk in a medium bowl until smooth and lump free. It will be thick. Transfer the icing into a piping bag and cut off a small opening at the tip. Pipe crosses over the buns, then serve. They are best eaten on the same day.

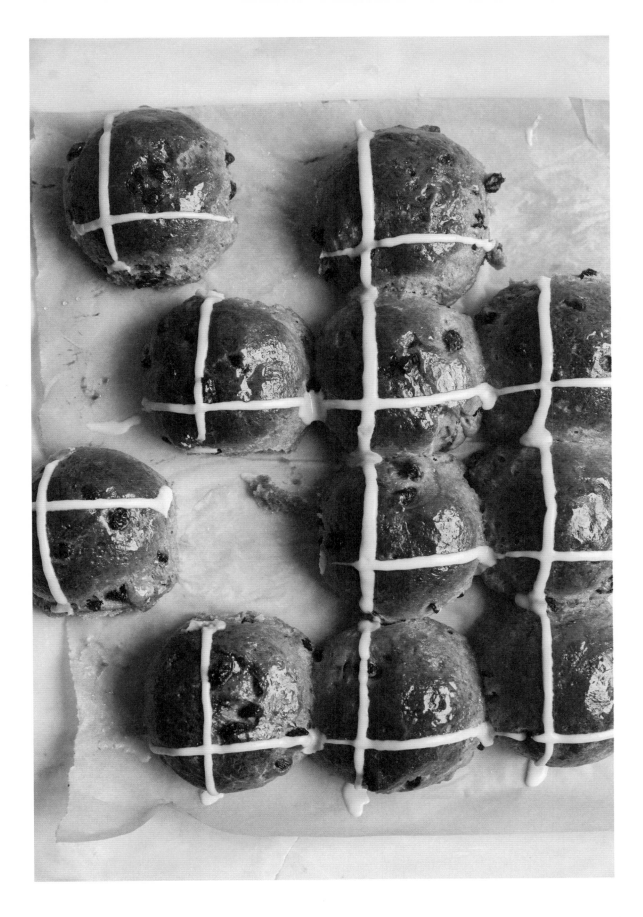

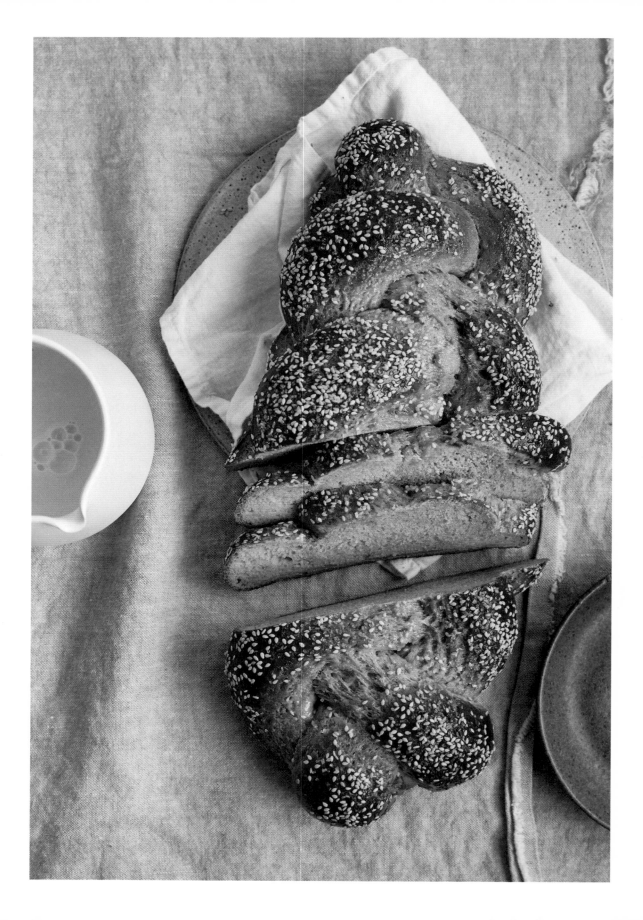

Braided Challah

1¼ cups plus 1 tablespoon (315 g) whole milk or oat milk, heated to 105 degrees F, plus more if needed

2½ teaspoons (10 g) active dry yeast

3 tablespoons (30 g) psyllium husk powder

1 cup (160 g) potato starch

1 cup (140 g) sweet white rice flour

1 cup (120 g) tapioca starch, plus more for dusting

½ cup (70 g) superfine brown rice flour

½ cup (100 g) sugar

1½ teaspoons kosher salt

1 teaspoon xanthan gum (optional)

Zest of 1 medium orange

¼ cup (55 g) extra-virgin olive oil, plus more for greasing and brushing

4 large eggs, divided

1 tablespoon raw sesame seeds or sparkling sugar

When we lived in Florida, many of our friends observed Sabbath and welcomed us to join them. Challah was always offered. I am often asked for a gluten-free challah recipe, and I am excited to share this with you. It is based on the Olive Oil Brioche (page 81) with added xanthan gum to give the dough more elasticity and support when braiding. You can omit it, but the dough will have less structure. Also, see the raisin and streusel variation on page 262.

I have never been able to master very complex braiding—the four-braid is my preferred method. (I highly recommend you watch challah-braiding tutorials online if you want to be mesmerized.) A note about shaping and proofing: The dough tends to expand to the sides when fermenting, which is OK. However, if you prefer a taller challah, I suggest you braid it, shape it into a crown, and ferment it in a 10-inch cake pan. This will provide a bit of extra support.

MAKES 1 LARGE OR 2 MEDIUM CHALLAHS

1   In a medium bowl, whisk together the milk and yeast. Proof until the yeast bubbles and a thin layer of foam forms on top, about 10 minutes. Whisk in the psyllium powder and let it gel for 5 minutes.

2   In the bowl of a stand mixer fitted with a dough hook, combine the potato starch, sweet white rice flour, tapioca starch, brown rice flour, sugar, salt, xanthan gum, and orange zest. Add the psyllium gel. Begin mixing on medium speed and add the olive oil and 3 of the eggs, one at a time. Mix the dough for 2 minutes or until it comes together and is lump free. It will be sticky. Add a bit more milk if the dough feels dry.

3   Grease a large bowl with olive oil and scrape the dough into it, shaping the dough into a ball as much as possible. Turn it over to coat with oil. At this point it won't feel as sticky and you should be able to shape it more easily. Tightly cover the bowl with a clean kitchen towel or plastic wrap and refrigerate at least 4 hours or up to 12 hours. Chilling the dough is an important step, so don't skip it. The dough needs to be very cold and hydrated to be braidable without the strands falling apart. ⟶

4   After the dough has chilled, lightly dust a work surface with tapioca starch and turn out the dough. If you are making a large challah, cut the dough into 3 or 4 equal pieces, depending on whether it will have three or four braids. If you are making 2 medium challahs, cut the dough in half, then cut each half into 3 or 4 equal pieces. Roll the dough pieces into balls, then into strands about 14 inches long (12 inches for medium challahs) and tapered at the ends. Arrange the dough strands vertically and pinch them together at the top. Braid each challah carefully and pinch again at the bottom. Tuck the ends under. Note that if your braid doesn't turn out correctly the first time, you can knead the dough back together and start over.

5   Line a baking sheet with parchment paper. Put the challah on it, cover with a clean kitchen towel, and proof for 45 minutes to 1 hour, or until nearly doubled.

6   Meanwhile, preheat the oven 375 degrees F. Lightly beat the remaining egg in a small bowl and brush the top and all the crevasses of the challah. Sprinkle the sesame seeds or sugar over the dough.

7   Bake for 35 minutes for a large challah or 30 minutes for medium ones, until golden brown. Let the challah cool completely before cutting into it. It will keep at room temperature tightly wrapped in parchment for 1 day or can be frozen for up to 3 months.

RAISIN CHALLAH WITH STREUSEL

Stir in ⅔ cup raisins after mixing the dough at the end of step 2. Once the braided dough has proofed, sprinkle it with ⅓ cup Streusel (page 49) instead of sesame seeds before baking.

Pantxineta

1 recipe Buttery Rough Puff
   Pastry Dough (page 180)
1½ cups Pastry Cream (page 34),
   chilled
¼ cup (25 g) almond flour
1 large egg, lightly beaten
⅓ cup (35 g) blanched almonds
   or hazelnuts, coarsely
   chopped
Powdered sugar, for dusting

Pantxineta is a traditional Basque tart: puff pastry layers filled with pastry cream and topped with almonds. The tart was made famous by Casa Otaegui in San Sebastián. My grandfather Angel was good friends with one of the Otaegui children. He never put *pantxineta* on the menu at his pastry shop as a sign of respect—it was his friend's to have—but he did make it for the family during holidays, always served warm out of the oven with flaky layers and creamy custard.

Pithiviers are similar to *pantxineta* but filled with frangipane. They are also called *galette des rois* and served on January 6 for Epiphany. You can find this variation below.

MAKES 8 INDIVIDUAL TARTS

1   Line a baking sheet with parchment paper. Cut the puff pastry dough in half. Roll out one of the halves to an ⅛-inch thickness. Using a 3½-inch round cookie cutter, cut 8 disks from the dough and place them on the baking sheet.

2   Put the chilled pastry cream in a medium bowl and fold in the almond flour, then spoon 1 tablespoon of the mixture into the center of each disk, leaving a ½-inch border all around. Don't overfill or the cream will ooze out when baked.

3   Preheat the oven to 375 degrees F.

4   Meanwhile, roll the remaining dough to an ⅛-inch thickness. Using a 4-inch round cookie cutter, cut 8 more disks of dough. Brush the exposed edges of the tart bottoms with the beaten egg, then gently lay the larger dough disks over the top. Lightly press the edges with a fork to seal. Make a small incision in the center of each tart using the tip of a knife, then put the baking sheet in the refrigerator for 15 minutes.

5   Brush the tart tops with egg and sprinkle generously with the almonds. Bake for 30 to 35 minutes, until golden brown and slightly puffed. Dust with powdered sugar and serve warm.

PITHIVIERS

Use Frangipane (page 38) in place of the pastry cream. Flavor the frangipane with 1 tablespoon dark rum and seeds scraped from ½ vanilla bean.

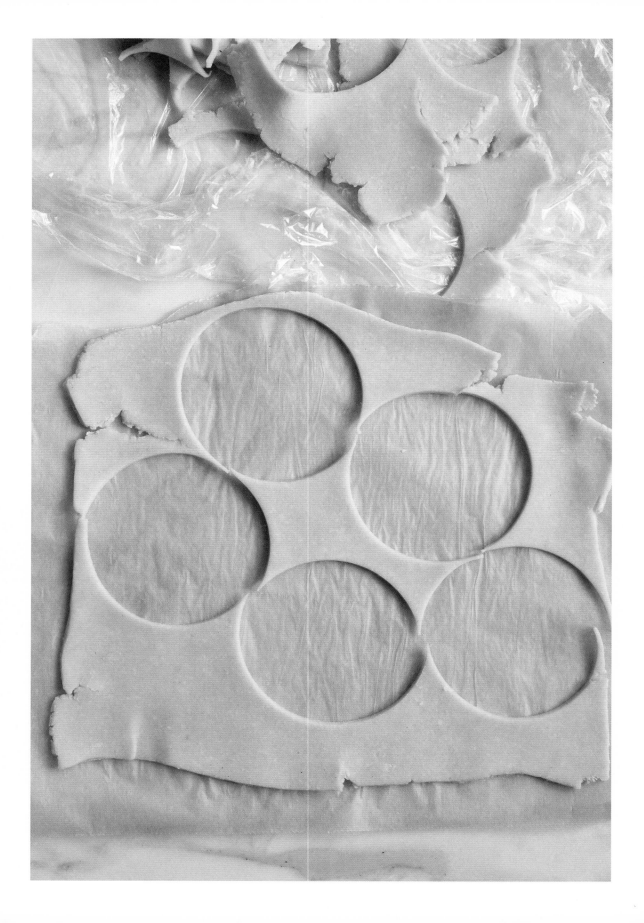

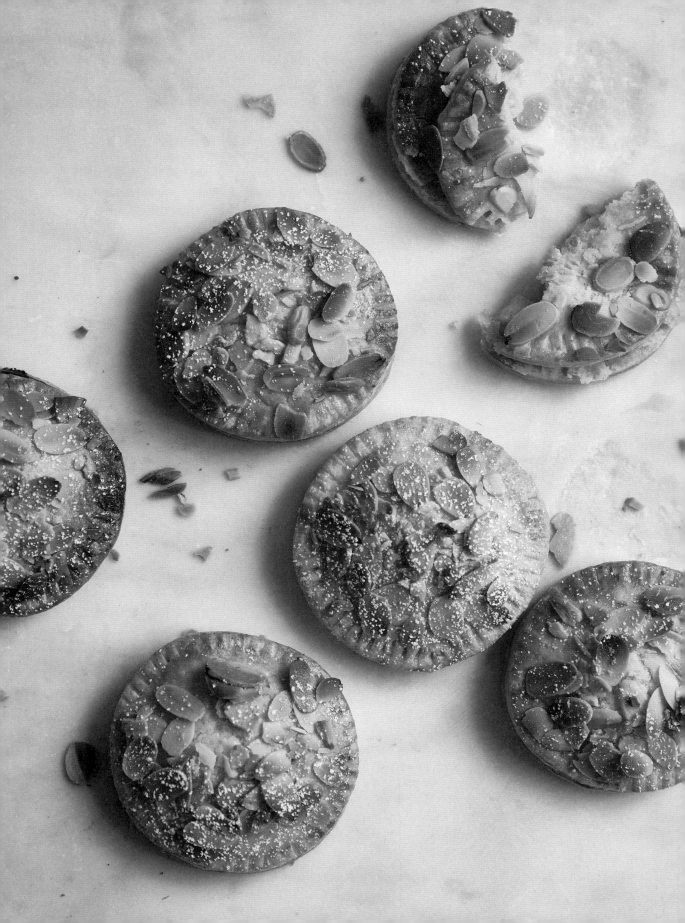

Pumpkin and Pine Nut Tart

1 recipe Date-Nut Crust
(page 267), made with
pine nuts
1 (15-ounce or 425-g) can
pumpkin puree
⅓ cup (70 g) sugar
¼ cup (70 g) maple syrup
1 teaspoon ground cinnamon
½ teaspoon ground ginger
½ teaspoon kosher salt
2 large eggs
1¼ cups (300 g) half-and-half or
canned full-fat coconut milk
3 tablespoons pine nuts,
toasted

Pumpkin pie seems to be one of those traditional desserts that some love, some detest, but it always makes an appearance on holiday tables. Personally, I adore traditional pumpkin pie. I learned to love it later in life because we had no pumpkin custard or even pumpkin baked goods when I was growing up. My version of pumpkin pie features a date-sweetened press-in pine nut short crust that you don't have to roll and is filled with a silky custard lightly sweetened with maple syrup.

If you want to make your own pumpkin puree, halve a pumpkin (Winter Luxury is my favorite variety for baking), put it cut side down on a baking sheet, and roast at 400 degrees F for 35 to 40 minutes, until the flesh is tender. Discard the seeds and skin, then puree the pumpkin flesh in a food processor until smooth.

MAKES ONE 9-INCH TART

1   Press the crust evenly into a 9-inch tart pan with removable bottom. Begin at the bottom center and move out and up the sides. Lightly press with your palm or the bottom of a measuring cup to ensure the dough is tightly packed and even. Put the pan in the freezer for 10 minutes before baking.

2   Preheat the oven to 375 degrees F. Place the prepared crust on a baking sheet and parbake for 15 minutes, until lightly golden brown. Let it cool slightly while you make the filling.

3   In a large bowl, whisk together the pumpkin puree, sugar, maple syrup, cinnamon, ginger, and salt until smooth. Whisk in the eggs and half-and-half until smooth.

4   Pour the filling into the crust and carefully slide the pan into the oven. Reduce the oven temperature to 350 degrees F and bake for 45 minutes or until the center of the tart doesn't jiggle when you lightly shake the pan. A knife inserted in the center won't come out completely clean—don't overcook it or the custard will crack. Remember that it will continue to set as it cools.

5   Let the tart cool completely. I prefer it chilled, so refrigerate for at least 4 hours before serving. Decorate the edges with toasted pine nuts. The tart keeps in the refrigerator for up to 2 days.

Date-Nut Crust

4 ounces (115 g) plump pitted
   Medjool dates (about 6)
¾ cup (105 g) superfine brown
   rice flour
⅔ cup (100 g) pine nuts or
   pecans
¼ cup (30 g) tapioca starch
¼ teaspoon kosher salt
6 tablespoons (85 g) cold
   unsalted butter, dairy-free
   butter, or virgin coconut oil,
   cut into ½-inch pieces

This crust can be made using a variety of nuts, including pine nuts, pecans, walnuts, or pistachios, and works really well with cream and fruit fillings, such as Pastry Cream (page 34), or even as a base for cheesecake.

MAKES ONE 9-INCH CRUST

1   Combine the dates, brown rice flour, nuts, tapioca starch, and salt in a food processor and pulse ten times until the dates and nuts are pulverized.

2   Add the butter and pulse five times, until the dough becomes a dry crumble. The dough should stick together when pressed. If it feels dry, add a teaspoon of ice water. Press the dough into a tart pan. It can be tightly wrapped and stored in the refrigerator for up to 2 days.

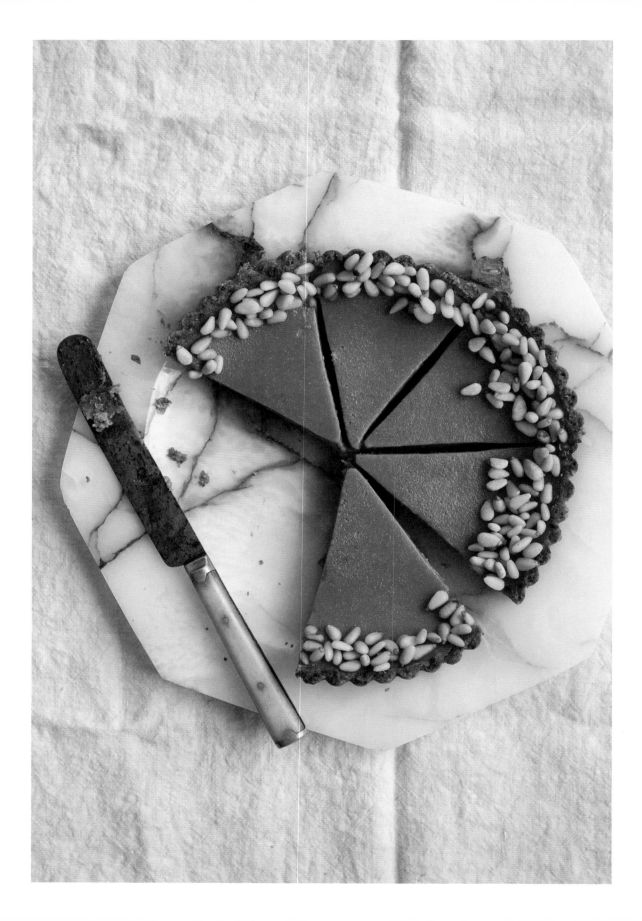

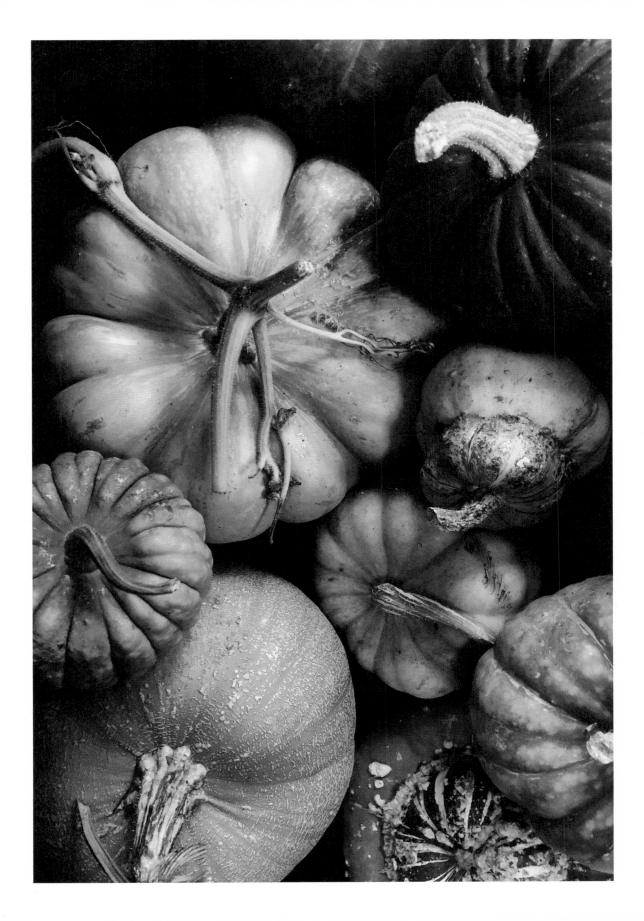

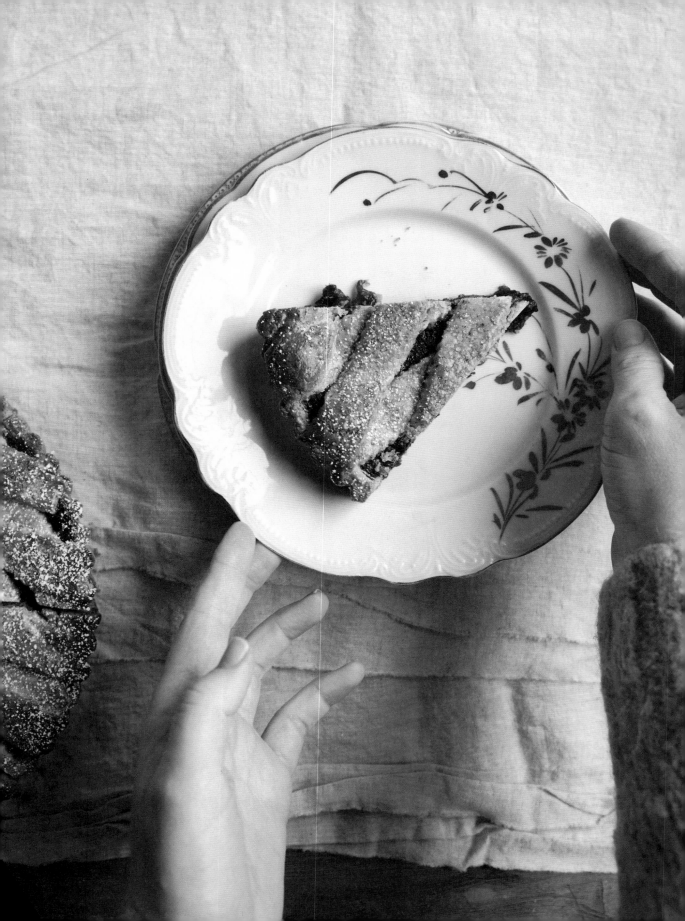

Cranberry Linzertorte

For the filling
1 pound (454 g) fresh or
    frozen cranberries
½ cup (160 g) maple syrup
¼ cup (55 g) freshly squeezed
    orange juice
1 tablespoon finely grated
    orange zest
¼ teaspoon kosher salt

For the crust and assembly
2¼ cups (225 g) hazelnut flour
1 cup (140 g) superfine brown
    rice flour
1 cup (120 g) powdered sugar,
    plus more for dusting
⅓ cup (40 g) tapioca starch,
    plus more for dusting
¼ cup (40 g) potato starch
1 teaspoon ground cinnamon
1 teaspoon ground cardamom
1 teaspoon ground cloves
¾ teaspoon kosher salt
½ teaspoon xanthan gum
    (optional)
1 cup (225 g) cold unsalted
    butter or dairy-free butter, cut
    into ½-inch pieces
2 large eggs, divided
1 large egg yolk
Coarse sugar, for topping

Linzertorte is a traditional Austrian tart with a buttery, nutty dough made from hazelnuts, a jam filling, and a lattice top. Cranberries are not a traditional filling, but I love their tartness with the rich crust. You could simply use raspberry preserves in their place if desired. Note that xanthan gum is optional here—since this is a dough that needs to be handled a bit, the xanthan gum adds a bit more elasticity. The dough needs to chill for at least 4 hours, so be sure to give yourself enough time. You will also have some leftover dough, which you can turn into cookies. Roll ¼ inch to ⅛ inch thick and cut into different shapes. It makes for a great sandwich cookie with some raspberry preserves in the middle.

MAKES ONE 9-INCH TART

1   To make the filling, combine the cranberries, maple syrup, orange juice and zest, and salt in a medium saucepan. Cover and cook over medium-high heat until the cranberries burst and the filling thickens, about 15 minutes. Transfer to a bowl to cool completely. The filling can be made 1 day in advance.

2   To make the crust, in a food processor, combine the hazelnut flour, brown rice flour, powdered sugar, tapioca starch, potato starch, cinnamon, cardamom, cloves, salt, and xanthan gum. Pulse a couple of times to aerate and mix the ingredients. Add the butter and pulse ten times, until it is cut into very small pieces (smaller than peas).

3   In a small bowl, lightly beat 1 of the eggs and egg yolk together and add to the processor bowl. Pulse until the dough comes together and resembles cookie dough. You will see very small pieces of butter throughout. Scrape out the dough onto a work surface. Cut it in half, shape it into a disk, and wrap each piece in parchment paper. Flatten the dough with your hands. Chill for at least 4 hours. ⟶

4   Once the dough is chilled, dust a work surface and rolling pin with tapioca starch. Place one of the dough disks on it and dust the top with a bit more tapioca starch. Roll out the dough ¼ inch to ⅛ inch thick. The dough will be quite soft, so work as quickly as possible and keep the room temperature cool. Gently lift the dough with both hands and drape it over a 9-inch tart pan with a removable bottom. Press the dough into the pan and scrape off any excess. You can reroll the excess dough once if needed.

5   Spread the cranberry filling inside the tart, then work on the decorations for the top.

6   Dust the work surface and rolling pin again with tapioca starch. Place the second dough disk on it and roll out ¼ inch to ⅛ inch thick. Using a pizza or pastry cutter, cut the dough into 13- to 14-inch-long strips about ¾ inch wide. Arrange half of the strips across the tart filling, leaving ¾ inch between strips. Turn the tart pan 90 degrees and arrange the remaining strips of dough perpendicularly over the others to create a lattice top. There is no need to weave the strips together. Press down on the edges of the tart pan to remove any excess dough. Put the tart in the freezer for 10 minutes to chill the dough.

7   Preheat the oven to 375 degrees F. Place the tart on a baking sheet. Lightly whisk the remaining egg in a small bowl and brush the lattice with it. Sprinkle some coarse sugar on top.

8   Bake for 35 to 40 minutes, until the filling is bubbly and the crust is golden brown. Let the tart cool completely before unmolding as it is fairly fragile. Just before serving, dust with powdered sugar. The tart will keep in the refrigerator for up to 3 days.

Profiteroles with Chocolate Glaze

½ cup (60 g) tapioca starch
⅓ cup (45 g) superfine brown rice flour
¼ cup (40 g) potato starch
½ cup (115 g) whole milk or oat milk
½ cup (115 g) water, at room temperature
½ cup (115 g) unsalted butter or dairy-free butter, cut into 1-inch pieces
½ teaspoon sugar
½ teaspoon kosher salt
4 to 5 large eggs, lightly beaten
2 cups Pastry Cream (page 34), for filling
1 cup Chocolate Glaze (page 46), or powdered sugar, for topping

Profiteroles, or *chuchus* as we call them in Spanish, are one of my family's signature pastries. I grew up helping my grandmother fill them, then coating the tops with ganache or liquid fondant. On holidays and special occasions, and by special order only, my grandfather made incredible towers of croquembouche, which are filled choux glued with caramel and topped with spun sugar. A masterpiece. Another favorite was the Paris-Brest (see page 274), which is a crown made with circles of choux that is baked, halved crosswise, and filled with mousseline.

Unfilled profiteroles can easily be frozen. Line a baking sheet with parchment paper and lay the profiteroles in a single layer. Freeze for 20 minutes. Once rock solid, transfer them into a freezer bag. To thaw, I simply leave them at room temperature for an hour.

MAKES ABOUT 30 PROFITEROLES

1   Preheat the oven to 400 degrees F. Position two racks in the center of the oven. Line two baking sheets with parchment paper and set aside.

2   In a medium bowl, whisk together the tapioca starch, brown rice flour, and potato starch.

3   In a medium pot, combine the milk, water, butter, sugar, and salt. Bring the mixture to a boil over medium-high heat, then add the dry ingredients all at once. Stir together with a wooden spoon. It will be a dry paste. Continue stirring until it comes together and starts sticking to the bottom of the pan, 1 to 2 minutes. As soon as the paste forms a ball, remove from heat and transfer into the bowl of a stand mixer.

4   Using the paddle attachment, mix the paste on high speed. It will release a lot of steam. Whisk 4 of the eggs in another medium bowl, reserving the fifth one in case it is needed. Wait until the steam subsides (an instant-read thermometer should read around 125 degrees F), then slowly add about 2 tablespoons of egg at a time, continuing to beat on medium speed between additions. It might look lumpy at times, but it will come together into a creamy and smooth paste at the end. $\longrightarrow$

The final consistency of the paste should resemble that of a thicker hummus, and it will be sticky, smooth, and stretchy. When you run your finger through it, the edges will begin to ripple back slowly. If after adding 4 eggs the paste still looks lumpy, whisk and add the fifth egg 1 teaspoon at a time, waiting after each addition, until the desired consistency is reached.

5   Fit a large pastry bag with a medium-size plain tip (number 5 or 6) and scoop the paste into the bag. Pipe the paste into 1½-inch circles on the prepared pans, leaving about 2 inches of space between. The paste might be sticky and hard to release from the pastry tip. Dip your finger in some water and help release it, if necessary. If the piped paste looks more like a Hershey's Kiss than a circle, simply press down the top with a wet finger. I like to keep a bowl of water nearby for this.

6   Put both baking sheets in the oven and reduce the temperature to 375 degrees F. Bake the profiteroles for 30 to 35 minutes, rotating them halfway through, until golden brown and puffed. The inside should be on the drier side so the choux won't collapse. If you're not sure, take one out, tear it open, and see if it's still too moist inside. If so, bake a few minutes longer. Let the profiteroles cool completely on the pan, then cut them in half crosswise using a serrated knife.

7   To assemble, fit a clean pastry bag with a medium-size plain tip (number 5 or 6) and fill it with the pastry cream. Pipe a dollop of pastry cream onto the bottom half of each profiterole shell, then replace the top. Drizzle with chocolate glaze or simply dust with powdered sugar. Serve immediately.

PARIS-BREST

Paris-Brest is a wreath made of choux paste and filled with lightly sweetened cream. It is a beautiful presentation.

Trace a 7-inch circle onto a sheet of parchment. Flip the parchment over and place it on a baking sheet. Follow the instructions to make the choux paste, then pipe 1¾-inch circles of the paste following the traced circle on your parchment. Bake at 375 degrees F for 30 to 35 minutes, until puffed up and golden brown. Cool completely, then cut it in half crosswise using a serrated knife. Fill with pastry cream and lightly dust the top with powdered sugar.

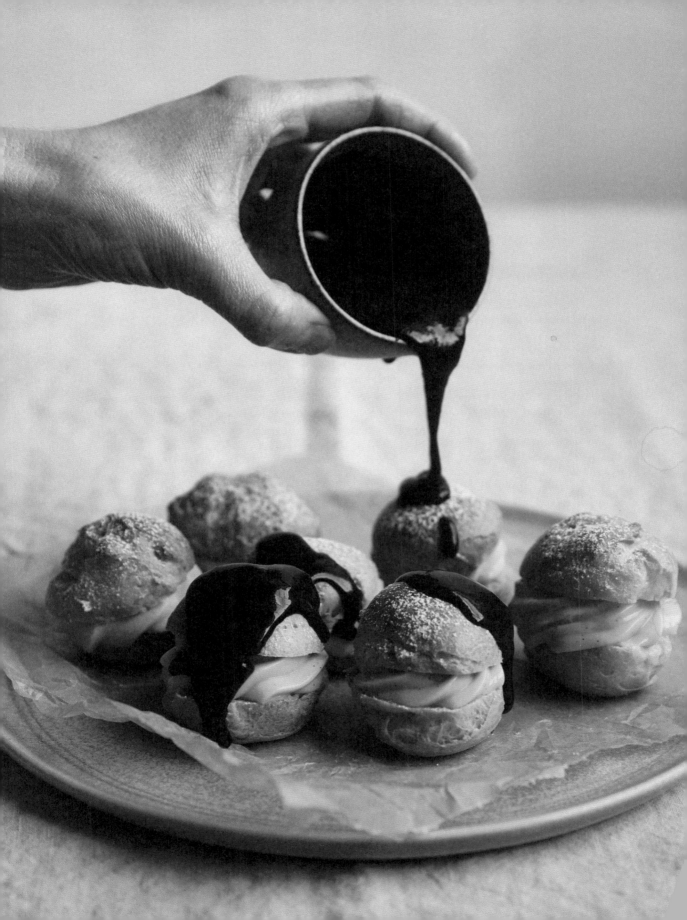

Chocolate Bûche de Noël

Cooking spray, for greasing

7 large eggs, separated

¾ cup plus 2 tablespoons (175 g) sugar, divided

2 teaspoons vanilla extract

¾ cup (75 g) unsweetened cocoa powder, divided

½ teaspoon ground cinnamon

½ teaspoon kosher salt

½ cup (60 g) plus 2 tablespoons powdered sugar, divided

2 cups (450 g) heavy cream or canned coconut cream

1 vanilla bean, split lengthwise and seeds scraped

2 cups Chocolate Swiss Buttercream (page 42) or Chocolate-Coffee American-Style Buttercream (page 45)

A *bûche de Noël* or Yule log might seem like a complicated dessert, but this simplified version comes together quickly. The chocolate cake is a flourless sponge that is leavened by whipping egg whites and yolks separately, then folding them together. The filling is chocolate whipped cream, and the entire cake gets covered with a thin layer of buttercream. It is a stunning dessert when decorated with chocolate branches and seasonal fruits—nothing fancy.

MAKES 8 SERVINGS

1 Preheat the oven to 350 degrees F. Grease a rimmed 12-by-16-inch baking sheet with cooking spray. Line the pan with parchment and grease that too.

2 Whip the egg whites in the bowl of a stand mixer fitted with the whisk attachment over medium-high speed. When they have doubled in volume, sprinkle in half of the sugar 1 table-spoon at a time. Whip until thick. Be careful not to overwhip or the mixture will become clumpy and hard to fold into the batter. Scrape into a large bowl.

3 Add the egg yolks, remaining sugar, and vanilla to the mixer bowl. Do not let the sugar sit on the yolks for long without whipping or they will curdle. Whip the yolks until very thick and pale, about 3 minutes. Add ½ cup (50 g) of the cocoa powder, cinnamon, and salt and whip for another minute, until smooth.

4 With a spatula, fold a third of the whipped egg whites into the yolk mixture. It's OK to be a bit vigorous. Add the remaining egg whites, folding carefully at this point to avoid deflating the batter too much. Fold until there are no visible streaks.

5 Spread the batter evenly on the prepared baking sheet and bake for 12 to 15 minutes, until the cake begins to pull away from the sides of the pan and the top springs back when gently pressed.

6 Lay out a clean thick kitchen towel on a work surface—making sure it is as flat as possible with no creases—and using a fine-mesh sieve, dust the entire towel surface with 2 tablespoons of the powdered sugar. Run a knife around the edges of the pan, then turn the cake out onto the towel.

7 Carefully peel off the parchment (do not pull too hard or the cake will tear), then roll the kitchen towel and cake together into a log, starting from the long end. Let the cake cool for 15 minutes. Do not let it sit wrapped in the towel for much longer or it may crack as it dries out.

8 Meanwhile, make the filling. In the clean bowl of a stand mixer fitted with the whisk attachment, whip the cream with the remaining ½ cup (60 g) powdered sugar, remaining ¼ cup (25 g) cocoa powder, and vanilla seeds until thick.

9 Unroll the cake and spread the filling over the inside, leaving a ½-inch border. Roll the cake back up, this time without the towel. It might crack in spots, which is OK, but be careful when handling as it is delicate. Transfer the cake to a serving platter, seam side down, and refrigerate for at least 2 hours, until firm. The cake can be made a day ahead and kept in the refrigerator.

10 To decorate the cake, first make sure the buttercream is very soft and aerated. If it is cold, it can tear the cake when frosting. Give the cake a crumb coat by spreading a thin layer of buttercream all over. Chill the cake for 15 minutes, until the buttercream hardens, then fully frost the cake, creating buttercream swirls with a spatula or using a fork to make lines that resemble wood bark.

11 Trim ½-inch pieces from both ends of the cake. At this point, you can slice the cake into 1½-inch pieces and serve. The cake will keep tightly wrapped in the refrigerator for up to 2 days.

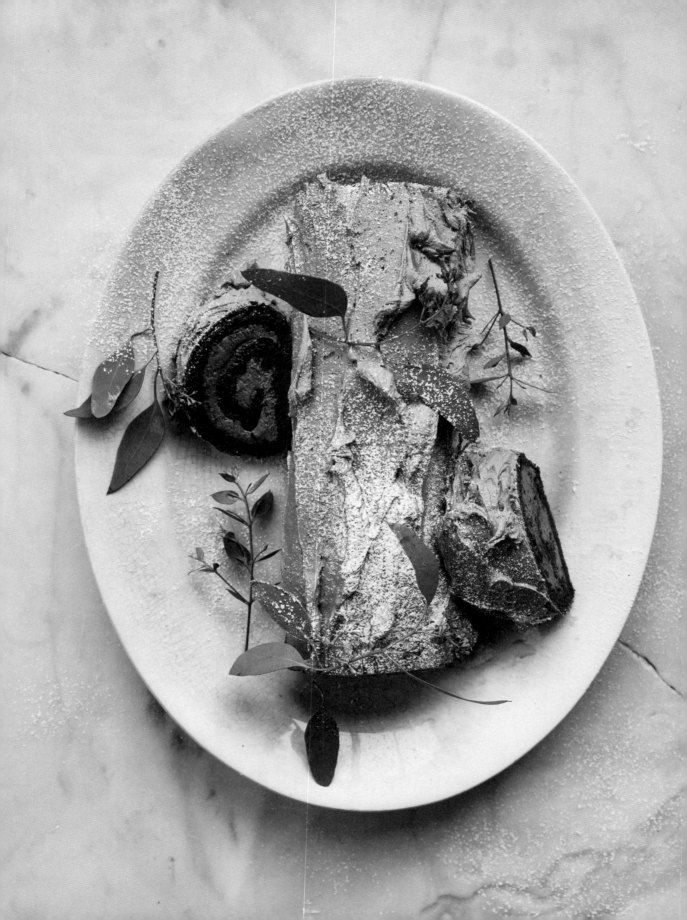

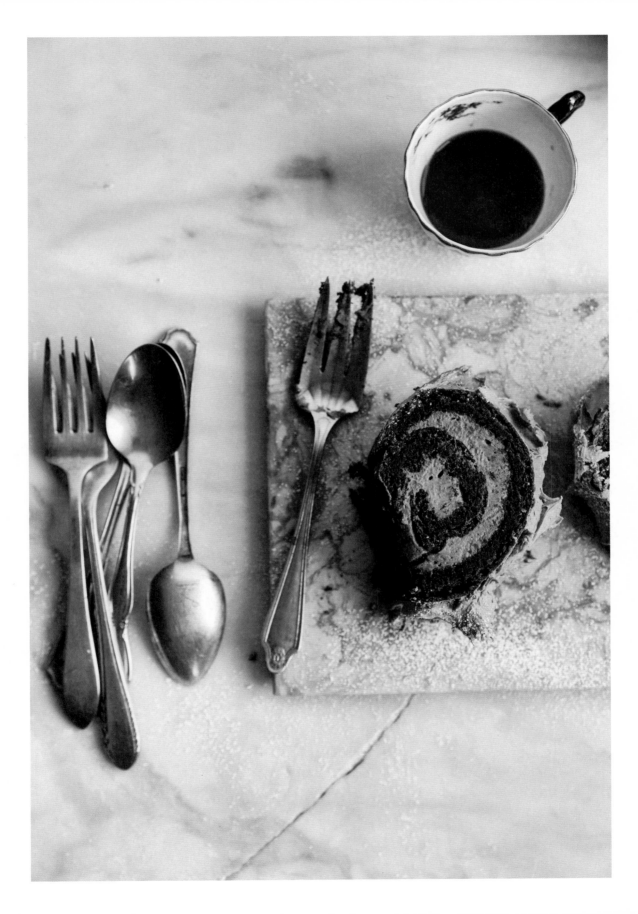

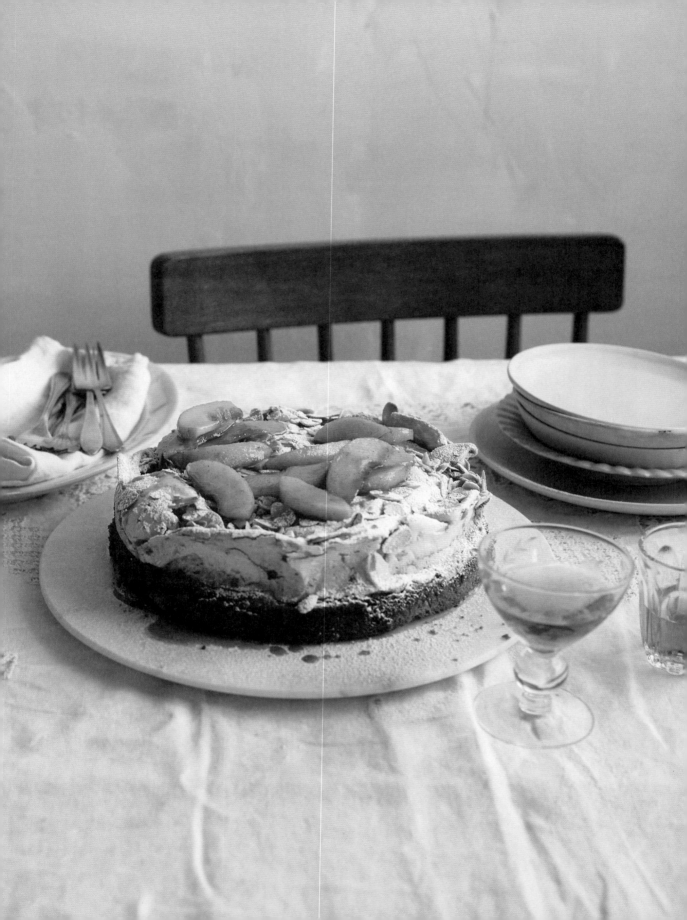

Meringue Cake with Roasted Apples

Baked meringue over a cake or swirled around an ice cream bombe will always be one of my favorite celebratory treats. There is something about that crispy topping covering a marshmallow interior. You could serve this cake with fresh berries, but the caramelized apples add another layer of sweetness and spice.

MAKES ONE 9-INCH CAKE

For the cake
7 tablespoons (100 g) unsalted butter or dairy-free butter, plus more for greasing
1 cup plus 2 tablespoons (225 g) sugar, divided
5 large egg yolks
⅔ cup (95 g) superfine brown rice flour
⅓ cup (40 g) tapioca starch
2 teaspoons baking powder
1 teaspoon ground cinnamon
¼ teaspoon kosher salt
¼ cup (55 g) whole milk or oat milk
4 large egg whites
⅓ cup (40 g) raw sliced almonds

For the caramelized apples
1 large firm and juicy apple, such as Granny Smith or Honeycrisp
3 tablespoons sugar
1 tablespoon unsalted butter or dairy-free butter
1 tablespoon apple cider vinegar
1 tablespoon vanilla extract
½ teaspoon ground cinnamon
¼ teaspoon ground ginger
¼ teaspoon ground cardamom

1   Preheat the oven to 325 degrees F. Position a rack in the lower half of the oven.

2   Grease the inside of a 9-inch springform pan or tube pan with butter. Alternatively, use a 9-inch cake pan: line the bottom and sides with parchment paper, leaving some overhang to help lift the cake out of the pan.

3   To make the cake, combine the butter and ½ cup (100 g) of the sugar in the bowl of a stand mixer. Using the paddle attachment, beat the butter and sugar over medium-high speed until pale and creamy, about 2 minutes. Reduce the speed to low and add the egg yolks one at a time until all are incorporated. Stop and scrape the sides of the bowl and paddle if needed.

4   In a small bowl, stir together the brown rice flour, tapioca starch, baking powder, cinnamon, and salt. Add the dry ingredients to the mixer and beat on medium speed until incorporated. Finish by adding the milk. Once the batter comes together, increase the speed to high and give it a good whip for 15 seconds or so to ensure everything is well incorporated.

5   Spread the batter into the prepared pan and set aside. Wash the mixer bowl, making sure there is no residue of batter in it.

6   Put the egg whites into the clean mixer bowl. Using the whisk attachment, whip them on medium speed until they begin to foam and increase in volume. Add the remaining ½ cup plus 2 tablespoons (125 g) sugar, 1 tablespoon at a time, and continue whipping until all the sugar is incorporated. ⟶

7   Increase the speed to high and whip the meringue into glossy, stiff peaks. Spread the meringue over the cake batter, creating swirl patterns with the spatula. Sprinkle the almonds on top.

8   Bake for 35 to 40 minutes, until a skewer inserted in the center comes out clean. The meringue will puff up and the almonds should be golden brown. Let the cake cool in the pan for 20 minutes, then run a knife around the edges to loosen the cake and remove it from the pan to cool completely. The top will have deflated slightly and cracked in spots.

9   Meanwhile, make the caramelized apples. Peel, halve, and core the apple. Cut each half into slices that are about ¼ inch thick.

10   Heat a medium sauté pan over medium-high heat. Sprinkle the sugar evenly over the bottom of the pan and cook until it melts and turns a light amber. Carefully stir in the butter, vinegar, vanilla, and spices, as the caramel may splatter.

11   Add the apple slices and toss to coat with the caramel. Reduce the heat to medium and cook for 5 to 7 minutes, turning the apples occasionally. Try not to mush them too much. They should be slightly soft and caramel colored. If the caramel thickens too much, add 1 tablespoon of water or orange juice. Let the apples cool for a few minutes before topping the cake. Store the cake, tightly wrapped, in the refrigerator for up to 2 days.

Pear
Marzipan
Cake

---

1 pound (454 g) ripe Bosc pears
1 cup (200 g) sugar
8 ounces (225 g) Marzipan
  (page 49)
1 cup (225 g) unsalted butter
  or dairy-free butter, at room
  temperature, plus more for
  greasing
4 large whole eggs plus
  1 egg yolk
1 teaspoon vanilla extract
½ cup (70 g) superfine brown
  rice flour
¼ cup (30 g) tapioca starch
1 teaspoon baking powder
½ teaspoon kosher salt
¼ cup (30 g) raw sliced almonds
Powdered sugar, for dusting

This recipe is inspired by many of the traditional marzipan and almond cakes I grew up with, such as *pain de Gênes* or *tarta de Santiago*. The cake is tremendously moist with butter and marzipan, plus layers of thinly cut pear that melt in your mouth. It is perfect for a winter treat or a holiday dessert table.

MAKES ONE 9-INCH CAKE

1 Preheat the oven to 325 degrees F. Grease the bottom and sides of an 9-inch springform or cake pan with butter. Line the bottom with parchment paper and grease that too.

2 Peel the pears. Slice them in half lengthwise and core them. Cut them into very thin slices from stem to base. Arrange the pear slices in tight concentric circles starting from the edge until the entire bottom of the pan is covered.

3 In a food processor, pulverize the sugar into a fine powder. Add the marzipan and process until the mixture resembles sand. Add the butter and pulse to a very creamy, smooth paste.

4 Add the eggs, egg yolk, and vanilla extract and pulse until the mixture is airy. Scrape the sides and bottom of the bowl to make sure the ingredients are well incorporated. Add the brown rice flour, tapioca starch, baking powder, and salt, and pulse until the batter is airy and smooth. It will be runny. Pour the batter over the pears and scatter the almonds all over the top.

5 Bake the cake for 55 to 65 minutes, until golden brown and a toothpick inserted in the center comes out clean. The cake will be very tender, moist, and delicate, so let it cool completely in the pan. If you used a cake pan, run a sharp knife around the edge to release the cake, then invert it onto a plate. Invert again onto a serving plate so the pears remain at the bottom. Dust the top with powdered sugar and serve. Store in the refrigerator for up to 4 days.

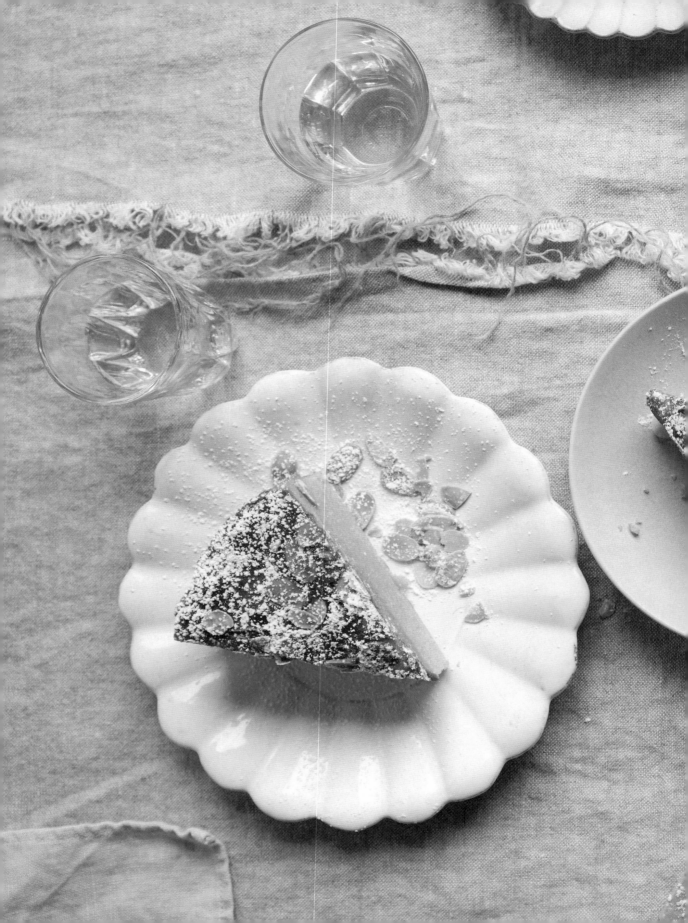

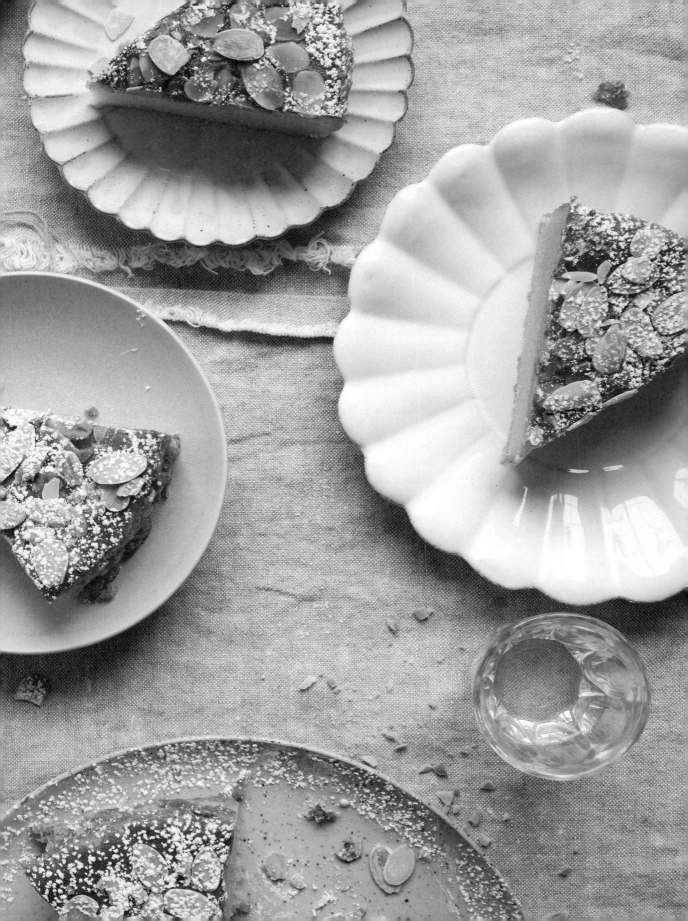

Spiced Sweet Potato Cake with Cream Cheese Frosting

This is a tall spiced snack cake to serve during autumn and winter days alongside hot tea or a cup of coffee. The cake, which is naturally dairy free, comes alive when paired with the tangy cream cheese frosting. If you want to make the frosting dairy free as well, note that you might have to refrigerate it after whipping, as plant-based cream cheeses tend to be much softer than their regular counterparts. You can make the cake batter with roasted pumpkin or canned pumpkin puree in place of sweet potato.

MAKES 1 LOAF CAKE

For the frosting
8 ounces (225 g) cream cheese or dairy-free cream cheese spread, at room temperature
1 cup (120 g) powdered sugar
½ vanilla bean, split lengthwise and seeds scraped, or 2 teaspoons vanilla extract
½ cup (115 g) unsalted butter or dairy-free butter, at room temperature
¼ cup (55 g) whole-milk sour cream or dairy-free sour cream

For the cake
1 large sweet potato
⅔ cup (150 g) neutral-tasting vegetable oil, such as grapeseed, plus more for greasing
4 large eggs
1 cup (200 g) light brown sugar
1 tablespoon finely grated orange zest
1½ cups (210 g) sorghum flour
1½ cups (150 g) almond flour
¼ cup (35 g) finely chopped candied ginger, plus more for topping

1 To make the frosting, in the bowl of a stand mixer fitted with the paddle attachment, beat the cream cheese, powdered sugar, and vanilla seeds together on medium-high speed until the mixture is airy, soft, and creamy, about 3 minutes. Make sure there are no large lumps of cream cheese.

2 Add the butter and continue beating on medium speed until very airy, about 2 minutes. Scrape the paddle and sides of the bowl to make sure all ingredients are well incorporated, then add the sour cream and continue beating until the frosting is creamy and fluffy. It will keep in an airtight container in the refrigerator for up to a week. Before using, bring the frosting to room temperature for a couple of hours and beat again until light.

3 To make the cake, put the sweet potato in a medium sauce-pan, cover with cold water, and cover with a lid. Bring the water to a boil over medium heat and cook the sweet potato until the center can be easily pierced with a knife, about 25 minutes. Drain and let the sweet potato cool until it is safe to handle. Peel and mash the flesh with a fork, then measure 1½ cups (340 g) of the puree. Keep the rest for another use.

4 Meanwhile, preheat the oven to 350 degrees F. Position a rack in the lower third of the oven. Grease the inside of an 8½-by-4½-inch loaf pan with vegetable oil, then line with a piece of parchment paper large enough to hang over the sides. This will help you lift the cake out of the pan after baking. Because this is a tall and hefty cake, be sure to use a 1-pound loaf pan.

1 tablespoon ground cinnamon
1 teaspoon baking soda
1 teaspoon kosher salt
½ teaspoon ground nutmeg
½ teaspoon ground cardamom

5   In a large bowl, whisk together the sweet potato puree, vegetable oil, eggs, brown sugar, and orange zest until smooth.

6   In a small bowl, stir together both flours, candied ginger, cinnamon, baking soda, salt, nutmeg, and cardamom. Add the dry ingredients into the sweet potato mixture and whisk to combine.

7   Pour the batter into the prepared pan and bake for 75 to 85 minutes, until golden brown and a toothpick inserted in the center comes out clean. If the cake begins to brown too much, cover the top with a piece of aluminum foil. Let the cake cool in the pan for 20 minutes, then invert onto a wire rack. Let the cake cool completely, then spread the frosting all over the top and sprinkle candied ginger over it. The cake will keep tightly wrapped in the refrigerator for up to 3 days.

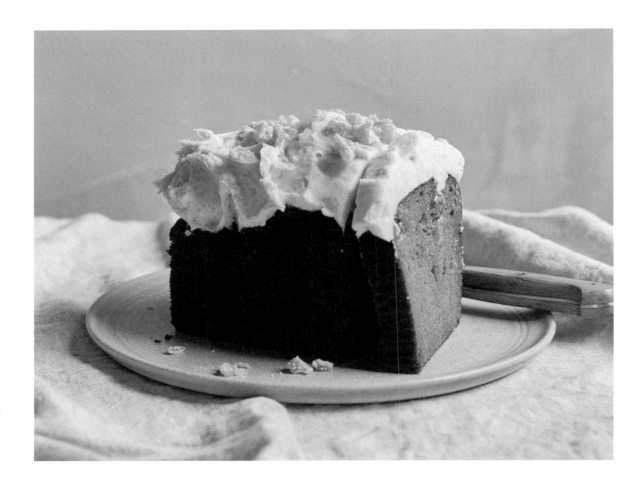

Honey Cake with Seed Brittle

For the brittle

¾ cup (100 g) mixed seeds and nuts (sesame, sunflower, pumpkin, pine nuts, chopped almonds or hazelnuts)

½ cup (170 g) raw honey

¼ cup (50 g) sugar

2 tablespoons unsalted butter or dairy-free butter

2 tablespoons water, at room temperature

½ teaspoon kosher salt

For the cake

Unsalted or dairy-free butter, for greasing

1½ cups (210 g) sorghum flour, plus more for dusting

¾ cup (70 g) gluten-free oat flour

⅓ cup (45 g) tapioca starch

¼ cup (40 g) potato starch

1½ teaspoons baking powder

1 teaspoon ground cinnamon

1 teaspoon xanthan gum

½ teaspoon ground ginger

½ teaspoon kosher salt

¼ teaspoon ground allspice

½ cup (115 g) brewed espresso or very strong coffee

½ teaspoon baking soda

2 large eggs

1 cup (340 g) honey

1 cup (200 g) sugar

½ cup (100 g) light brown sugar

When writing this book, I knew I wanted to include a recipe for Rosh Hashanah. I admire the Jewish tradition of New Year that honors renewal and forgiveness. My friend Jacque Altman shared some of her family's favorite honey cake recipes, which contained gluten, of course. She tested various adaptations for me and provided helpful feedback based on her expectation of what a perfect honey cake should be, and this version passed the test with flying colors. A big thank-you to Jacque.

This is a rich cake that, when wrapped, will last on your kitchen counter for days. In fact, it gets better as it matures—the flavors will intensify, and the crumb will be moist and not as crumbly. I also include instructions for making a honey glaze, as well as honey-seed brittle. Neither is mandatory but they will make your cake a festive standout. Make the cake and brittle anywhere from two to five days in advance and the glaze just before serving.

MAKES 1 BUNDT CAKE

1   To make the brittle, first line a baking sheet with parchment paper and set aside.

2   In a medium sauté pan over medium heat, toast the seeds and nuts until fragrant, about 2 minutes.

3   In a small saucepan, combine the honey, sugar, butter, water, and salt. Cook the mixture over medium heat until a candy thermometer reads 300 degrees F, about 15 minutes. Remove the pan from the heat and stir in the nuts and seeds.

4   Pour the brittle over the parchment paper and use a spatula to spread it into a thin layer. Let the brittle cool completely, then break it into pieces. Store the brittle in an airtight container for up to 7 days.

5   To make the cake, preheat the oven to 350 degrees F. Grease the inside of a 9-inch tube pan or 9-cup Bundt pan with a generous amount of butter, then dust with sorghum flour. Shake off excess flour. The cake tends to stick to the pan, so pay attention to any crevices.

¾ cup (170 g) grapeseed oil
  or other light vegetable oil
1 tablespoon freshly squeezed
  orange juice
2 teaspoons finely grated
  orange zest

For the glaze
1½ cups (180 g) powdered
  sugar, sifted
2 tablespoons honey
1 to 2 tablespoons whole milk
  or oat milk
1 teaspoon vanilla extract

6 In a very large bowl, whisk together the sorghum flour, oat flour, tapioca starch, potato starch, baking powder, cinnamon, xanthan gum, ginger, salt, and allspice.

7 In a medium bowl, whisk together the coffee and baking soda.

8 In a large bowl, whisk together the eggs, honey, both sugars, oil, and orange juice and zest. Pour this and the coffee mixture over the dry ingredients and whisk until you have a very liquid and smooth batter. Pour it into the prepared pan, but don't fill it more than three-quarters full or it will overflow when baking.

9 Bake for 55 to 65 minutes, until the cake is a deep golden brown and it springs back nicely when touched. You can also test by inserting a toothpick in the center and making sure it comes out clean. The cake might sink a little in the center while baking; this is OK. Let the cake cool in the pan completely, then invert onto a plate.

10 Once the cake is cool, wrap it tightly in plastic wrap. Let it mature at room temperature for 2 to 5 days. The honey will keep the cake moist and all the flavors will intensify.

11 Just before serving, make the honey glaze. In a medium bowl, whisk together the powdered sugar, honey, milk, and vanilla until it becomes a thick, pourable consistency.

12 To serve, place the cake on a cake stand or platter and drizzle the glaze over the top, letting it drip down the sides. Decorate the top and sides with pieces of brittle.

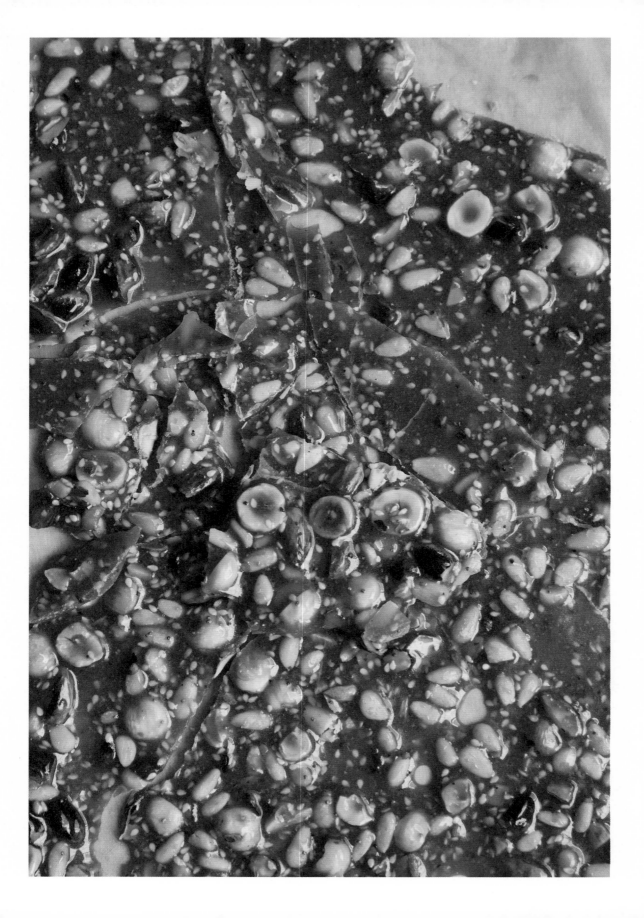

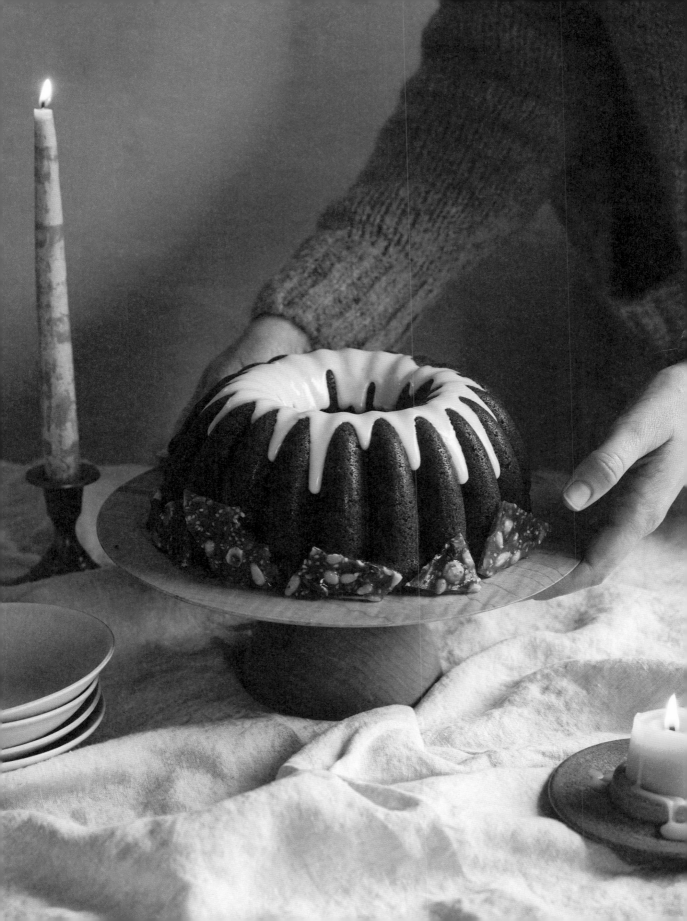

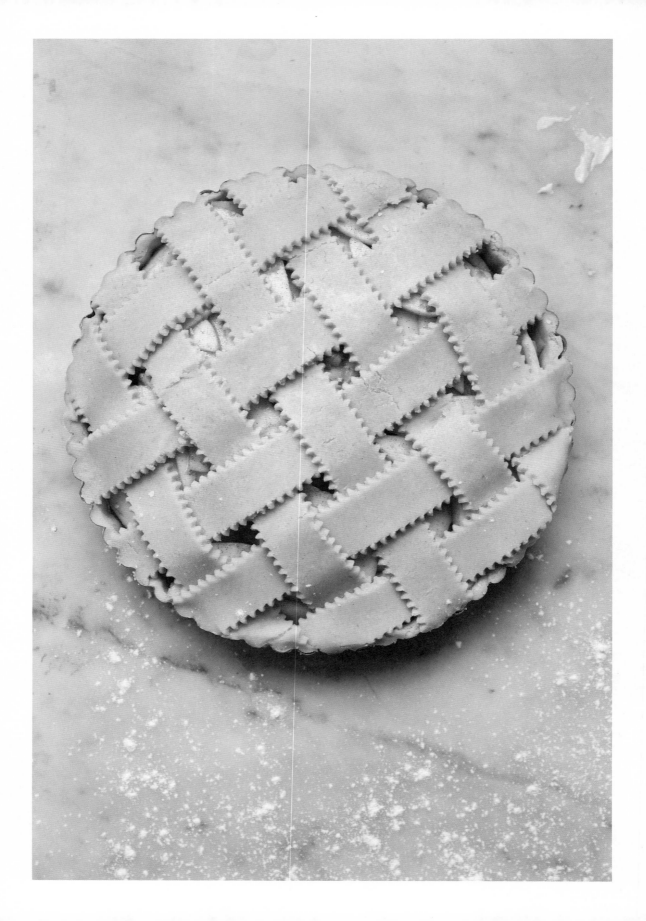

Acknowledgments

To my editor Susan Roxborough and to designer Anna Goldstein—thank you for carrying out my vision so beautifully. Huge thanks also to production editor Bridget Sweet, copyeditor Rachelle Longé McGhee, director of marketing Nikki Sprinkle, publicist Molly Woolbright, and the entire team at Sasquatch Books for your support. To my agent of over ten years, Judy Linden, thank you for keeping things real and always having my back.

Thank you to my generous friends Dorothée Brand, for the most beautiful portraits; Jenn Elliott-Blake, for sprinkling your styling magic; and Hardie Cobbs, for letting me escape to your beautiful island home.

Thanks to all the recipe testers that invested time and resources to help me perfect the recipes and make sure every word written on the page worked beautifully: April Boyer, Ashley May, Becky Dale, Beth King, Carley Knobloch, Carrie McCleary, Danica Rog, Deborah Zener, Hardie Cobbs, Hilary Bovay, Jacque Altman, Jacqueline Bendrick, Jenny Choi, Jill Haapaniemi, Kara Hoey, Karen Torres, Kate Marks Roseiro, Katy Ionis, Kelsi Leitz, Kiersten Kirschman, Klara Heuscher, Lizzy Ervin, Mary Piepmeier, Nikki Gaffaney, Rena Williams, Sally Shintaffer, Tanya Protasenya, Terisa Means, Tonya Veilleux, Vanessa Palomo, and Victoria Thomas.

Thank you to all of you who have followed me and have bought my books. Your support has carried me through the years and has allowed me to continue pursuing what I love the most.

And most importantly, thank you to my family. This book exists only because of your constant support and love. My family in the Basque Country: *amatxu*, *aitatxu*, Jokin eta Jon, and the whole Ayarza clan. And my family in Seattle: Chad, Jontxu, and Mirentxu. Love you all.

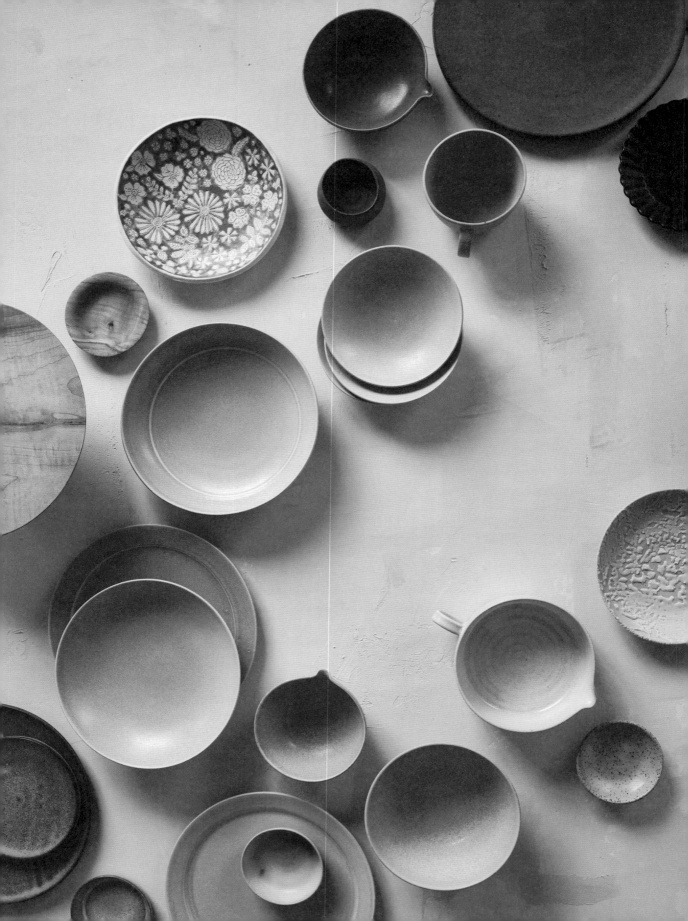

Online Resources

Below are some of my favorite sources for ceramics, pantry items, and baking tools. Some are widely available, others are small-batch makers, but all are brands I use in my daily life.

CERAMICS

Akiko's Pottery
AkikosPottery.com

Dorotea Ceramics
DoroteaCeramics.com

Henry Street Studio
HenryStreetStudio.com

Janaki Larsen
JanakiLarsenCeramics.com

Natasha Alphonse Ceramics
AlphonseStudio.com

PANTRY

Anthony's Goods
AnthonysGoods.com

Authentic Foods
AuthenticFoods.com

Bob's Red Mill
BobsRedMill.com

Diaspora Co.
DiasporaCo.com

ILA
ILA-Shop.co

Thrive Market
ThriveMarket.com

Wonder Valley
WelcometoWonder Valley.com

TOOLS

KitchenAid
KitchenAid.com

Lodge
LodgeCastIron.com

Nordic Ware
NordicWare.com

Staub
Zwilling.com/us/staub

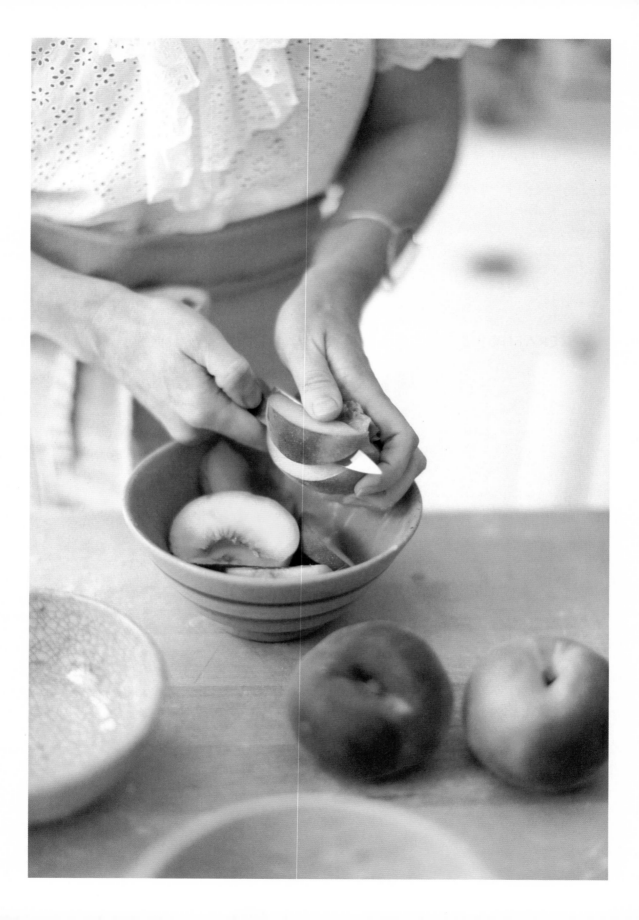

Index

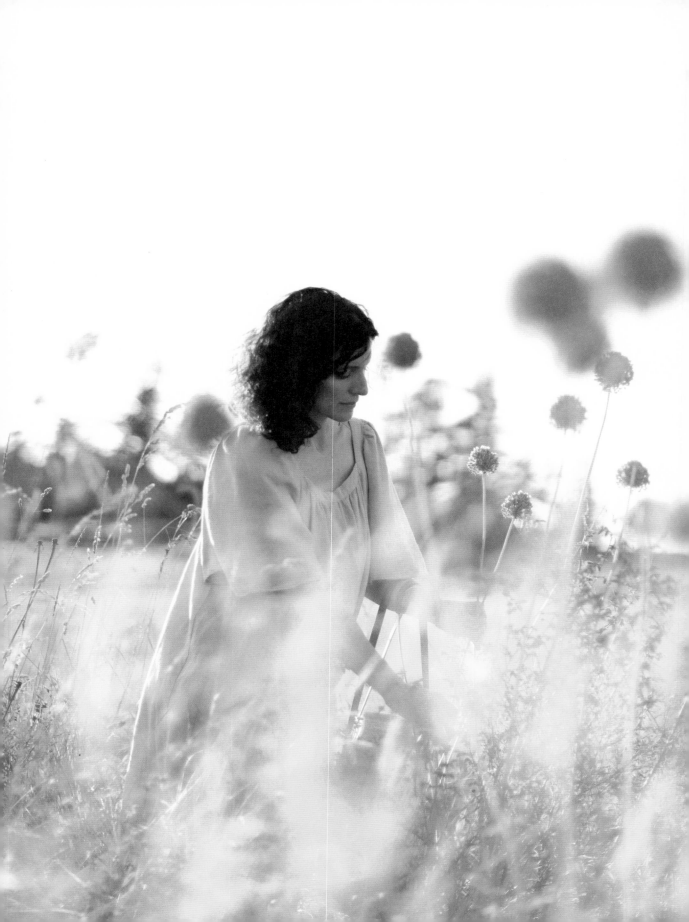

About the Author

ARAN GOYOAGA is a cookbook author, food stylist, and photographer. Aran was born and raised in the Basque Country in northern Spain, where her maternal grandparents owned a pastry shop and her paternal grandparents lived off the land. Aran is a three-time James Beard Award finalist. She currently lives in Seattle with her husband and two children.

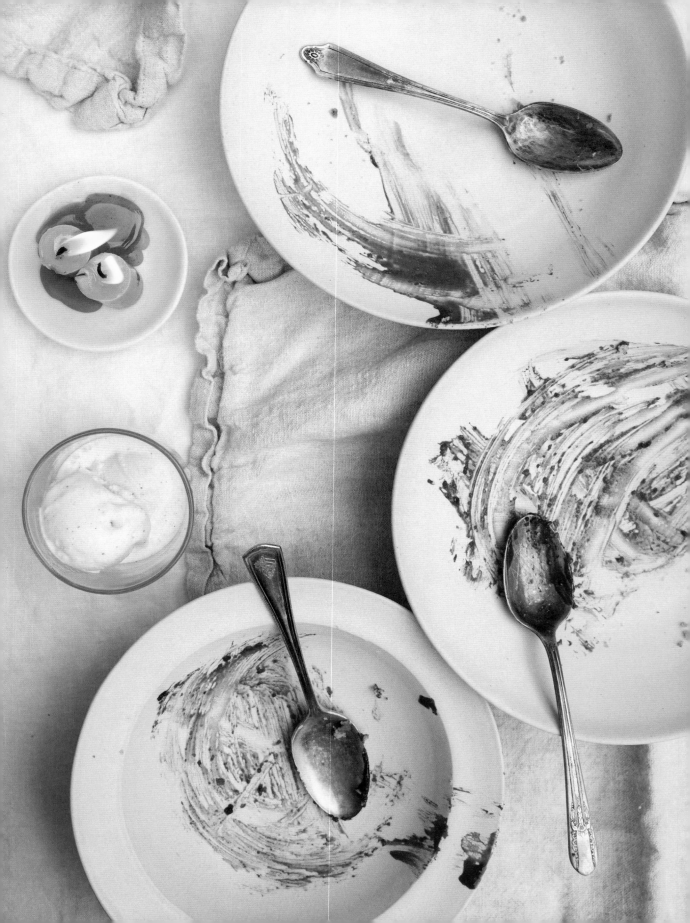

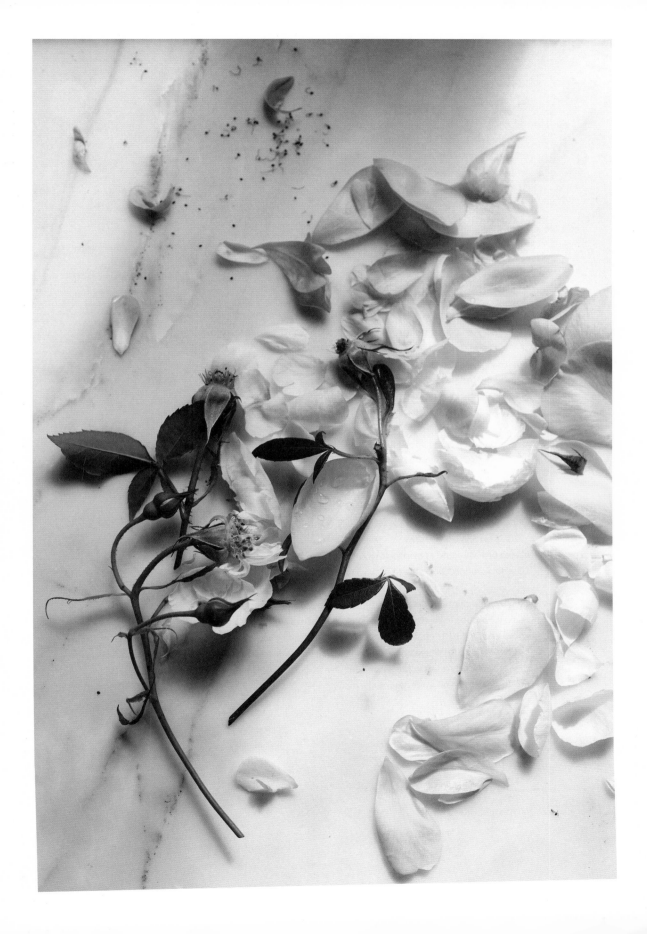

Printed in China

SASQUATCH BOOKS with colophon is a registered trademark
of Penguin Random House LLC

25 24 23 22 21   9 8 7 6 5 4 3 2 1

Editor: Susan Roxborough | Production editor: Bridget Sweet
Designer: Anna Goldstein | Photography: Aran Goyoaga, except for pages iv,
18–19, 41, 134, 156, 163–165, 242, 296, and 304 by Dorothée Brand/Belathée

Library of Congress Cataloging-in-Publication Data
Names: Goyoaga, Aran, author.
Title: Cannelle et Vanille bakes simple : a new way to bake gluten-free /
  Aran Goyoaga.
Description: Seattle : Sasquatch Books, [2021] | Includes index.
Identifiers: LCCN 2020054938 (print) | LCCN 2020054939 (ebook) | ISBN
  9781632173706 (hardcover) | ISBN 9781632173713 (ebook)
Subjects: LCSH: Gluten-free diet--Recipes. | Baking. | Gluten-free foods. |
  Cannelle et Vanille. | LCGFT: Cookbooks.
Classification: LCC RM237.86 .G678 2021 (print) | LCC RM237.86 (ebook) |
  DDC 641.5/639311--dc23
LC record available at https://lccn.loc.gov/2020054938
LC ebook record available at https://lccn.loc.gov/2020054939

ISBN: 978-1-63217-370-6

Sasquatch Books
1904 Third Avenue, Suite 710
Seattle, WA 98101

SasquatchBooks.com

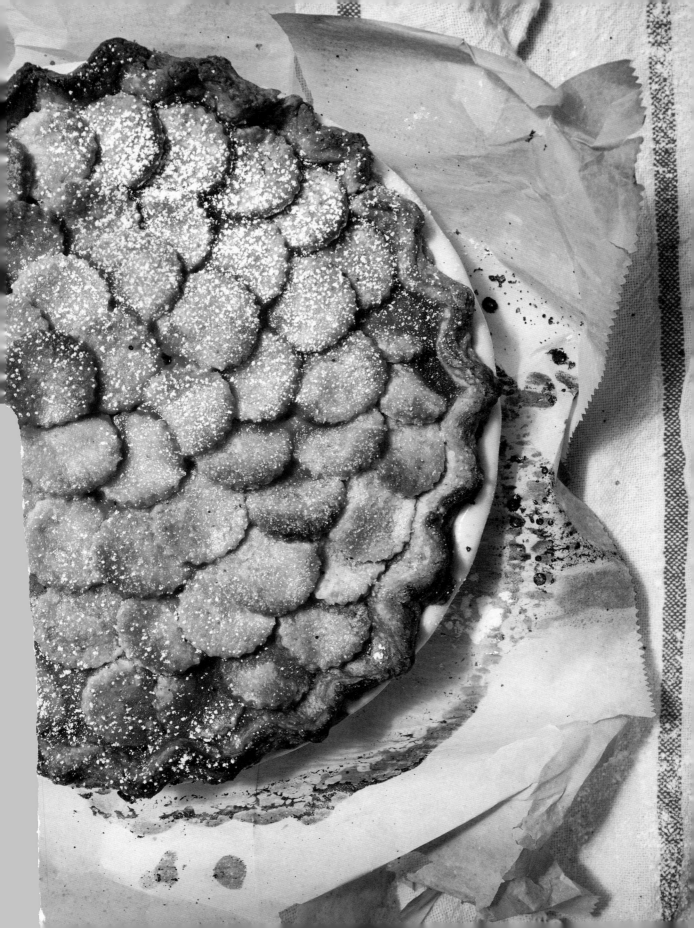

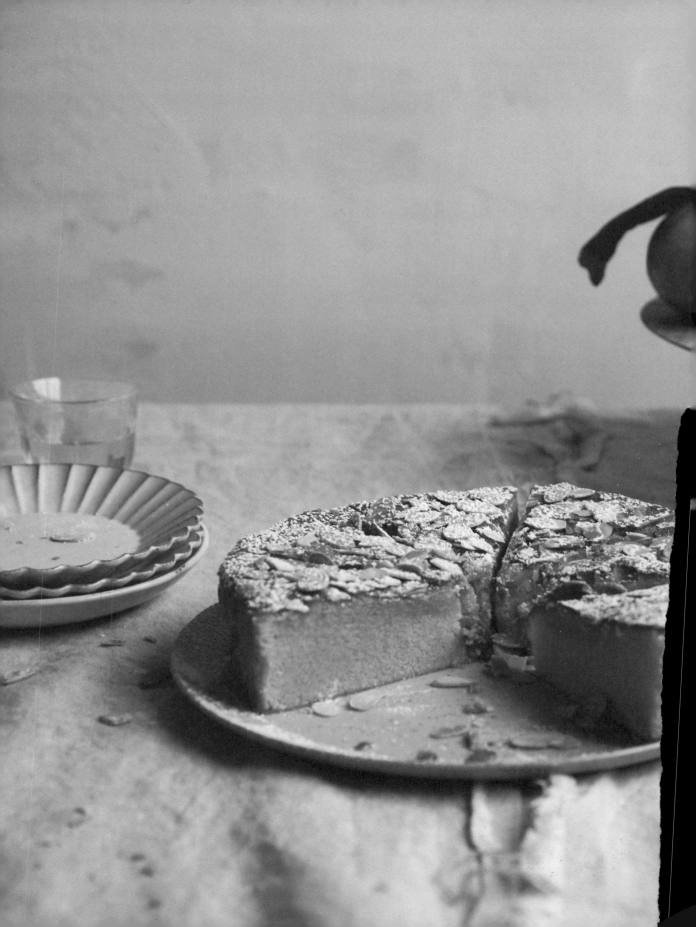